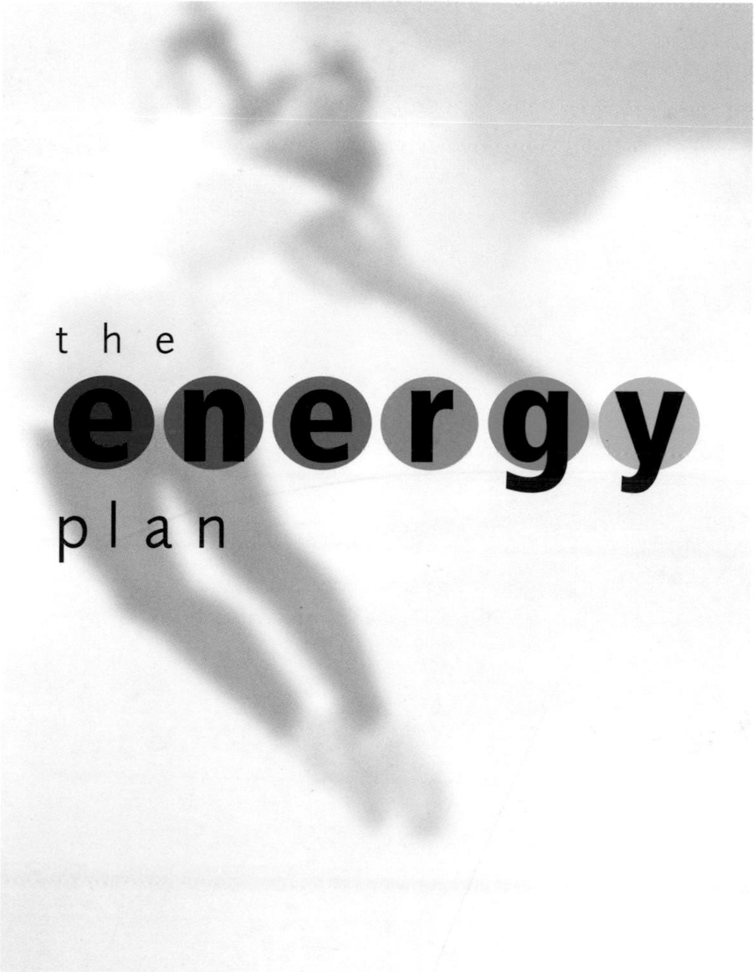

# the energy plan

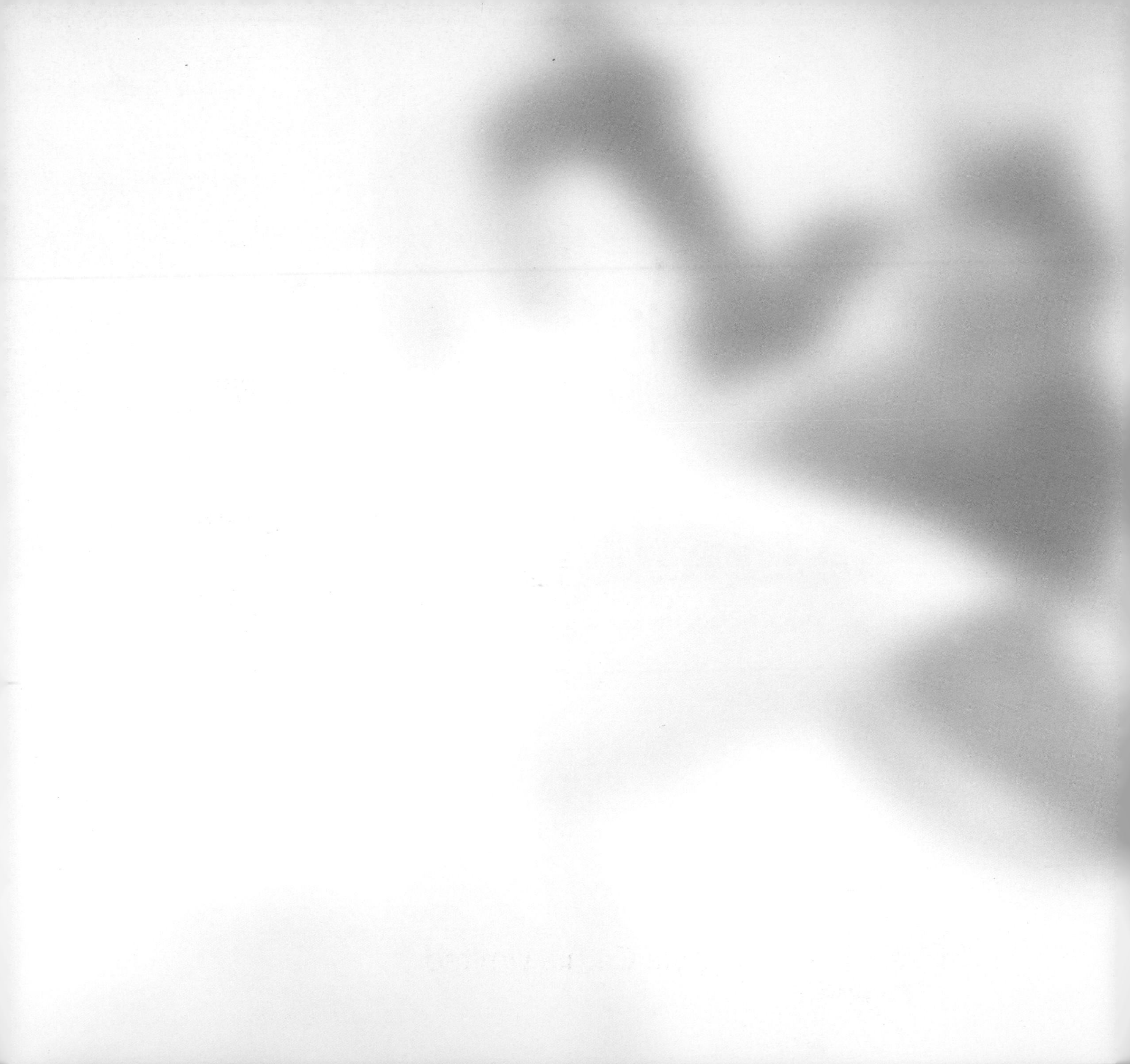

# the energy plan

## step-by-step plans to increase your energy levels

Aliza Baron Cohen

Kyle Cathie Limited

First published in Great Britain 2002 by
Kyle Cathie Limited
122 Arlington Road
London NW1 7HP
general.enquiries@kyle-cathie.com
www.kylecathie.com

ISBN 1 85626 442 4



Senior Editor: Helen Woodhall
Copy Editor: Anne Newman
Editorial Assistant: Esme West
Designer: Mark Buckingham
Production: Sha Huxtable and Lorraine Baird
Index: Helen Snaith



A Cataloguing In Publication record for this title is available from the British Library.

Colour separations by Sang Choy International
Printed in Singapore by Kyodo Printing Co.

# Contents

# Foreword

## *Pete Cohen, Life Strategist, author and health and fitness professional*

Energy is something that we all talk about and desire in our lives. Everyone has been in a position in their life where they have craved more energy – the energy to concentrate, the energy to get well, the energy to stay awake, the energy that enables us to be healthy and live a long life.

But what exactly is energy and where do you get it from? The mere mention of the word to some people makes them uncomfortable, as it calls to mind connotations of mysticism or spirituality.

We really do not know that much when it comes to understanding how the human mind and body work. We are made up of over 10 billion cells and modern science only knows and understands about 5 percent of how we work.

Conventional medicine has been slow to catch on to some of the principles that have existed for thousand of years in other cultures. For example, the manifestation of energy and its flow through the body is the foundation of Chinese medicine. Conventional medicine is based on scientific understanding and proof of how things work.

I once heard about a research project on acupuncture. The study wanted to prove scientifically how it works, exploring the body's meridians and energy points. When I heard about this and the huge amount of money that had gone into it I thought how much more useful the study would have been if it had simply researched acupuncture's effectiveness as a treatment by giving it to people and monitoring their progress.

This book will guide you through a transformation process in which you begin to experience a deeper and more practical understanding of energy. By following the practical and simple exercises you will learn to manifest more energy than you ever thought possible.

My philosophy in life is: if something works for you, then do it. This book will show you many simple but highly effective techniques and exercises that will really work to increase your energy.

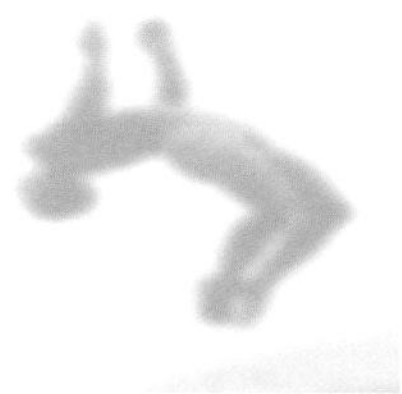

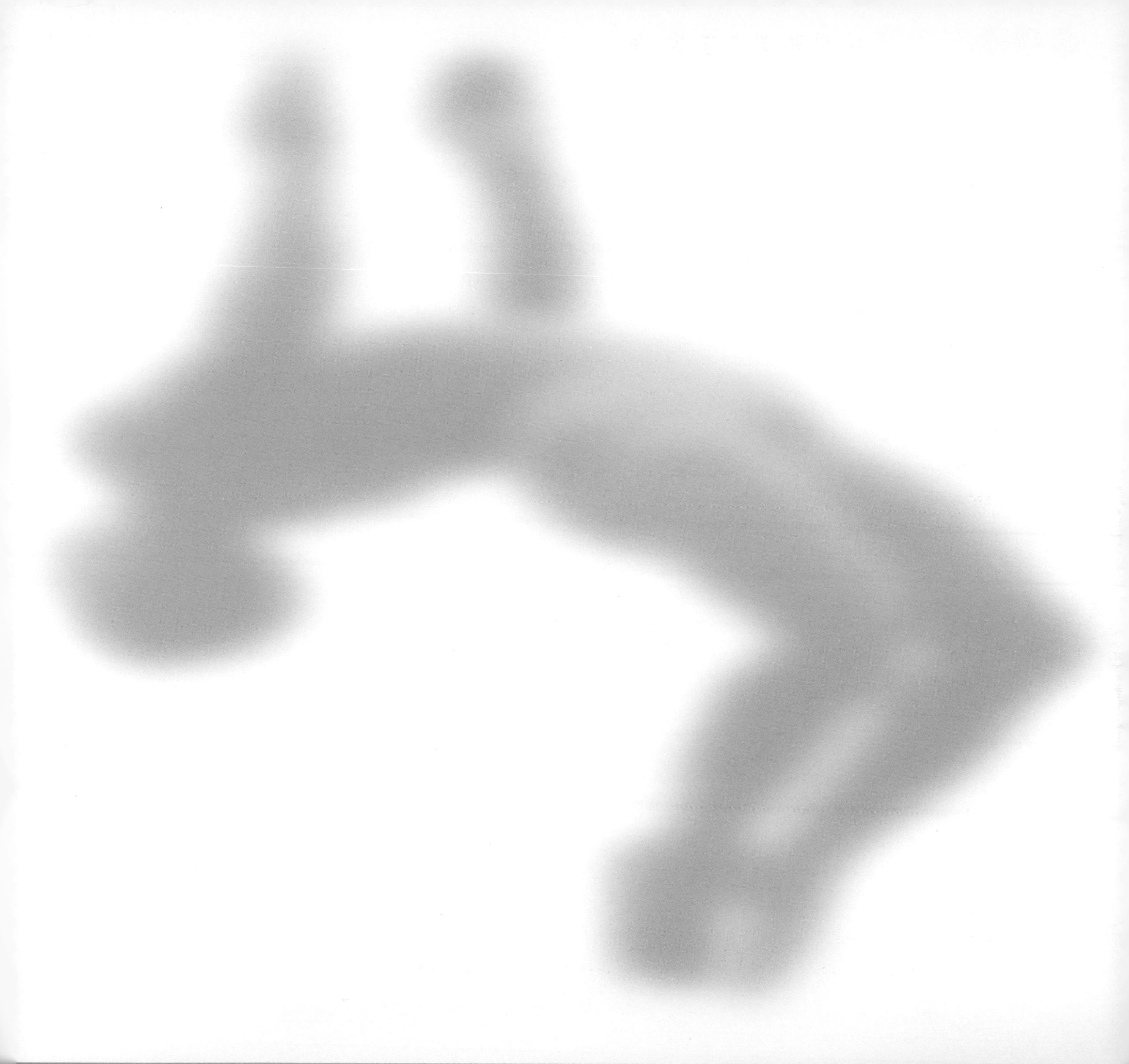

# Introduction

## *Do you wake up every morning wondering how you will find enough energy to get you through the day?*

Do you sometimes feel as though you've been tired for years and can't even remember when you last had any energy? Does it often seem to you that everyone else copes with the day-to-day hustle and bustle of life only too well, while you plod along at your own slow pace? Or perhaps you just find yourself sometimes wishing for a little more energy to allow you to take on a new hobby or activity?

If so, this book is for you, and for millions of others like you, since believe it or not, tiredness and lack of energy affect us all at one time or another, and in spite of outward appearances, there are very few of us who actually live life at an optimum energy level.

Of course, in some cases an underlying health problem may be causing feelings of tiredness and lethargy, and if you suspect that this is the case (see pages 22–7) it is essential for you to see your GP or health practitioner for a thorough check up before doing any of the energy plans.

As well as all of these, *The Energy Plan* looks at pregnancy and early parenthood, and why some people find themselves exhausted and barely able to cope after having a baby, while others in similar situations seem to glow with energy. Having had a baby myself a year ago I know only too well how

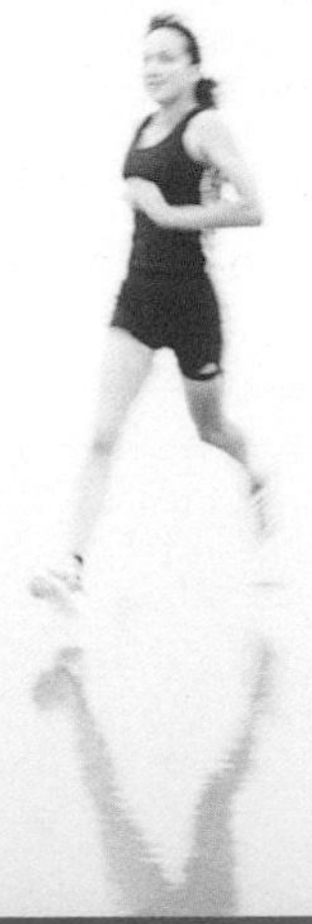

energy can dip during these times. The book offers advice on how to take care of yourself during emotionally or physically demanding times, and how to conserve and build your energy when you most need it. There is a section for older people (written by my own mum, a vibrant woman and mother of five), and general information on therapies, diet and exercise, as well as specific plans to follow.

*However, other factors such as late nights, stress at work or at home, or jet lag from travelling, can all conspire to make us function and feel below par some, or all, of the time.*

This book is designed to help you regardless of your age, or the stage of life you are at. It's about quality of life and how to improve it by giving you the energy and zest for life that you deserve.

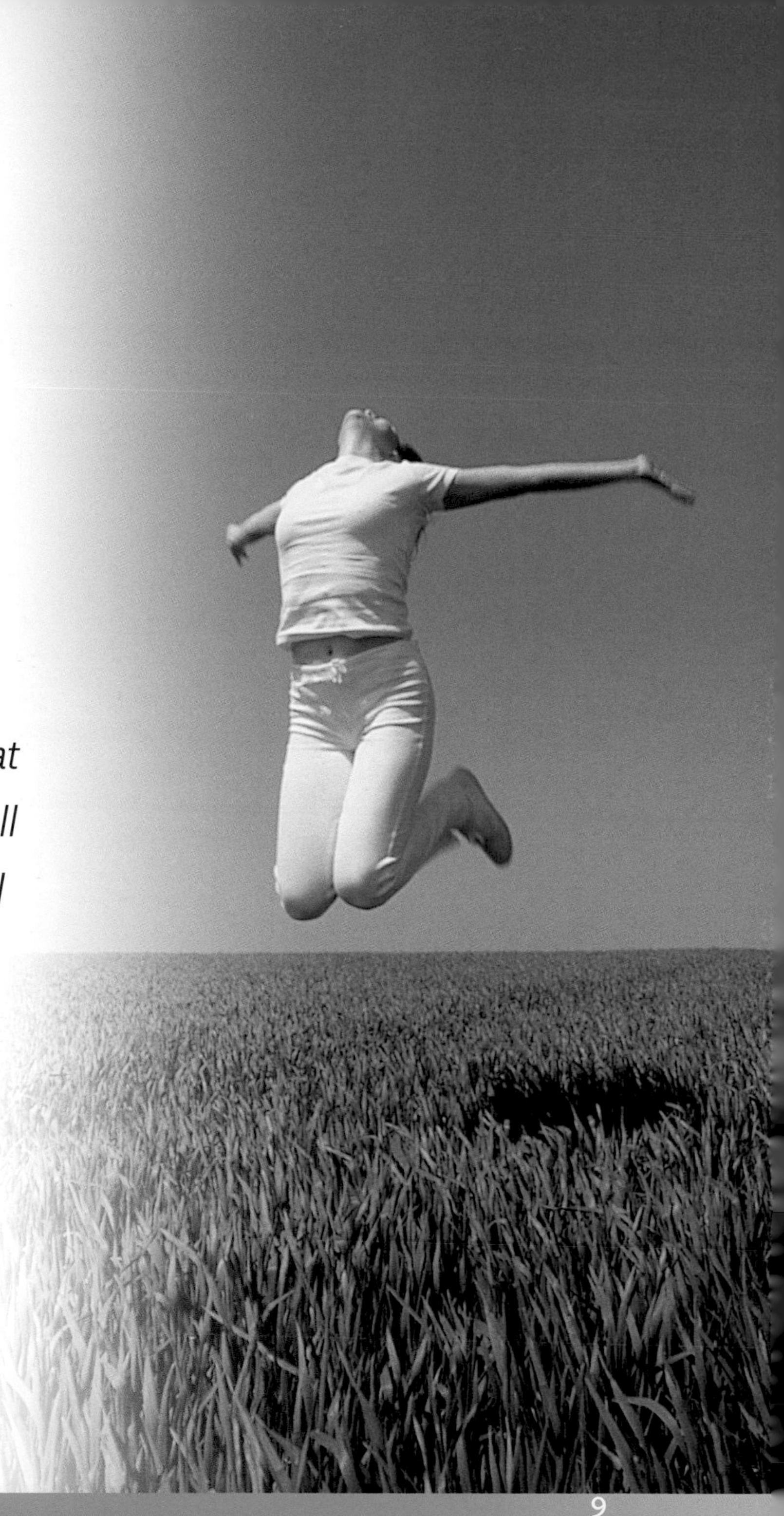

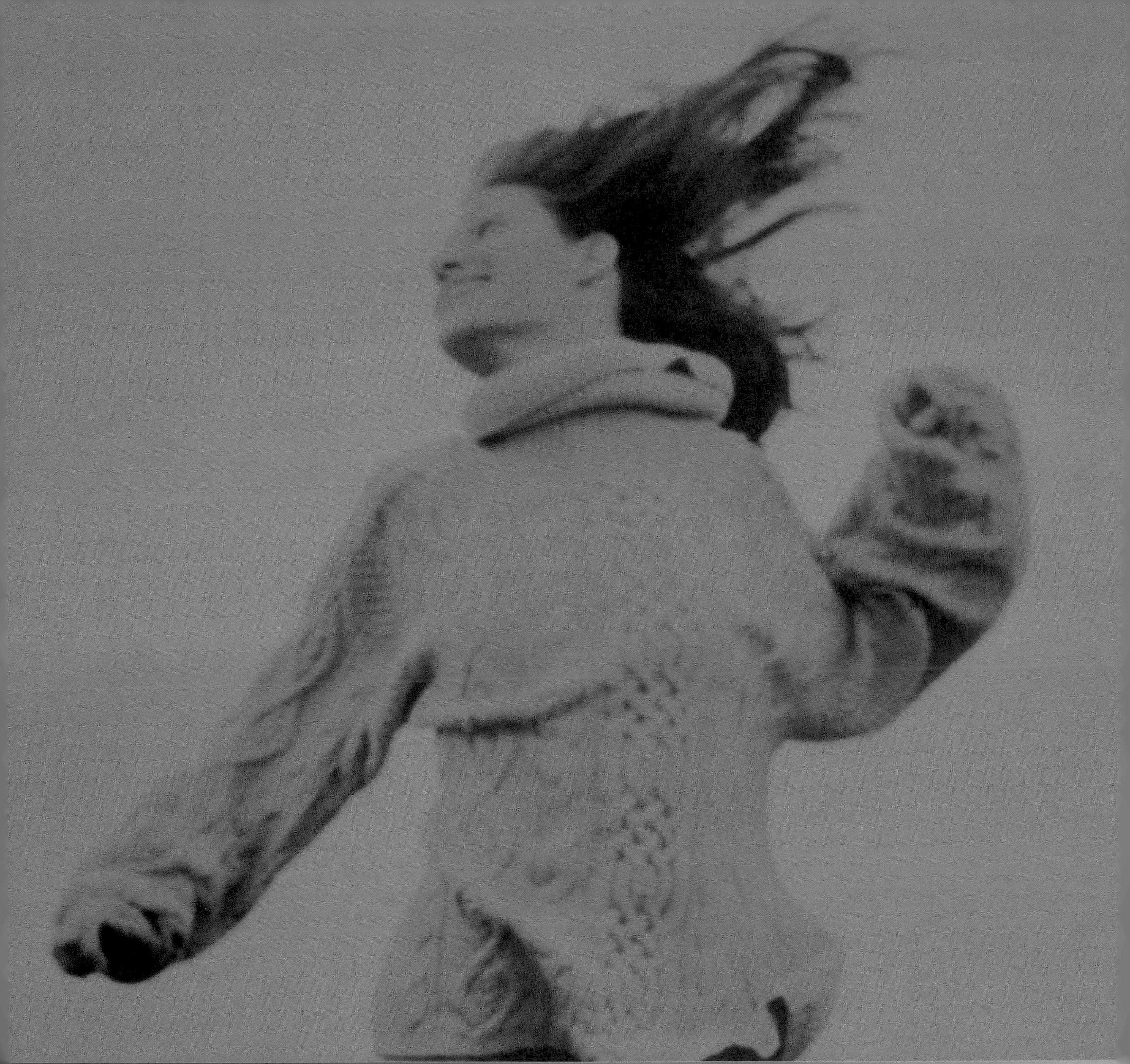

**CHAPTER 1**

# What is energy?

*In the West we tend to see energy in terms of how much we are able to do.*

From an early age we are taught that energy in (i.e. food) = energy out (i.e. being able to work hard and play hard). We take energy in through food and air, process it and pass it out again. The amount of energy we have depends then on us eating well, breathing correctly and not allowing ourselves to become overworked or over-stressed.

Imagine your energy levels as a bank account: if you keep taking energy out without putting something back in you will start to use up your savings or reserves. Therefore, in order to achieve optimum energy levels it is vital that we learn how to replenish our reserves through, for example, meditation, good diet, exercise and so on. We must also develop more of an awareness of our own energy levels so that we know when we are overdoing it, and take the opportunity to recharge our batteries.

Ancient civilisations believed that our bodies were made up not only of skin, muscle and bone, but an energy that cannot be seen even under a microscope. Most cultures and traditions see energy as the essence of life or our life force: the Chinese call it qi, the Japanese call it ki, the Indians call it prana, and in some parts of the Middle East it is known as quwa. Whatever it is called, healers from these different cultures all work with energy centres and pathways. Shamans use rituals and ceremonies to shift energies. Eastern traditions also believe in disciplines such as t'ai chi, qi gong and yoga to help stimulate energy flow. Clairvoyants and psychics also work with energy stemming from an aura that surrounds the body which they describe as many colours of light.

*Ultimately, it does not matter how you view energy – it is the same thing viewed from a different cultural perspective.*

*When someone feels that they are lacking in energy it can mean one of two things:*

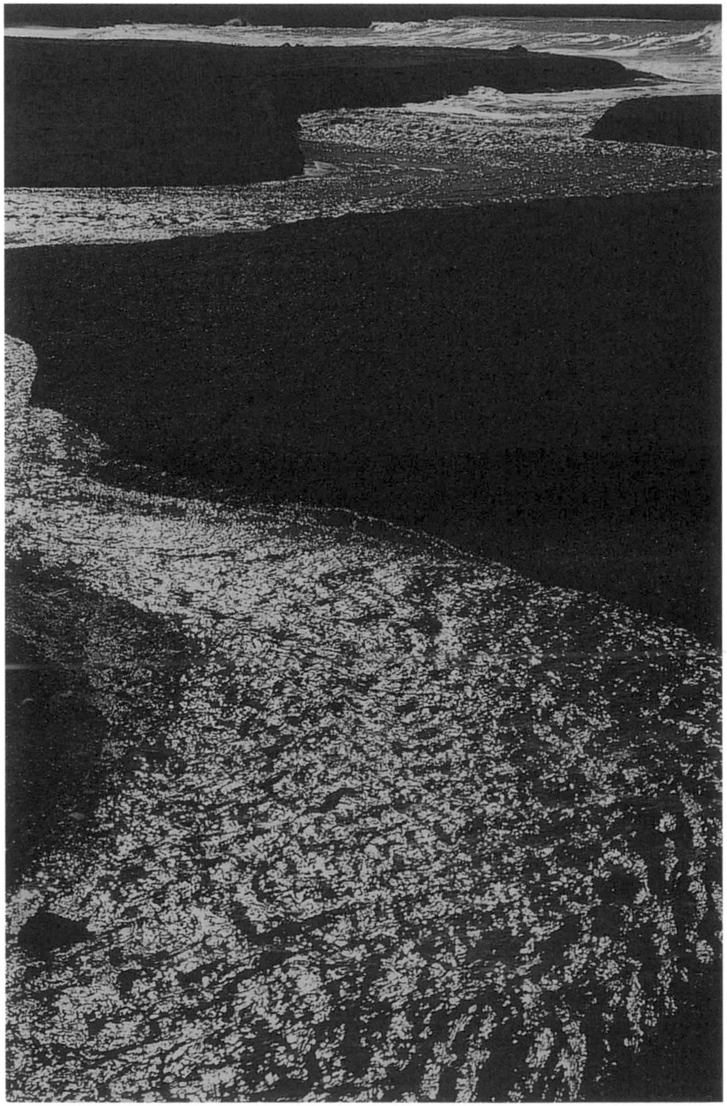

either there is a blockage preventing the free flow of energy (caused by factors such as stress, emotional or physical trauma, smoking and alcohol and drug abuse) or there was never enough energy in the first place. Imagine your body's energy as water in a river: if nothing is in its way the water can flow freely, but if there is an obstruction, it will become stagnant; equally, if there is not enough water in the river then it will dry up altogether. It is vital then to find ways to build up our energy supply whilst also making efforts to continually stimulate and balance its natural flow.

In order to better understand the underlying principles behind many of the exercises that will be used later in the book – such as qi gong (Chinese) and yoga (Indian) – let's take a look at their meaning, and their relevance when trying to work on our energy levels.

# Qi

Qi is a key concept in traditional Chinese medicine, similar to prana in Indian philosophy (see page 14) and ki in Japanese. Chinese medicine views the mind and body as working due to the interaction of vital substances. It sees the body and mind as a combination of energy (our get-up-and-go energy) and vital energy (the energy needed for all our systems to function). These energies interact to make a person. At the basis of all of this is qi. All the other vital substances such as blood, body, fluids or shen (mind) are all also qi manifested in different forms.

*Qi is a vital essence found in all things. It is the force that drives every cell of our bodies, without which we would die.*

Qi supports, nourishes and defends us against mental, emotional and physical problems. It is an invisible electromagnetic energy that modern research in the West interprets as energy.

The Chinese believe that inner harmony is dependent upon a healthy, balanced and unobstructed flow of qi. A smooth, uninterrupted flow will mean that you relax easily, feel energetic, happy and able to cope with difficult situations, sleep well, wake up rejuvenated and, and have the ability to fight off disease with an efficient immune system.

Acupuncturists work with the qi that moves through the meridians or channels. Qi is also used in the practice of feng shui, where the energy of a house may be studied and furniture and other objects placed in certain positions in order to improve the flow of qi.

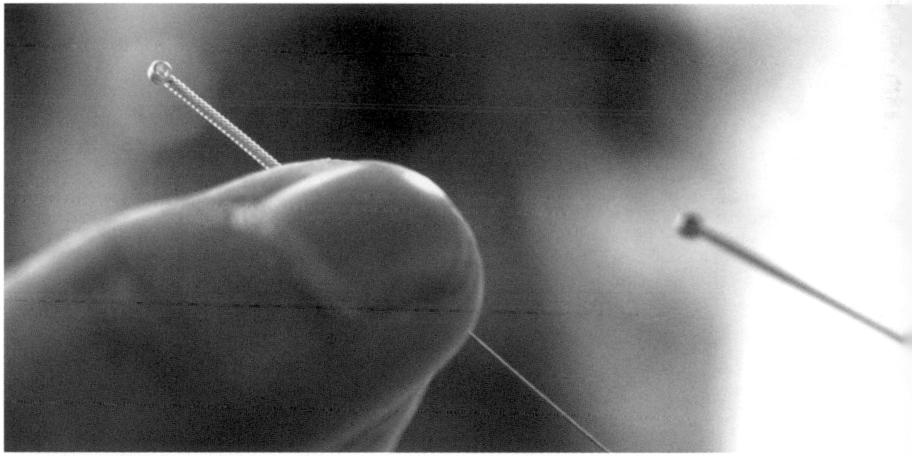

# Prana

*Prana is a Sanskrit word meaning the energy which sustains all life and creation.*

It is thought to be all the energy that exists in the universe, and strength, power, vitality, life and spirit are all forms of prana. It is used in Indian medicine and the practice of yoga. Ayurvedic medicine (the ancient system of medicine practised in India) also talks of prana, using it to denote the living energy that fills our food, bodies and our relationships.

**The philosophy of energy** While many ancient philosophies consider the concept of universal energy, it also plays a part in modern philosophies such as quantum physics which holds that everything that exists in the universe is made up of patterns of energy (for example atoms). Like atoms, people and objects are made up of groups of vibrating energetic particles (also known as prana/qi). Indian medicine teaches that we take prana into our bodies through the nadis. These are subtle energy channels that feed our chakras. Nadis are very similar to the subtle energy channels or meridians in Chinese medicine, and as in that discipline, it is important to ensure that prana flows smoothly. Yoga postures, a healthy diet, sunlight, fresh air, meditation and correct breathing techniques can all encourage this.

Yoga practitioners teach that by using yoga techniques, prana can be controlled, directed and stored at will, and that by learning to tap into it you can acquire endless energy. Some of these techniques will be looked at later in the yoga and breathing sections of this book (see pp. 102 and 120). Yoga, like Chinese medicine, teaches that a balance of masculine and feminine energy makes for balance of the whole. This can be brought about through the physical postures often referred to as hatha yoga (ha meaning sun and tha meaning moon). Yoga also teaches that masculine and feminine energy can be balanced through correct breathing: the right nostril carries the nadi for the sun or masculine energy, while the left carries the nadi for the moon or feminine energy. Both energies then connect and travel down the spine which is the main nadi.

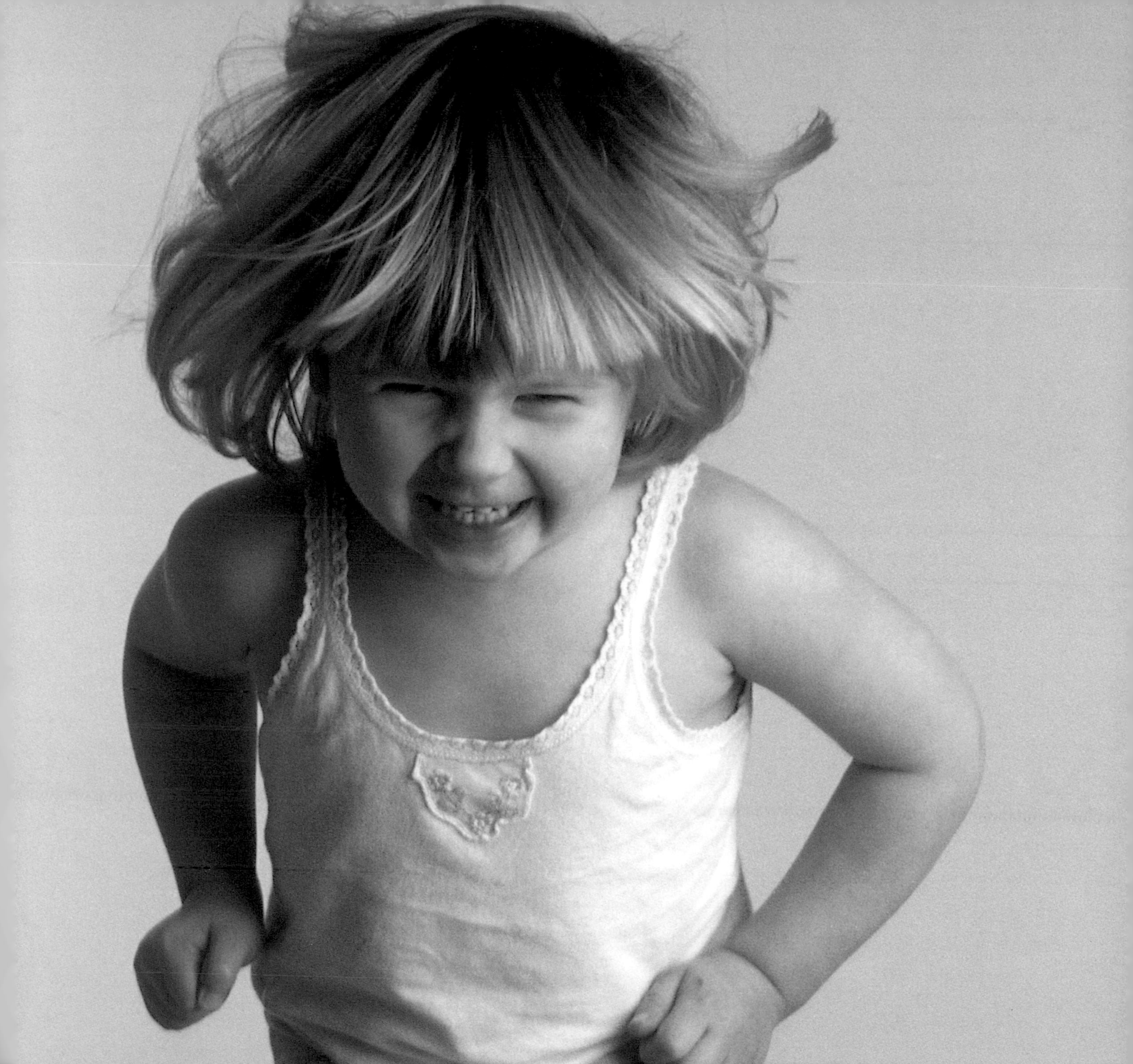

**HOW MUCH ENERGY DO YOU HAVE?** When I ask patients at my acupuncture practice, 'How much energy do you have?', many of them find it a difficult question to answer. A lot of people will gauge their own energy levels in terms of their friends': some will measure themselves against a friend who is often lethargic and lacking in motivation, and feel that they have lots of energy in comparison, while others might think that because they cannot keep up with a friend who can seemingly do everything without ever complaining of tiredness, they must therefore have low energy.

This sort of reasoning is not helpful when trying to assess your own energy levels. It is therefore essential, before going any further, to learn to never compare yourself to others in this respect. Everybody's energy needs are different and vary at different times in their lives which is why it is so important to think about yourself as an individual. (For example, your partner might only be able to go out and party every evening because they work more flexible hours than you do, and can therefore catch up on sleep when you can't.) Concentrate on your own lifestyle and expectations of what you might like it to be, in order to achieve the optimum energy to fulfil it.

To help you to formulate a fair assessment of what your energy levels might be, answer the following questions as truthfully as possible. They should help to give you an awareness of those areas of your life in which you are spending too much energy or not replenishing it, and help you to devise some realistic goals to address this.

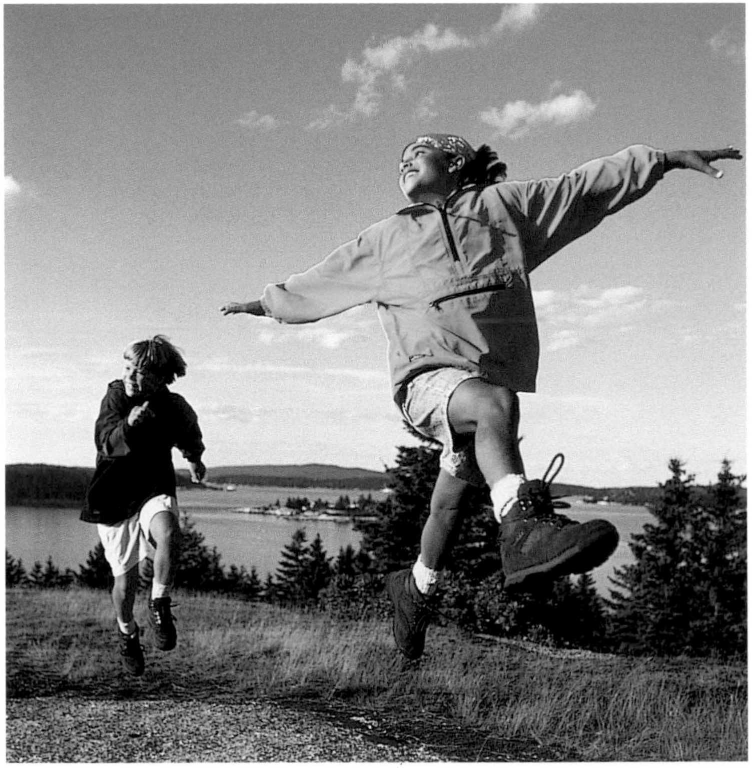

## GAUGING ENERGY LEVELS

Here are some examples of how some people say they feel living with and without optimum energy levels:

**With**

- wake up in the morning feeling refreshed and ready for the day ahead
- bursting with the joys of life
- motivated
- powerful
- confident and outgoing
- full of get-up-and-go
- very active, with an extra spring in their stride

**Without**

- wake up in the morning feeling tired
- simple day-to-day living feels like a huge effort
- everything is a hassle, even getting up from a chair is an effort
- dips of energy occur throughout the day
- feel aches and pains.

By answering the questions below you will establish what it is that you would like to achieve and what might be standing in your way. Now turn the page and let's take a closer look at some of the factors that could be taking your energy away from you.

### What would you like to achieve?

- Do you have enough energy for your current lifestyle?
- If not, what realistic goals would you like to set for your energy levels? (Remember, don't compare yourself to other people.)
- Why do you not have 'enough' energy? (Don't worry if you can't pinpoint the answer to this one, but there will be some people who know the cause – for example poor diet, not enough sleep – and choose to ignore it.)
- How are you losing your reserve energy (the energy that the body has inherited or made and stored since birth)? (Perhaps you are going out late even when you are tired?)
- What are you doing to prevent yourself from replenishing your reserves?

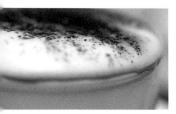

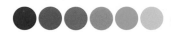

## ENERGY ZAPPERS AND FAKE ENERGY

*Energy zappers are things that rob us of our energy.*

They include:

- stress
- feeling low
- depression
- anxiety
- blood deficiency (mild) – anaemia (severe)
- vitamin deficiency/poor diet
- sedentary lifestyle/no exercise
- dehydration, low sugar levels
- overwork
- eating meals on the run
- being overweight
- lack of fresh air
- insufficient sleep
- emotional strain, worry
- negative thoughts (your own or other people's)
- stimulants (coffee, tea, sugary fixes like sweets, fizzy drinks, chocolate, alcohol, cigarettes, recreational drugs).

False or fake energy is the energy you get from a stimulant: you feel a rush of energy but this is not real and is, in fact, stolen from your reserve energy. After the energy rush you feel even more tired than before and need more of the stimulant to get any energy hit at all, thus creating an addictive effect. Adrenaline, or emotions such as anxiety, can have a similar effect by generating the same 'rush' that an 'energetic' person has naturally all the time.

Trying to manipulate our energy levels by drinking coffee and alcohol, smoking, taking social drugs and sleeping pills can never work in the long term. Because the 'rush' these can give you is activated by a stimulant, the energy generated is not real and will leave you feeling exhausted because you will have used up your reserve without realising it. Comfort foods and sugary drinks have the same effect: they create a temporary adrenaline increase similar to that used in the body's response to stress.

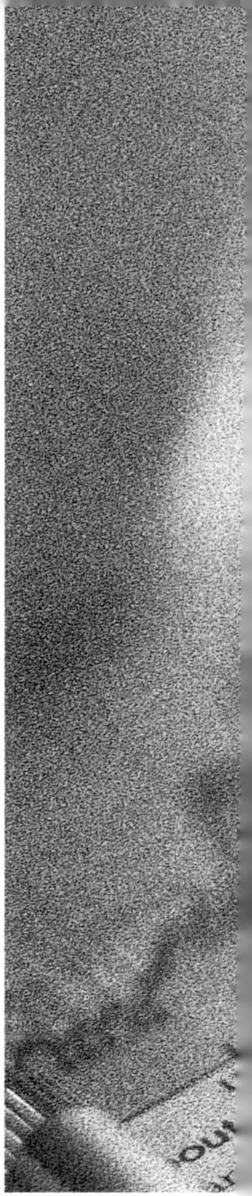

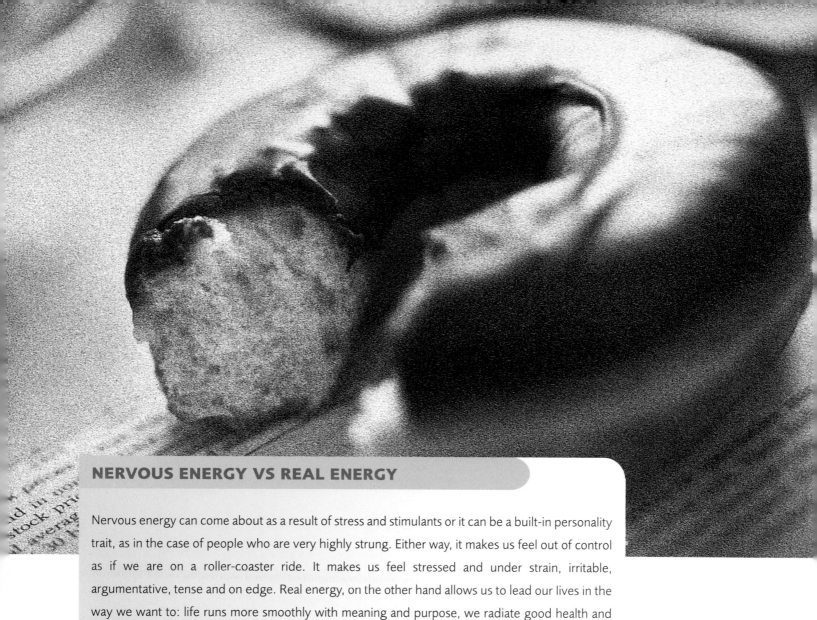

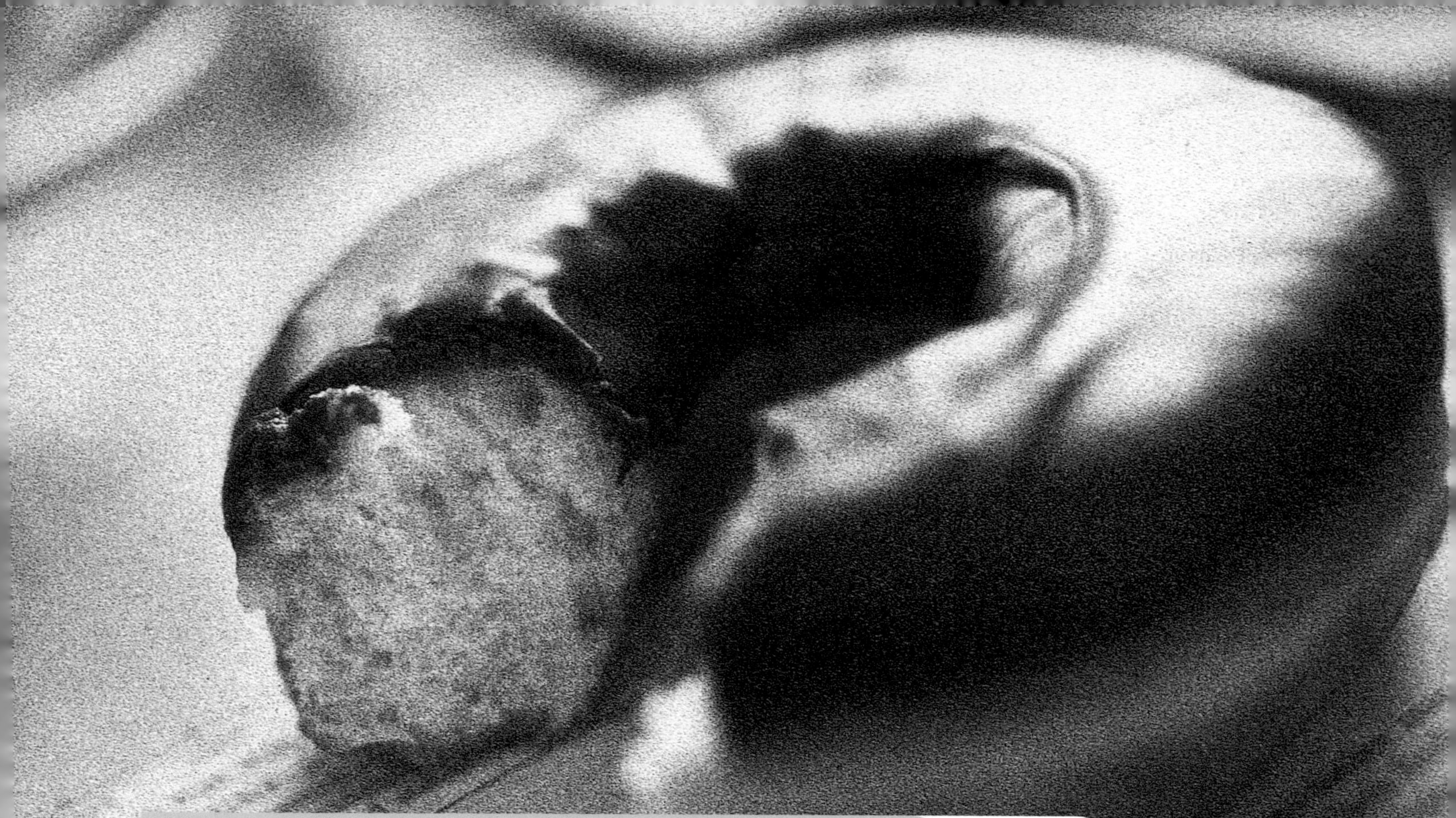

## NERVOUS ENERGY VS REAL ENERGY

Nervous energy can come about as a result of stress and stimulants or it can be a built-in personality trait, as in the case of people who are very highly strung. Either way, it makes us feel out of control as if we are on a roller-coaster ride. It makes us feel stressed and under strain, irritable, argumentative, tense and on edge. Real energy, on the other hand allows us to lead our lives in the way we want to: life runs more smoothly with meaning and purpose, we radiate good health and move with ease, with each day feeling like a new adventure or experience. And at those times when everything doesn't feel quite right, real energy gives us the patience to work through whatever it is that is bothering us.

## LISTEN TO YOUR BODY QUESTIONNAIRE

1.Do you wake up feeling tired? YES ◯ NO ◯

2.Are you always saying 'I am so tired and I don't know why?' YES ◯ NO ◯

3.Do you sigh a lot? YES ◯ NO ◯

4.Do you find life a big effort? YES ◯ NO ◯

5. Is it an effort just to go to another room or floor in your house just to get something? YES ◯ NO ◯

6.Do you look at other people and wonder how they have the energy to do so much with their lives.? YES ◯ NO ◯

7.Is just getting up off the chair a big effort? YES ◯ NO ◯

8.Do you have dips of energy throughout the day where you find yourself reaching for tea, coffee or chocolate for help? YES ◯ NO ◯

9.Do people always say that you look tired? YES ◯ NO ◯

10. Are you stopping yourself living the life you would like to live because you always or often feel tired? YES ◯ NO ◯

11. Do you feel tired behind the eyes? YES ◯ NO ◯

12. Do your shoulders feel too heavy? YES ◯ NO ◯

13. Do you find it difficult to concentrate? YES ◯ NO ◯

14. Do you have a muzzy head? YES ◯ NO ◯

**LISTEN TO YOUR BODY** Finding an endless source of energy need not be that difficult, and listening to your body is a key step in achieving this. So if you are always saying, 'I'm so tired', listen – your body is telling you to take action. If you are not exhausted all the time but sometimes feel tired, you may be running below your optimum energy and in need of a boost.

The questionnaire opposite will help you assess how much energy you have (or lack), and to determine which energy plan would be most suitable for you. If you answer mainly 'Yes', then your energy is very low, and one of the longer energy plans would be best for you.

If you answer some questions 'Yes' (less than half), one of the shorter plans would be helpful. More specifically, when you know you have a particularly taxing week ahead, you might use the seven-day plan to prepare yourself for it.

Once you increase your energy levels, all other aspects of your life will improve: physically – you will look and feel better and fitter; mentally – you will feel more alert and able to concentrate; emotionally – you will be more relaxed and happy. You will also notice that your work will improve, as you will be less stressed and able to focus better.

**Finding Energy** So how do you find energy for all the things you want to do in life, and not just what you have to do? Let's start by looking at what gives us energy and what takes it away.

| GIVES US ENERGY | TAKES ENERGY AWAY |
|---|---|
| Living healthily | Illness |
| Keeping fit | Being unfit |
| Relaxation | Tension/stress |
| Drinking water | Dehydration |
| Good posture | Poor posture |
| Healthy, balanced diet | A poor diet |
| Good sleep | Lack of sleep |
| Good quality air | Poor quality air |
| Positive emotions | Negativity |

# Ill health

Depleted energy can sometimes be the result of a long-term illness, but often we may not even be aware of having the illness in question, having grown used to weariness and fatigue without ever looking into the cause.

The following are just a few of the main illnesses that can cause you to have no energy. I have included stress in this list because being under tremendous amounts of stress on a regular basis can eventually cause you to be run down and even ill. If you do think you might be suffering from one of the illnesses below it is important to seek professional medical advice.

**Allergies** These days allergies seem to be more and more common because we put our bodies under much more stress than we used to. Antibiotics, additives, pesticides, stimulants, poor nutrition, alcohol and drugs all put a big strain on our immune systems and this has a direct impact on our energy levels.

The immune system responds to an allergen (any substance that causes an allergic reaction) by not recognising it and treating it like an enemy: it releases histamine to attack it. Allergic reactions take many forms, typical examples being:

- skin rash
- breathing problems such as wheezing
- streaming eyes, itchy throat and a runny nose
- tiredness/fatigue
- bowel problems such as irritable bowel (often known as IBS), colitis and Crohn's disease
- joint problems such as arthritis.

Tiredness comes as a result of your immune system's constant fight against the allergen or allergens in question, and if this continues over a long period of time you will gradually feel more and more exhausted.

If you can pinpoint the cause of your allergy to and avoid coming in contact with it you will find that your energy levels will increase dramatically. This may not always be easy as often we actually crave the foods we are allergic to because eating them causes an adrenaline rush as the body tries to fight the reaction. Afterwards you will inevitably feel unwell and tired again.

*A lack of energy and tiredness can be the body's signal that it is run down, and can eventually lead to ill health.*

An electro diagnosis machine (the quantum QXCI machine), kinesiology, or blood, urine, stool or hair test can help you to establish what you are allergic to. Homeopathy can also help to desensitise you to the allergen.

**Blood Deficiency/Anaemia** Anaemia or blood deficiency as it is known in Chinese medicine, is the medical term for a deficiency of red blood cells or haemoglobin. Haemoglobin carries oxygen around the body and contains iron.

Symptoms of anaemia can include the following:

- increasing tiredness until you find you are exhausted all the time and feel quite run down
- hair and skin lacking life and lustre, dry skin, and nails that split more easily
- looking pale, with pale nails and tongue
- pins and needles or numbness in your limbs
- dizziness
- floaters in front of your eyes.

If you think you have anaemia/blood deficiency it is vital that you get a blood test to confirm this. Supplementing your diet with vitamins C, B12, folic acid and iron are recommended, and you should also eat foods containing these. A good naturopath or nutritionalist can give you more specific advice on doses and diet. A herbalist or acupuncturist can also help you to 'build' the blood. Once your haemoglobin levels pick up again so too will your energy.

**Candida albicans** is a yeast-like fungus that inhabits the gut, mouth, throat, genital tract, intestines and oesophagus. It lives in all of us normally but is kept in balance by other friendly bacteria and yeasts in the body. When that balance is disrupted, candida multiplies and weakens the immune system resulting in candidiasis. Things that might disrupt the balance include:

- overuse of antibiotics which, over time, weaken the immune system and destroy the friendly bacteria that usually keep candida under control
- taking oral contraceptives (candida thrives when progesterone is high)
- taking steroids regularly
- an already weak immune system
- too much stress
- too much sugar, alcohol, dairy products, fried food
- pregnancy.

Candida can also lead to leaky gut syndrome, which occurs when undigested food is allowed to pass into your bloodstream causing allergies. This can cause even more tiredness.

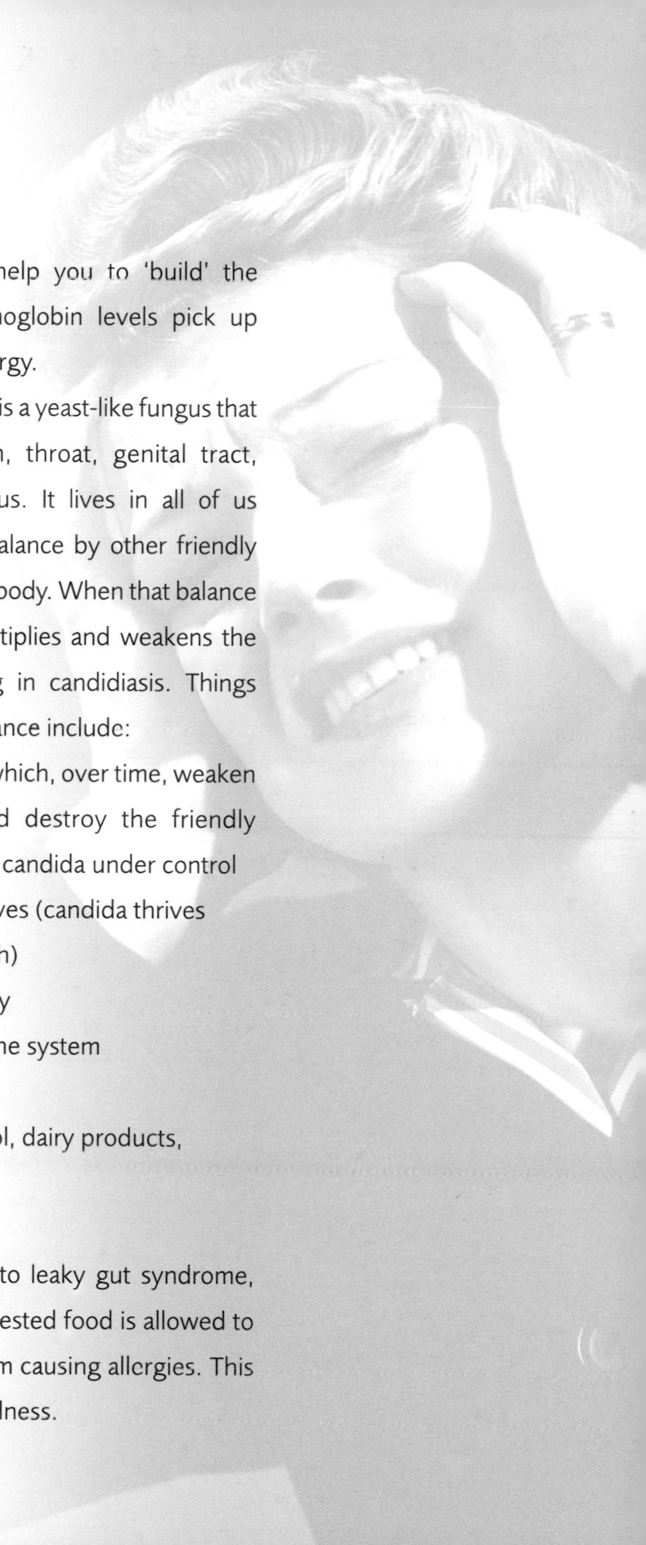

Because candida can affect many different parts of the body it can cause a multitude of symptoms, including: exhaustion, diarrhoea, abdominal pain, bloating, constipation, gas, irritable bowel, persistent heartburn, itchy anus, thrush, bad breath, headaches, mood swings, difficulty in concentrating, food cravings, allergies, athlete's foot, muscle and joint pain, sore throat, nagging cough, clogged sinuses, pre-menstrual syndrome (PMS), and kidney and bladder infections

Because there are so many different symptoms, candida often goes undiagnosed. Killing off the candida involves following a strict diet with no sugar, yeast or alcohol and supplements that help to redress the balance of the friendly bacteria. The actual process can make you feel very unwell as toxins are released into the body, but afterwards you will feel re-energised. Always seek the help of a health practitioner if you think you have candida.

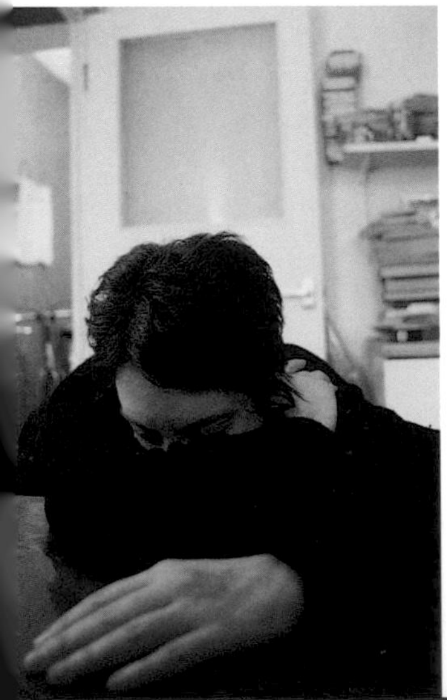

**Chronic Fatigue/ME (myalgic encephalitis)** Chronic fatigue/ME is completely different from just feeling tired all the time. It can occur as a result of a viral illness such as flu, or after a shock, exposure to an environmental toxin, or a vaccination. If the body is put under more stress than it is able to cope with the adrenals become exhausted – this is also thought to be a common cause of chronic fatigue.

Chronic fatigue causes complete mental and physical exhaustion for six months or more, sometimes even for years, along with symptoms such as muscle aches and pains, sensitivity to light and noise, muzzy-headedness and difficulty in concentrating. Most chronic fatigue sufferers have to give up work and many social activities.

If you are, or if you think you might be suffering from chronic fatigue/ME you must seek the advice of a medical practitioner before starting any exercise routines or energy plans in this book. A herbalist, acupuncturist or naturopath can be of great help.

**Depression** Depression is a very common cause of tiredness, and something that most people don't like to admit to. People often become depressed when their expectations of life don't actually match up to reality. Depression can also occur as a result of being under too much stress. Many people don't even realise that they are suffering from depression as it can creep up on them quite slowly and it is not until the world feels like a hopeless place that they finally realise that something is wrong.

Symptoms of depression can include:

- having no energy
- feeling anxious all the time
- putting on weight or losing weight
- loss of interest in life/people
- feelings of worthlessness; feeling like a failure
- feeling bored and dissatisfied all the time
- finding it difficult to get to sleep/insomnia
- having low self esteem and no confidence, being self critical
- difficulty getting out of bed; sleeping all the time
- being very detached from the world.

If you are depressed it is vital to get help from a medical practitioner or counsellor. Therapy and counselling can help you to see the world is not such an awful place and help you to regain the confidence that you may have lost. Dealing with the depression will in turn help with the symptoms, including tiredness.

**Hormone Imbalance** There are many different types of hormone, which are mainly controlled by the pituitary gland in the brain. When one hormone is out of balance it will usually have a knock-on effect on all the others, and when an imbalance occurs, symptoms such as tiredness and mood changes can follow.

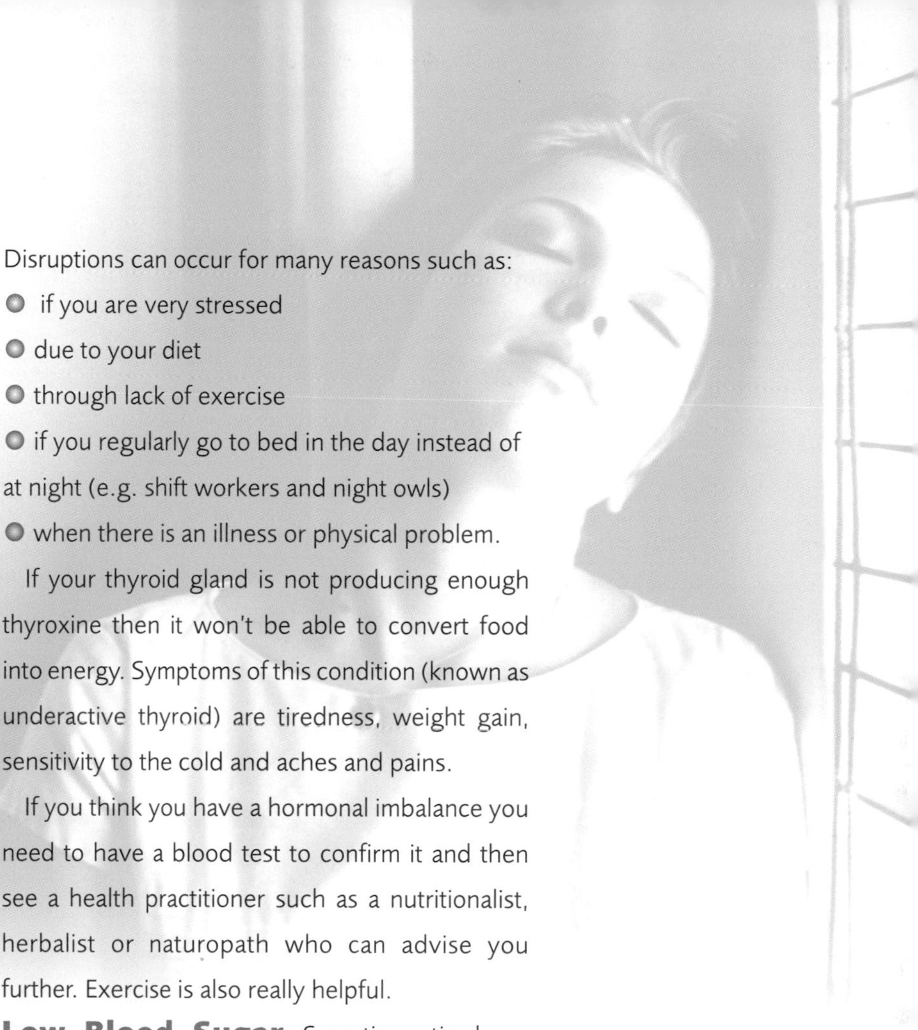

Disruptions can occur for many reasons such as:

- if you are very stressed
- due to your diet
- through lack of exercise
- if you regularly go to bed in the day instead of at night (e.g. shift workers and night owls)
- when there is an illness or physical problem.

If your thyroid gland is not producing enough thyroxine then it won't be able to convert food into energy. Symptoms of this condition (known as underactive thyroid) are tiredness, weight gain, sensitivity to the cold and aches and pains.

If you think you have a hormonal imbalance you need to have a blood test to confirm it and then see a health practitioner such as a nutritionalist, herbalist or naturopath who can advise you further. Exercise is also really helpful.

**Low Blood Sugar** Sometimes tiredness can occur as a result of low blood sugar, known as hypoglycaemia.

Energy comes from food when the body converts it into glucose, which we need not only for energy but also for the brain and nervous system. When you eat, this glucose makes your blood sugar level rise temporarily, after which it should then go back to normal. However, if you

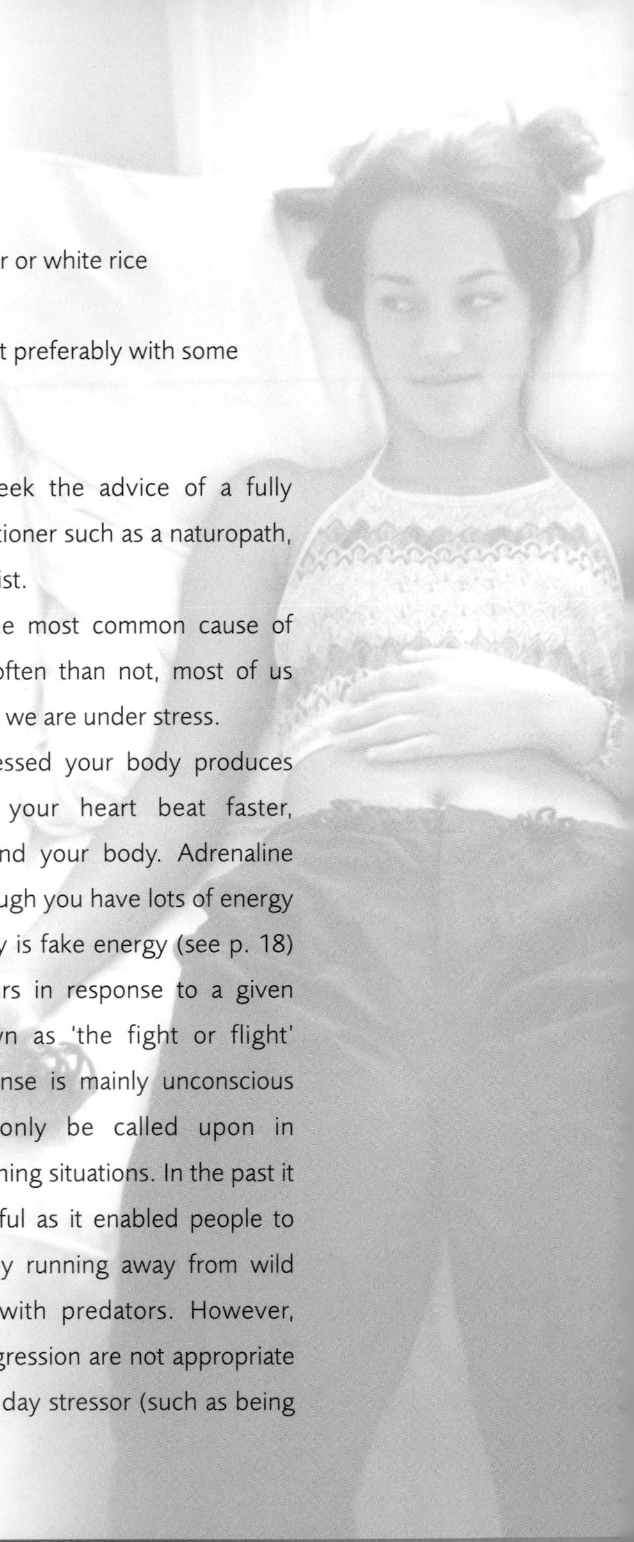

eat lots of sugary foods, or fast-releasing carbohydrates such as white bread, cakes or biscuits your blood sugar level rises too high too quickly. The pancreas then releases insulin to try and compensate for this. Insulin tries to make the sugar level go back down again, but it can then sometimes drop below its normal level causing:

- tiredness and shakiness
- irritability and mood swings
- nausea and dizziness
- difficulty in concentrating
- regular headaches
- sugar cravings.

These symptoms occur mainly between meals or if you skip a meal. This is when most people will reach for a sugary snack to help lift their energy, but in fact, this is the worst thing you can do as your blood sugar level will afterwards drop again, sometimes even lower than before and you will feel exhausted.

It is important to break the cycle of high and low blood sugar levels. To help you do this:

- make sure you eat every three to four hours
- snack on things such as nuts and seeds
- avoid sugar and sugary drinks, caffeine and alcohol.
- don't eat white flour or white rice
- never miss meals
- always eat breakfast preferably with some protein in it
- exercise regularly

You should also seek the advice of a fully qualified health practitioner such as a naturopath, nutritionalist or herbalist.

**Stress** Stress is the most common cause of tiredness and more often than not, most of us don't even realise that we are under stress.

When you are stressed your body produces adrenaline, making your heart beat faster, pumping blood around your body. Adrenaline makes you feel as though you have lots of energy but this sort of energy is fake energy (see p. 18) because it only occurs in response to a given situation. It is known as 'the fight or flight' response. This response is mainly unconscious and should really only be called upon in emergency or threatening situations. In the past it would have very useful as it enabled people to respond to danger by running away from wild animals or fighting with predators. However, running away and aggression are not appropriate responses to modern day stressor (such as being stuck in a traffic jam, trying to meet deadlines or struggling financially) and the physical effects that they generate – increased heart rate, blood pressure and breathing – will leave you feeling exhausted. Regularly stimulating the fight or flight response will cause your body to function less efficiently than it usually would.

Constant pressure means that the nervous system cannot calm down enough to re-establish the body's status quo. The body then finds it difficult to relax at all, and after a while you become 'stressed out'.

People who are under stress all the time tend to do everything quickly, whether it's eating, talking, walking, or any other day-to-day activity. This is very tiring as the body is being repeatedly depleted of its natural energy reserves. Once the adrenals start to become stressed, the adrenaline will not be able to cope with demands that stress is putting on the body's energy levels, and will no longer be able to maintain blood sugar levels. The immune system may then suffer, and illnesses such as high blood pressure, digestive disorders, depression, anxiety, irritability can all occur, as well as mood swings, headaches and sleep problems.

This is when most people reach for stimulants to help cover up the tiredness /burnout and give them a false sense of having some energy. Stimulants like coffee, cigarettes, alcohol, sugary foods and drugs may all feel like they are helping but in fact they are simply putting further pressure on the adrenals.

Because you become used to functioning at this pace you may not even realise just how stressed you really are. In order to assess if you are stressed, ask yourself questions like: am I doing too much?; do I need more 'space'?; do I need more time for rest and relaxation?; do I feel under pressure/anxious/irritable?; do I find it difficult to relax/sleep? If you answer 'yes', to all or most of these questions, you need to take positive steps to relieve yourself of some stress.

Following the simple relaxation and posture, breathing and exercise routines later in the book will give you the tools to help your body to unwind and deal with stress. Regular treatments of massage, acupuncture, meditation, healing can also be very beneficial. A qualified health practitioner will also be able to help you to highlight those areas in your life that you have learnt to consider 'normal' but which are in fact major stress factors.

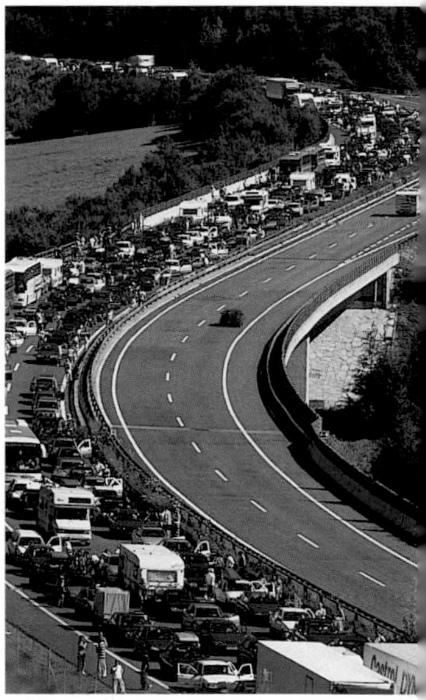

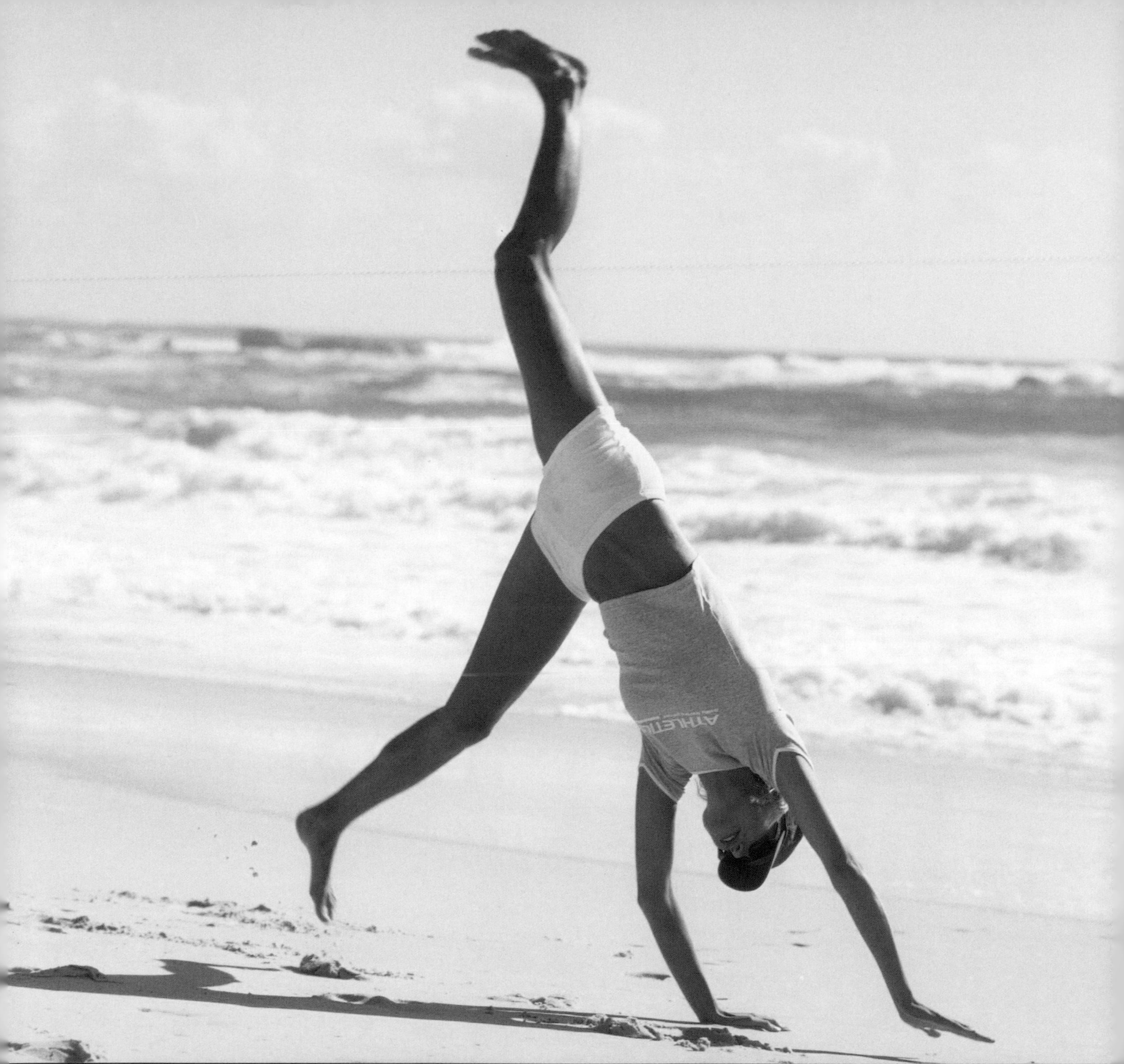

CHAPTER 2

# Increase your Energy

*So far we have looked at why we feel tired and how tired we really are but we haven't yet looked at ways to treat and beat this constant fatigue.*

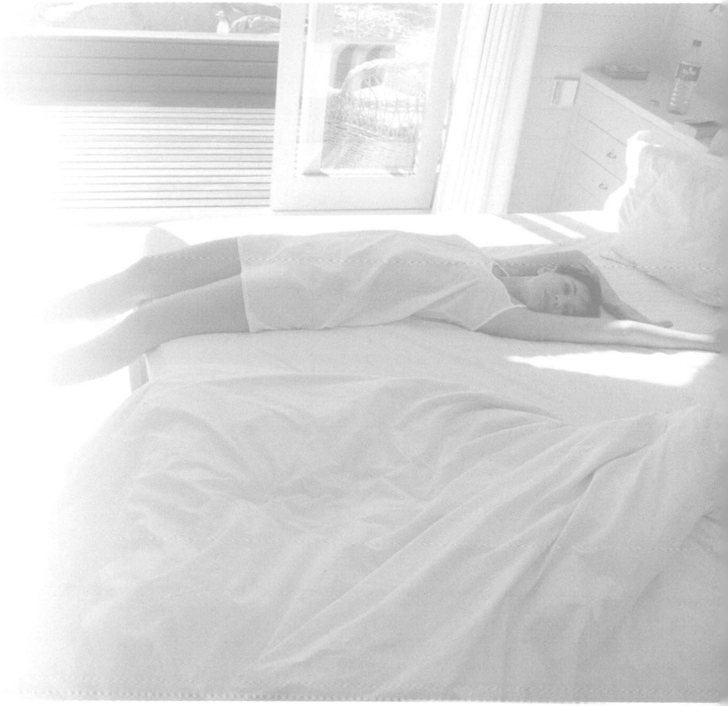

The following therapies can either be practised at home, or with the help of a qualified practitioner (see page 216 for a list of relevant councils, or ask your doctor for a referral). They can help treat fatigue by treating the underlying physical, emotional and spiritual causes.

Before going to any therapist always make sure that they are fully qualified and recognised (i.e. that they are members of a body or council), and that they have the necessary insurance. It is also very important that you like the therapist you choose and that you feel comfortable talking to him or her about personal matters.

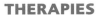

THERAPIES

# Acupuncture

*Acupuncture (meaning, literally needle-piercing) is an ancient form of medicine over two thousand years old, and it is still the main medical system used in China today.*

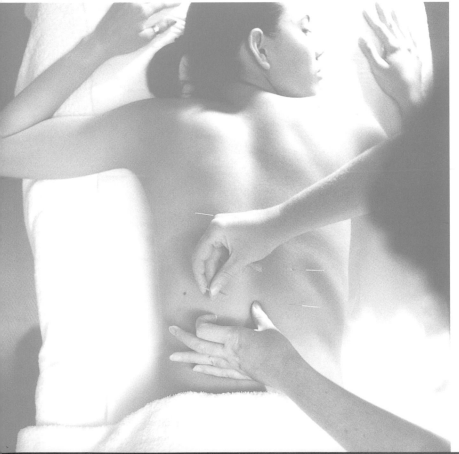

It is based on the insertion of fine needles into specific points along the channels of the body. Its exact origins are unknown, but one theory is that when the ancient neighbouring tribes were warring, men who were wounded in battle found that injuries in specific points seemed to help various illnesses that they suffered from.

Acupuncture is used to treat disease, for pain relief and for anaesthesia during surgery. Yin and yang, which form the basis of Chinese medicine, are essentially about balance and harmony. Yin represents things like cold, rest, and the feminine, while yang represents active, light, hot and masculine. The two are opposites that make up a whole, and one cannot be without the other. They exist in varying degrees in everything, and when they are in harmony we feel good, but if one dominates it creates an imbalance and we feel unwell. There are twelve main channels in the body, each of which relates to a particular organ. They are divided into six pairs so that there are yin meridians which flow up the inside of the legs and body and down the inside of the arms as they gather energy up from the earth, and yang meridians that run oppositely up the outside of the arms to the shoulders, head and body and down the outside of the legs as they gather energy down from the sky.

Through these channels flows qi (pronounced chee) which is the body's energy or life force. There are three types or sources of qi:

- congenital qi: this is given to us by both parents at conception and is the measure of our overall vitality. It is stored in the kidneys and can be depleted by lack of sleep, stress and too many stimulants. Dark rings around the eyes are often a sign of depleted congenital qi.
- protective qi: as its name suggest this qi helps to protect the body by surrounding it and helping to maintain its thermostat so that we don't suffer excessive cold or heat. It also strengthens the immune system. If protective qi is weak then resistance is lowered and the likelihood of illness is increased, which we in the West would recognise as being 'overtired' or 'run down'.
- nutritive qi: this is made from the air we breathe and the food that we eat. Breathing correctly, eating natural foods and drinking lots of fresh water helps to strengthen the nutritive qi. Whereas a nutritionalist might say that a particular food is high in vitamins and nutrients an acupuncturist would say that food was rich in qi. In the West we would recognise someone whose nutritive qi was weak if they ate a poor diet and were therefore more susceptible to illness and feeling tired.

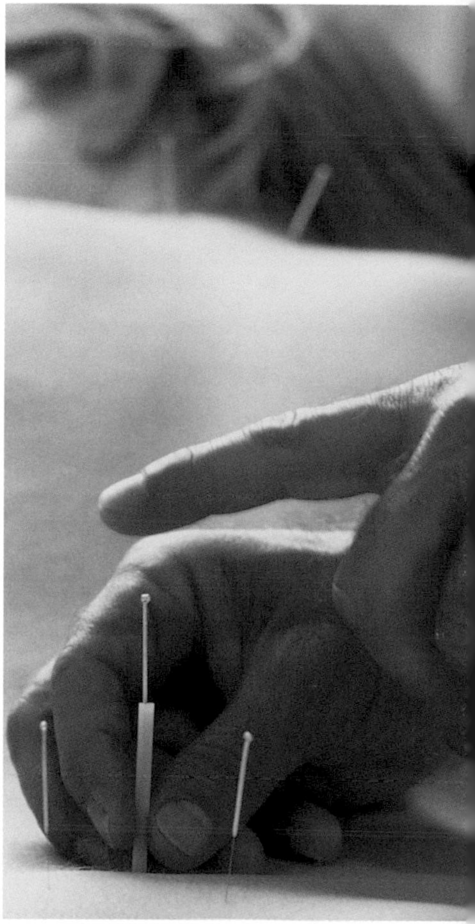

Acupuncturists believe that if a person is lacking in energy it can be for many different reasons including:

- blood deficiency (which in its most extreme form can present as anaemia, see page 23)
- qi deficiency
- qi stagnation (where the energy has become blocked and therefore stagnant due to illness or stress etc.)

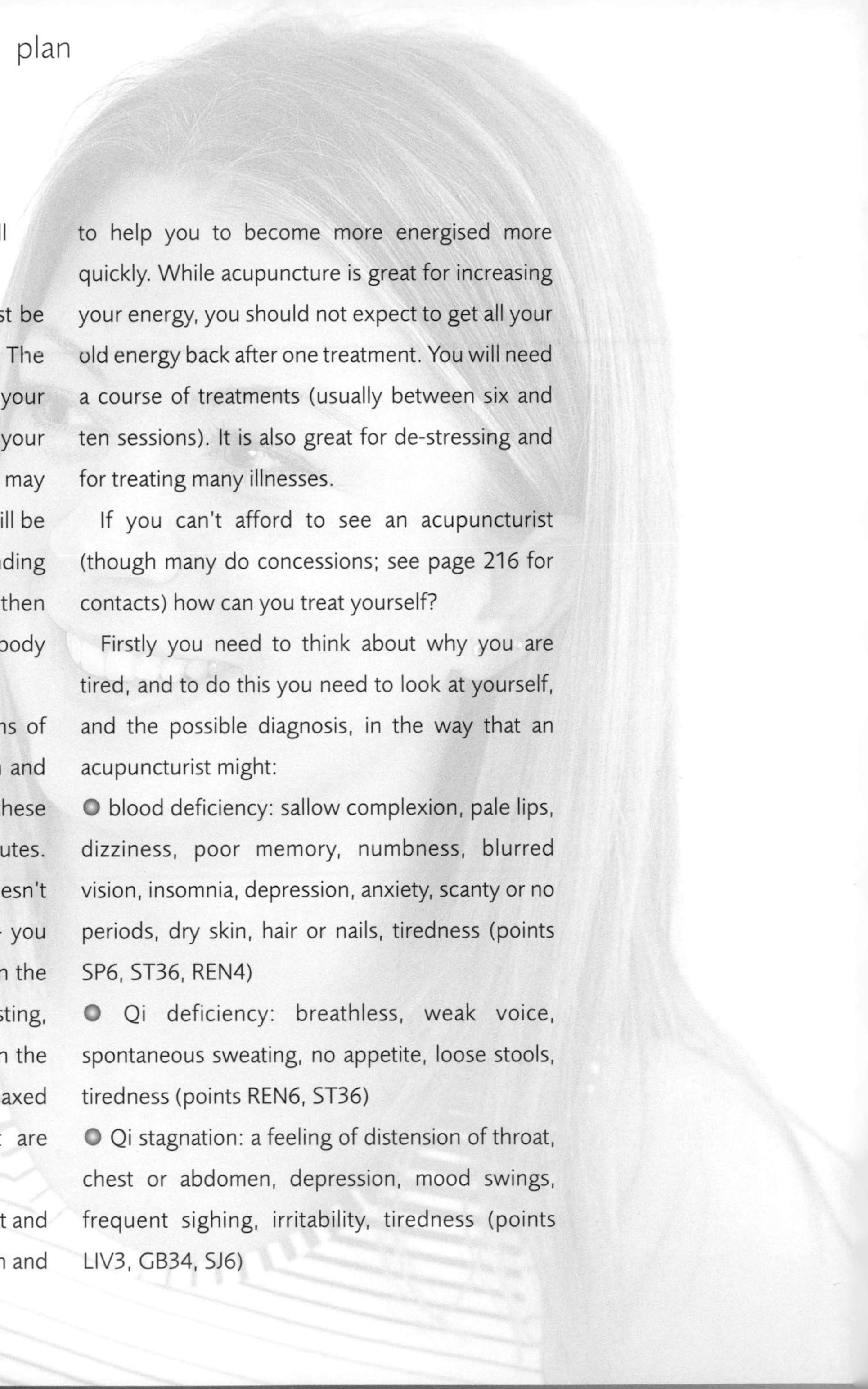

- yang deficiency (where people feel cold all the time, lack energy etc.)

The specific reason for your tiredness must be established before treatment begins. The acupuncturist will look at your tongue, check your pulse and ask you many questions about your medical history, diet and lifestyle. These may seem irrelevant to you and your illness but will be very relevant in forming a diagnosis. Depending on the diagnosis, the acupuncturist will then choose specific points to work on along the body to help treat the tiredness.

You will be asked to remove certain items of clothing in order to reach the points chosen and then very fine needles will be inserted into these points and left there for about twenty minutes. People always ask if acupuncture hurts. It doesn't actually hurt but you can definitely feel it – you will most likely feel a strange sensation when the needle is inserted like a dull ache or a bee sting, and this is the qi arriving at the point. When the needles are taken out you will feel very relaxed and happy due to the endorphins that are released during acupuncture.

Most acupuncturists will also advise on diet and lifestyle changes as part of the treatment plan and to help you to become more energised more quickly. While acupuncture is great for increasing your energy, you should not expect to get all your old energy back after one treatment. You will need a course of treatments (usually between six and ten sessions). It is also great for de-stressing and for treating many illnesses.

If you can't afford to see an acupuncturist (though many do concessions; see page 216 for contacts) how can you treat yourself?

Firstly you need to think about why you are tired, and to do this you need to look at yourself, and the possible diagnosis, in the way that an acupuncturist might:

- blood deficiency: sallow complexion, pale lips, dizziness, poor memory, numbness, blurred vision, insomnia, depression, anxiety, scanty or no periods, dry skin, hair or nails, tiredness (points SP6, ST36, REN4)
- Qi deficiency: breathless, weak voice, spontaneous sweating, no appetite, loose stools, tiredness (points REN6, ST36)
- Qi stagnation: a feeling of distension of throat, chest or abdomen, depression, mood swings, frequent sighing, irritability, tiredness (points LIV3, GB34, SJ6)

- yang deficiency: pale/bright white face, cold, listless, clear abundant urine, cold limbs, no thirst, loose stools, desire for hot drinks, sore back, sensation of cold in the back (points REN4/REN6, KID7).

Once you have decided which of the above best matches your symptoms (and there may be more than one), you can follow the points suggested (see diagram for location of acupressure points) and do some acupressure on yourself. Using your thumbs, gently massage the acupressure points making small circular movements; they may feel sensitive but this is quite normal. When diagnosing don't worry if you don't have all the symptoms of a particular category as long as you have a few of them.

Note: pregnant women, or anyone suffering from any serious illness should always consult a qualified acupuncturist before attempting any acupressure on themselves.

When visiting an acupuncturist make sure that they are fully qualified, insured and that they use sterilised or disposable needles only (see page 216 for contacts). Nobody should ever use needles on themselves; only ever allow someone who has a full qualification in acupuncture to do so.

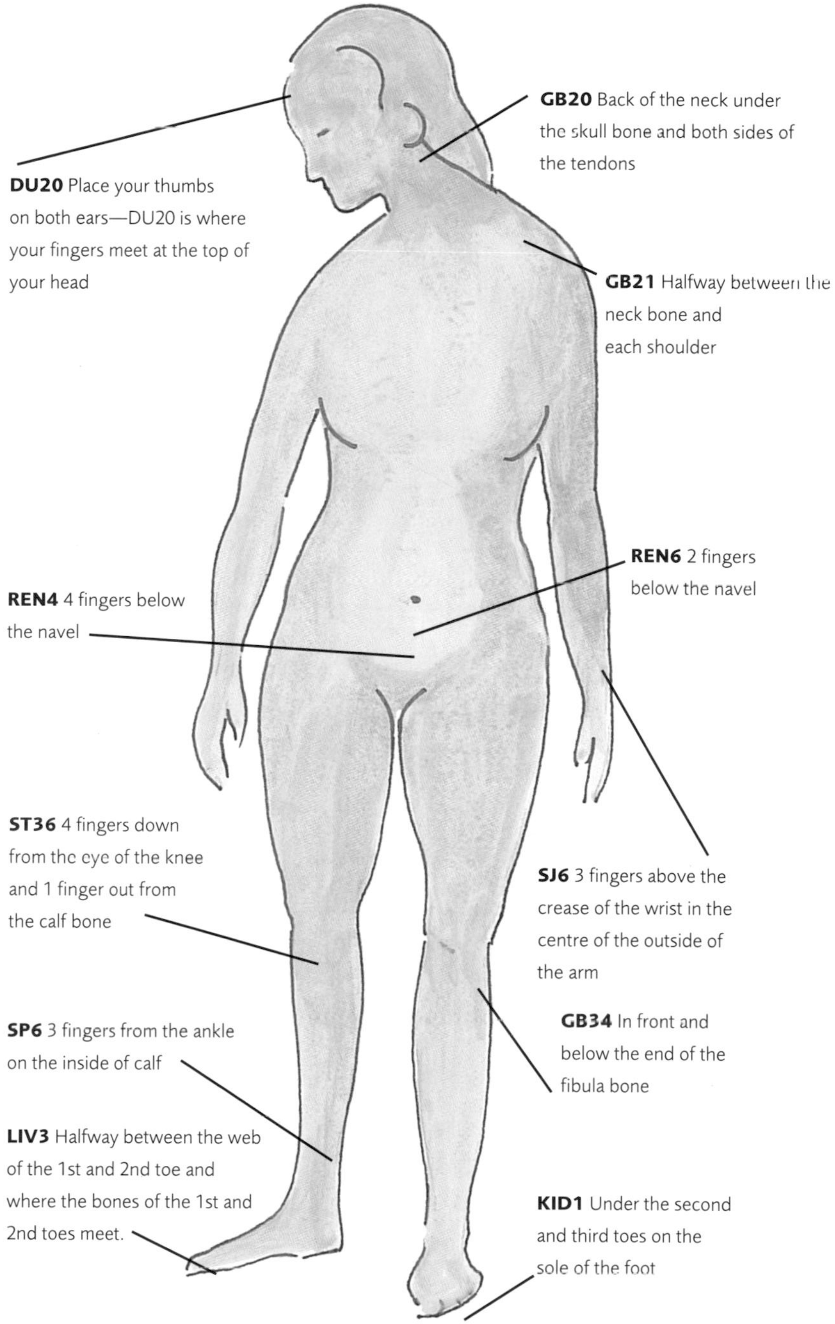
**GB20** Back of the neck under the skull bone and both sides of the tendons
**DU20** Place your thumbs on both ears—DU20 is where your fingers meet at the top of your head
**GB21** Halfway between the neck bone and each shoulder
**REN6** 2 fingers below the navel
**REN4** 4 fingers below the navel
**ST36** 4 fingers down from the eye of the knee and 1 finger out from the calf bone
**SJ6** 3 fingers above the crease of the wrist in the centre of the outside of the arm
**GB34** In front and below the end of the fibula bone
**SP6** 3 fingers from the ankle on the inside of calf
**LIV3** Halfway between the web of the 1st and 2nd toe and where the bones of the 1st and 2nd toes meet.
**KID1** Under the second and third toes on the sole of the foot

# Aromatherapy

Many people think of aromatherapy as a pampering treatment but it is also very useful for treating medical conditions and great for helping with de-stressing and tiredness. It is a therapeutic treatment that uses essential oils and massage. The beauty of aromatherapy is that it is easy to use at home on your own, though a massage with a qualified aromatherapist is advised at least once a week, as a regular treatment can help you to stay relaxed, balanced, energised and in harmony. Hippocrates said, 'The way to health is to have an aromatic bath and scented massage every day.' But what exactly is aromatherapy, how does it work and how can you incorporate it into your routine if you can't afford to see a professional?

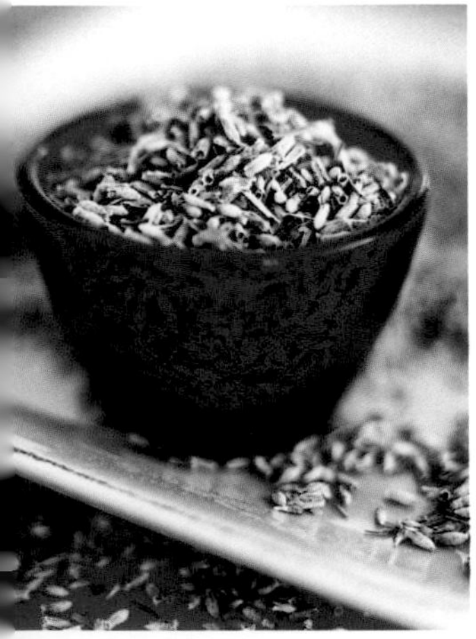

Aromatherapy uses the essences of plants for healing and the maintenance of vitality, through their unique character, smell and healing properties. The essences are known as essential oils and are extracted from a wide variety of plants. They are very concentrated, to the extent that it takes the petals of thirty roses to produce one drop of rose essential oil, and several kilos of lavender to make a small bottle of lavender oil. So you can imagine how potent they are. Essential oils are obtained either by steam distillation or, for the more fragile flowers, by solvent extraction.

Each oil has its own healing property which can be psychological as well as physical in its effects, and several may be used together to help to heal on a mental, physical and emotional level. They can be used in a bath, massage, compress or inhalation, but must never be used orally.

Essential oils work by absorption through the skin or by inhalation of the aroma. When they are inhaled they have an immediate effect on our hormonal and autonomic nervous systems which govern our emotions as well as our response to stress. The scents of different essential oils bring about different responses. For example, lavender can soothe and relax whereas rosemary can revive and energise, and basil can clear the head. The oils can also work by entering the bloodstream, through the lungs when they are inhaled, or through the skin when they are used in massage, made into a compress, or used in a bath. When the blood circulates the oils are transported around to all the organs. The oil molecules are small enough to be absorbed by the skin, and any that are not used are excreted through sweat, urine and faeces. The oils remain in the body for a few hours but they trigger a response that can last for days which is why people say they feel energised, relaxed and brighter for several days after an aromatherapy treatment.

The Romans used essential oils for massage and to make the home smell nice, while in the seventeenth century oranges and cloves were used to ward off the Black Death. At the time of the plague in Athens Hippocrates urged everyone to burn aromatic oils to protect themselves, and centuries later Charles II did the same. Doctors who treated plague victims wore protective clothing comprising a leather gown, gloves and a beaked mask filled with cloves, cinnamon and other spices. Sponges were also made with these spices and put under the noses of the sick.

In 1937 a chemist called René-Maurice Gattefosse coined the phrase 'aromatherapy', following an incident in which, when working in a perfume laboratory, he badly burnt his hand. He promptly plunged it into the nearest bowl of liquid which happened to be lavender essential oil, and when his hand healed quickly and with virtually no scarring he realised that lavender essential oil had better healing and antiseptic properties than any synthetic equivalent. Dr Valnet, a medical surgeon in the Second World War, added to Gatefosse's research by using oils when medical supplies were short. Since the war aromatherapy has grown in many ways so that now even the lay person knows about essential oils and how to use them.

Some oils can invigorate and stimulate while others calm and relax us. Modern research has shown that all of them are natural antiseptics, while some are antibiotic, antiviral, anti-inflammatory, antibacterial, expectorant, diuretic, antispasmodic, antineuralgic – all very much more than just a pampering treatment.

Note: essential oils should be stored in a cool, dark place and in a dark bottle. Most oils will keep for up to two years, but will evaporate if left open in the air. Never take essential oils internally or use them undiluted on the skin.

Always seek the advice of a qualified aromatherapist before using oils on babies and children, pregnant women, or people with any serious medical condition (under supervision of their GP).

**Massage with oils** Massage has been found to be one of the most effective ways of using essential oils, as the oils enter the body through

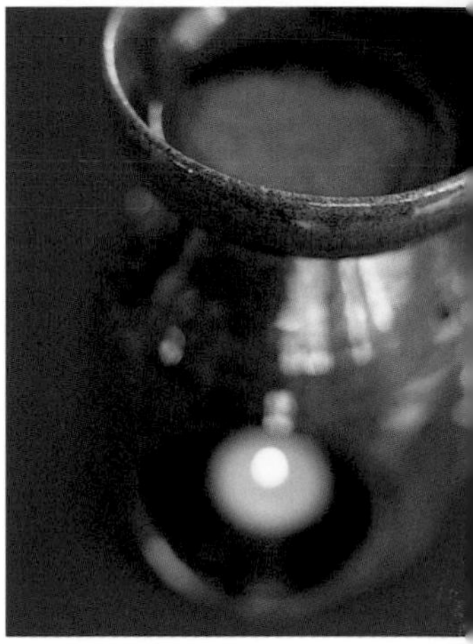

contact with every area of the body. The oils are blended with a base oil such as sweet almond, grapeseed, apricot kernel, sunflower, avocado or wheatgerm oil (the latter being particularly good for people with dry skin). Always dilute the oils with a base oil as they are very concentrated in their undiluted form and can cause irritation if applied directly to the skin.

Massage of the hands and feet is a good way to stay in good health and help to balance the body's energy flow as this stimulates all the zone points of the body. For best results it is important to leave the oils on the skin for six to eight hours to allow total absorption into the system (see pp 50–57 for how to do massage).

**Bathing with oils** After massage, bathing is the next most effective way of using the oils. Simply run a warm bath, add five drops of oil, agitate the water and then bathe for ten to fifteen minutes. This can be done daily to help you relax and revitalise.

**Inhalation of oils** Inhalation is best used for congestion, during a cold for example. Pour two pints of boiling water into a bowl, add ten drops of oil, agitate the water, put a towel over your head, close your eyes and inhale for up to ten minutes. Repeat several times a day if required. You can also put a few drops of oil on a tissue and inhale wherever you are.

**Oil burners** are available at most health food shops. Put five drops of oil in the water in the bowl of the burner. As the oil you choose gradually evaporates it not only makes the room smell nice but also has beneficial effects on your health. For example, lavender makes for a relaxing atmosphere and also helps you to sleep better. Burning an oil such as eucalyptus can also help in the prevention of illnesses such as colds and flu.

If you do not have a burner, try putting a few drops of oil on a cold light bulb: as the bulb gets warmer the oil will vaporise. Alternatively you can put a few drops in a saucer of water and put it on top of the radiator to vaporise and humidify at the same time. You can also put oils on a handkerchief or tissue.

**Compresses** are a very comforting and soothing way of using essential oils, particularly if you have any aches, strains, or cramps. Fill a bowl with hot water, add about six to eight drops of oil and then soak a piece of cotton gauze in the liquid. Apply to the appropriate area, cover with towels that have been warmed on the radiator and leave for about fifteen minutes. The compress may be hot or cold depending on what it is being used for, though heat helps the oils to be absorbed.

## Oils to help increase energy

Choose the oils that best suit, or whose smell most appeals to you from the list below:

- physical exhaustion – clary sage, lavender, orange
- mental exhaustion – basil, rosemary, peppermint
- insomnia – clary sage, lavender, camomile
- nightmares – frankincense
- tiredness – rosemary
- apathy (emotional/spiritual) – jasmine; (mental/physical) – rosemary
- listlessness – clary sage, sandalwood
- sluggishness – lemon, cypress, rosemary
- stress – cedarwood, clary sage, neroli, lavender, orange, chamomile
- lack of confidence – rose, orange, bergamot, chamomile
- depression with lethargy – lavender, melissa, clary sage, orange
- jet lag (to help regulate sleep patterns) – clary sage, lavender, geranium, rose; (to awaken the body and mind) – bergamot, melissa, orange, peppermint, rosemary.

When you go to see a qualified aromatherapist always check that they are fully insured and registered with the relevant body or council. The first treatment will usually last from one to one-and-a-half hours. The aromatherapist will take a detailed history of any symptoms that you have and of your medical history and choose the oils accordingly, taking into account the smells that you are drawn to. They will then mix a blend designed especially for your treatment or massage, and you will need to remove your clothes and lie on a couch in your underwear covered by towels for the massage to begin. After the massage you will be left to get up in your own time and get dressed. You will feel very good, both relaxed but also refreshed and energised. Your aromatherapist might suggest further treatments and/or give you a blend to take home. He or she will probably also offer advice on diet and lifestyle.

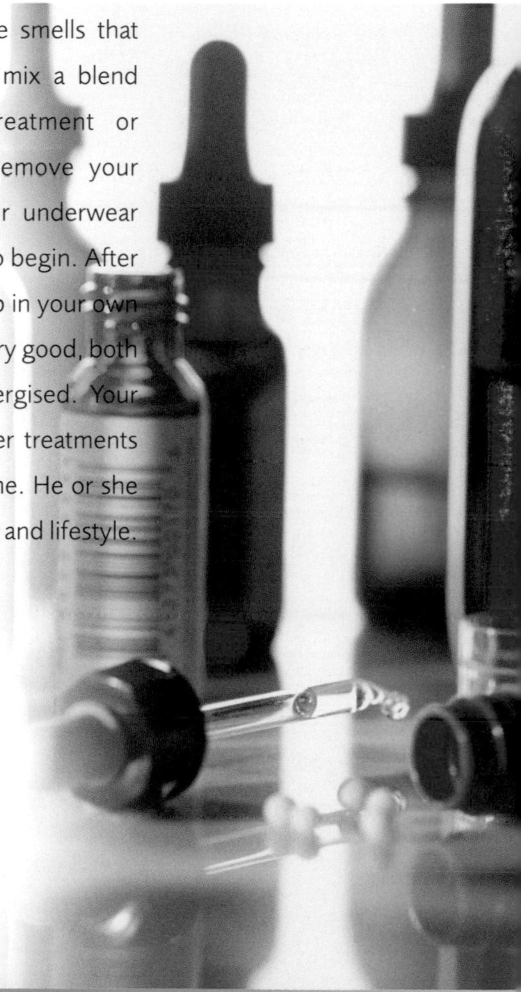

# Ayurvedic Medicine

*Ayurveda is a Sanskrit word meaning 'the wisdom or science of life'.*

It is an ancient Indian medicine system which has been practised for over five thousand years. It embodies science and philosophy and looks at our physical, mental, emotional and spiritual aspects for good health. Ayurveda evolved from the Atharva Veda, an ancient Hindu book of knowledge containing wisdom about the universe and the secrets of sickness and health.

Like Chinese medicine, Ayurvedic medicine is a complete healthcare system, and is more than just medicine; it is a way of living. According to Ayurveda living with your optimum energy can only come about when body and mind are in harmony and when we are in tune with our soul and the universe. It involves advice on diet, exercise, yoga, detoxification and aromatics, and uses therapeutic tools including bathing, massage, herbs, mantras, rituals and meditations to prevent maintain good health and wellbeing.

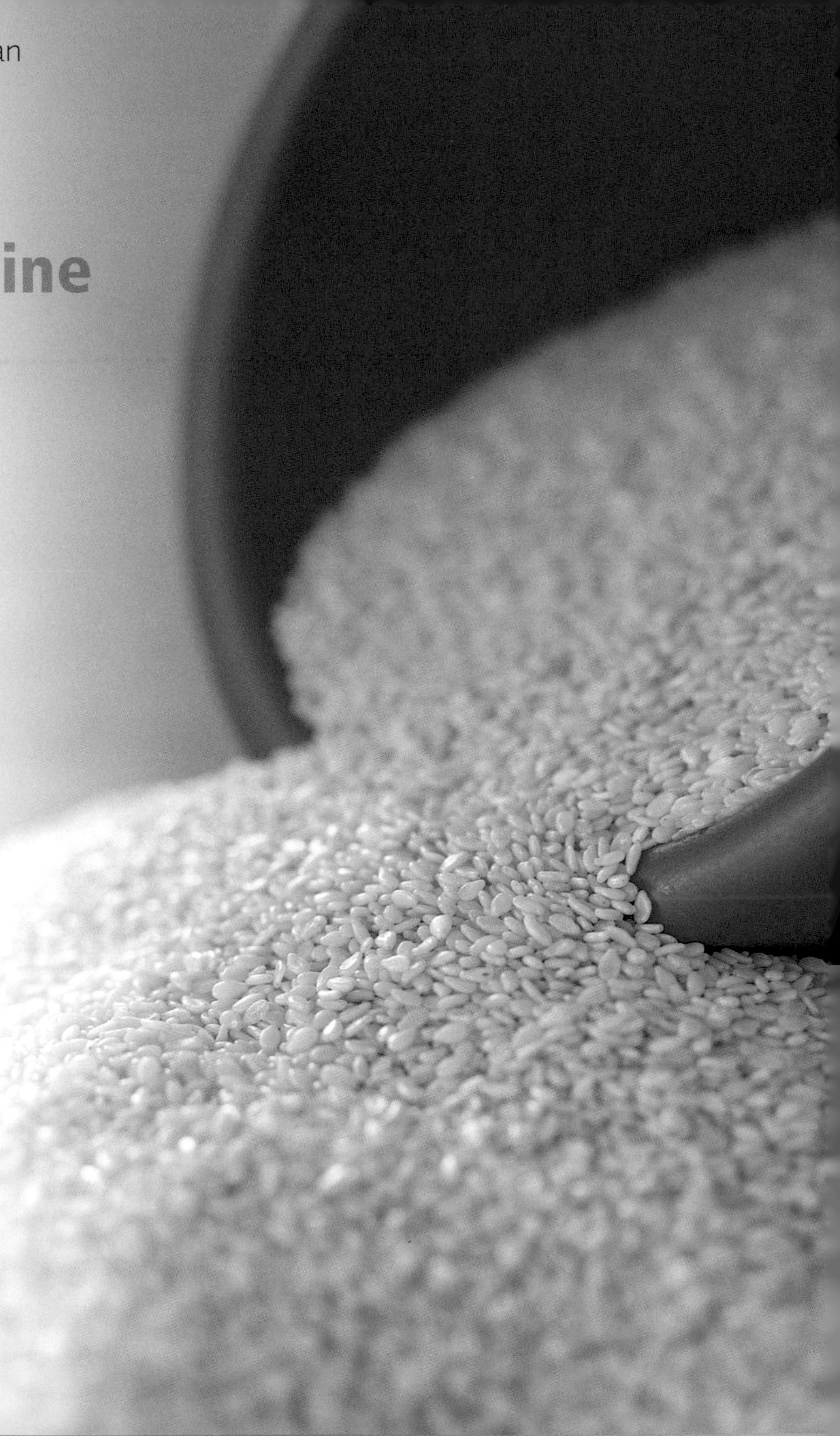

Ayurveda teaches that every cell in our body is controlled by energy, or prana, the life force of the universe that flows in all people, all living things, and all objects. Prana also controls our thoughts, emotions and actions, so that conversely, every aspect of our lives affects the quality of our energy and therefore our health.

Ayurveda aims to prevent disease by working with your body rather than trying to change it. It looks at the elements (earth, water, fire and wind) and their related energies: vata (wind/air), pitta (fire) and kapha (earth/water) and believes that health and vitality come from the balance of these energies. These elements determine our constitution, illnesses we might suffer from, our temperament and the type of foods we should eat and so on. However, in most of us one element tends to get out of balance more easily than the others due to weather, poor diet, emotional upsets like stress, and when this happens it can lead to tiredness, emotional imbalance and poor health.

## What do the elements stand for?

- Vata: thin build; cold, dry skin; very active and restless/curious; creative.

Unbalanced vata can cause anxiety and nervousness.

- Pitta: moderate build; fair, warm, soft skin; intelligent; maybe aggressive; clear-sighted; courageous.

Unbalanced pitta can cause frustration, anger and impatience.

- Kapha: solid build; prone to weight gain; cool and moist skin; calm with a receptive mind; loving and stable;

Unbalanced kapha can cause laziness, lack of motivation, depression.

If you are tired due to stress it is most likely to be your vata or pitta that is out of balance whereas if you are lethargic and lazy it is more likely to be your kapha. You can buy specially made teas to balance your type from most health food shops.

**Breathing in Ayurveda** According to Ayurveda, without inner bliss (ojas) we cannot find vitality. Ojas fills our cells with energy, or, as Deepak Chopra, Californian health writer and doctor of Ayurvedic medicine says, it 'enables the cells to "feel happy", to experience the cellular equivalent of bliss'. To this end, correct breathing is very important. When we are stressed or upset or angry we can often forget to breathe. Deep breathing helps to deal with stress and emotional upset and also helps to oxygenate the body.

Ayurveda teaches that when our circulatory channels become blocked by emotions or undigested food it causes stagnation which creates toxins making us feel tired and lethargic .

**Diet in Ayurveda** In Ayurvedic medicine, what you eat is also very important, and ojas is only taken from food once it is properly digested. Ancient sages observed how their bodies, minds and spirits reacted to different foods. They even observed the vibrational energy of a food and noticed how its energy changed from when it was growing, to once it had been picked, and finally cooked. Food is classified in three ways in Ayurvedic medicine:

1 *Sattvic*: foods that promote life, health, satisfaction and happiness. They help us to be content and calm and they balance our energies. The sattvic diet includes foods that are usually light, sweet in nature, medium in portion size and easily digestible. They are calming, soothing and comforting. They are also fresh, organic and grown locally. Examples of sattvic foods are: milk (which should be boiled before drinking so that it does not encourage the formation of mucus; turmeric and ginger may also be added before boiling), ghee (clarified butter), fruits (and their juices), sesame seeds, rice, honey, wheat, mung beans, coconut, dates, spring water.

A strict sattvic diet is usually only followed by people who spend most of their time meditating or doing yoga and not participating in the stresses of the Western world. However, if you are lacking in energy because your lifestyle is highly stressed, you can easily help by eating more sattvic foods and by practising some yoga, meditation and other relaxation techniques.

2 *Rajasic*: these are very powerful foods; they are pungent, sour, and burning (hot) and make our energy aggressive and overactive.

3 *Tamasic*: these are considered to be dead foods, and are tasteless and stale, for example, leftovers or over-processed foods like takeaways. These foods make us feel sluggish and lazy.

In order to increase your energy Ayurvedic tradition teaches the following:

- enjoy meal times make them relaxed, calm and pleasurable
- never eat when you are angry and upset
- set aside a time to eat and always sit down
- concentrate only on eating (i.e. do not read or watch television while eating) and eat at a calm moderate pace

- try to always eat fresh, organic and grown locally food (as in sattvic diet)
- try to avoid stale, processed, convenience and junk food (tamasic foods)
- avoid ice-cold drinks and food
- eat only small amounts of raw food as it is harder to digest
- drink warm drinks and preferably not with your food
- only eat if you are hungry
- don't eat so much that you feel you might burst; try to leave a quarter of your stomach empty to aid digestion
- try to have all of the six tastes in every meal (i.e. sweet, sour, salty, pungent, bitter and astringent)
- when you have finished eating, always sit for a while to allow your meal to be digested.

The first session with an Ayurvedic practitioner usually lasts about an hour. You will be asked for an in-depth medical history, not only of yourself, but also your immediate family. You will be asked about your diet, lifestyle, emotions and stress levels, your work, likes and dislikes. They will look at your appearance: your size, colour, shape, eyes, lips, tongue and nails. They will also take your pulse. Treatment will be with massage, steam baths, herbs as well as advice on diet, exercise, meditation and lifestyle.

If you can't afford to see an Ayurvedic practitioner, see the meditation (see page 76) and yoga exercises (see page 102) for self-treatments.

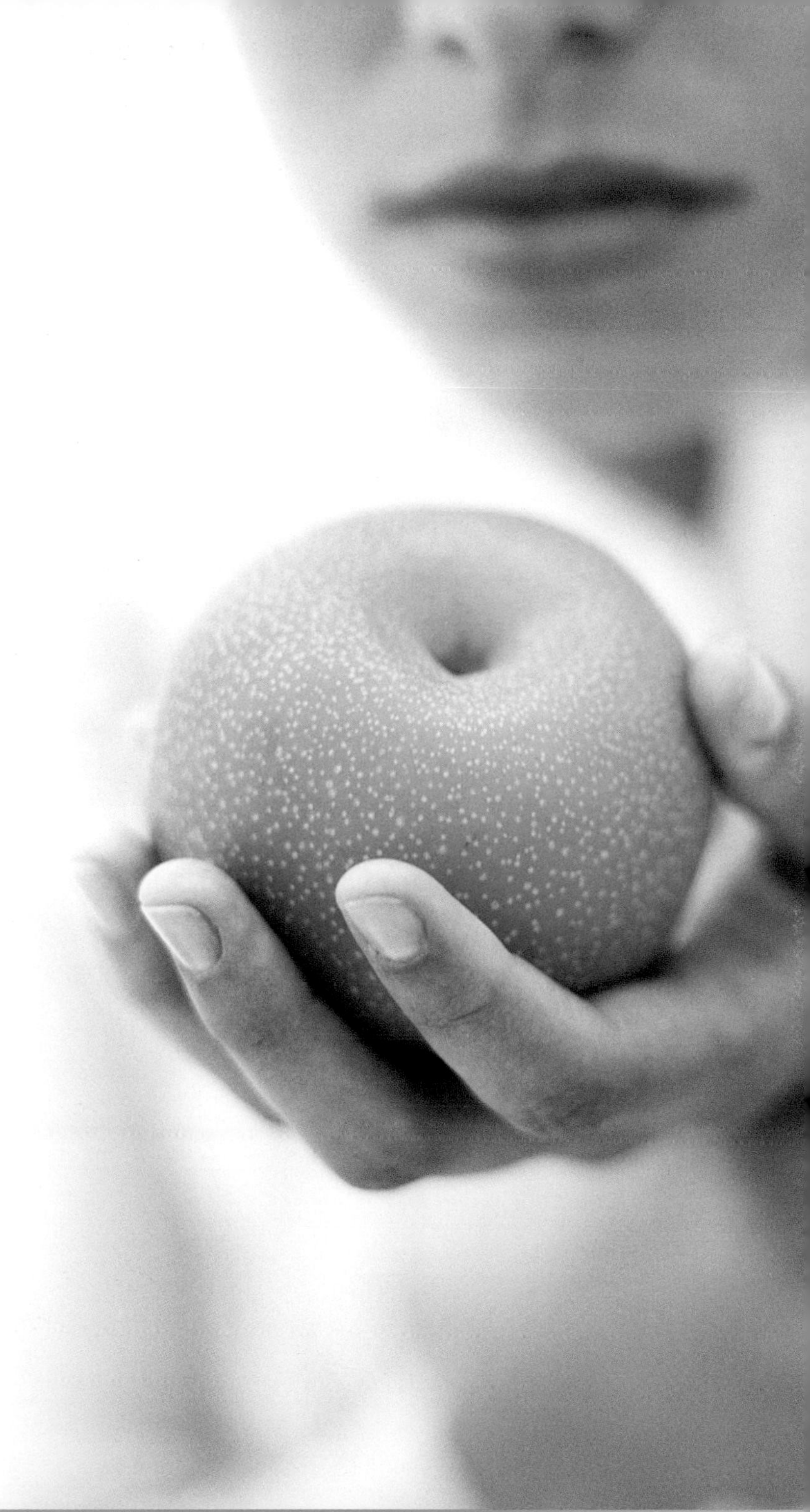

# Colour Therapy

Colour can have a massive effect on our mood. The colours with which we choose to surround ourselves, those that we wear, even the colours of the food that we eat, all affect our lives and the extent to which we feel healthy, happy, confident and full of energy. Certain colours can even influence how relaxed we feel, the quality of our sleep, and whether we have a good sex life. Red, for example can cause aggression, whereas pink creates calm.

Research has found that looking at a specific colour can actually have a physical effect on different parts of the body. Red, for example, stimulates the glandular system and increases heart rate, blood pressure and respiration. It has been found that people with high blood pressure can actually lower their blood pressure just by visualising the colour blue (whereas if they visualise red their blood pressure soars back up again).

When I was pregnant I visited a hypnotherapist and together we worked with colours in a visual way. I was asked to think of pain and observe it from the outside looking in. I was then asked to describe the pain in terms of colour, texture, smell and so on. For me, pain is red and very all-consuming. I was then asked which colour would mean not being in pain; for me this was blue. I then had to observe the pain, turning the red into blue. When I actually went into labour the pain was strong but manageable. My husband softly whispered in my ear, 'Think blue, breathe blue ...', and it definitely helped me.

## What do different colours mean and how can they help us?

- Red – good for circulation, problems with blood, sexual problems, conditions that are worse with the cold (numbness etc.). Red is a very strong colour, so when you are feeling tired it can make you feel more energised, and if you are feeling unconfident, wearing red can make you feel and come across as more powerful.
- Orange – good for depression, hernias, kidney stones and can also help milk to flow in breastfeeding mothers. Also good for sexual problems. Wearing orange is said to make your sexual energy more vibrant.
- Yellow – good for digestion, constipation, lymphatic system, diabetes, liver and kidney. Wearing yellow can help the solar plexus. It is

also recommended as a good colour with which to decorate the kitchen (as it has a benificial effect on the digestion).

- Green – good for nerves, colds, flu, ulcers, and hay fever. Green is the colour for the heart chakra, so if you are feeling low, or 'broken-hearted' it is a good colour to wear.
- Turquoise – good for throat problems and can be anti-inflammatory. When you wear turquoise you give off a strong healing energy. If you have throat problems or difficulty in communicating with people it is a good idea to wear a turquoise scarf or necklace.
- Blue – good for pain relief, bleeding, burns, colic, respiratory problems, skin problems and rheumatism. It is a very calming and soothing colour to wear. Blue is also great for the bedroom as it helps to induce good sleep.
- Indigo – good for migraine, ears and eyes, skin and nervous system.
- Violet – good for emotional problems, arthritis and can also help in childbirth. It is a good colour for healing.
- Magenta – good for heart and mental problems.

Colour therapists use coloured lamps, choosing the right colour, filtered in the right amount, to balance a patient as too much of one colour can cause imbalances. Each colour has a complementary colour and the therapist might use both to get the right balance. You will be given a white robe to wear and you will sit or lie under the coloured lamps.

The therapist takes a full medical history and speaks to you about your emotions and personality, best times of the day for you and favourite colours. Some therapists ask you to choose the three most appealing colours (to you) from cards, to reveal your mental, emotional and physical state. They might also make a colour diagnostic chart based on the vertebrae relating to mental, emotional and physical health. The first session lasts for up to two hours and follow-ups are around one hour long. If you can't afford to see a colour therapist use the colours in visualisations or wear or surround yourself with the colours you need.

# Flower Remedies

## *Flower essences have been used for thousands of years and in many different cultures.*

The Australian Aboriginals used to eat the whole flower to benefit from the essence. Or, if a flower was inedible they would sit in a group of flowers to absorb the healing vibration of that flower. Egyptians, Malayans and Africans also used flower essences to treat emotional imbalances. However, most of the knowledge of flower essences was lost until Dr Edward Bach brought them back into use around the 1930s.

Therapists believe that a flower remedy contains the energy, or imprint, of the plant from which it was made (the Doctrine of Signatures), and that the shape, colour, scent or taste of a plant help to indicate its healing properties. Dr Bach believed that you did not need to take the whole of the herb but just the essence of the plant. The essence then goes to work, mainly on an emotional level rather than the physical, thus helping to balance the psyche. From knowledge passed down through generations of his ancestors, Ian White discovered Australian Bush flower remedies. I enjoy working with these and have found them to be very powerful.

There are fifty Australian bush flower remedies at present; they are very safe to use, even on babies and animals, and they work as a catalyst for people to start healing themselves. You can self-prescribe, however if you have a serious illness or find it hard to self-prescribe it is well worth consulting someone who specialises in flower remedies. The first consultation usually lasts for one hour during which you will be asked about your medical history, your emotional state and the ways in which you might react to various situations. At the end of the session the practitioner will recommend the flower essences she or he thinks are best for you and prepare a mix for you. A follow-up treatment will usually be arranged for around two to three weeks later.

It is fine to take more than one remedy at a time. For Bach flower remedies just add two drops of each to 30ml of fresh spring water, then take four drops four times daily either in water or directly in your mouth. For the Australian Bush flower remedies take seven drops under the tongue morning and night or add the same number to water and drink throughout the day.

## Bush flower remedies

- banksia robur/swamp banksia (for feeling low in energy, disheartened, weary and frustrated)
- mulla mulla (for rejuvenation)
- old man banksia (for feelings of sluggishness, being low in energy, disheartened, weary, frustrated)
- macrocarpa (a 'pick-me-up' for tiredness, exhaustion, burnout, convalescence)
- crowea (for continual worrying and feeling 'not quite right', lack of vitality)
- black-eyed Susan (for impatience, being on the go, using up all your energy, striving all the time)
- kapok bush (for people who give up easily, whose immune system is deficient and/or who feel constantly exhausted)
- alpine mint bush (for physical and emotional exhaustion)
- dog rose (for treating fears which can be a drain on the immune system and impair the free flow of the vital force)
- jacaranda (for people whose energy is scattered – they have a tendency to start too many things without seeing them through and eventually feel exhausted)

## Bach flower remedies

- hornbeam (for lack of energy, listlessness and uncertainty)
- olive (for exhaustion and burnout)

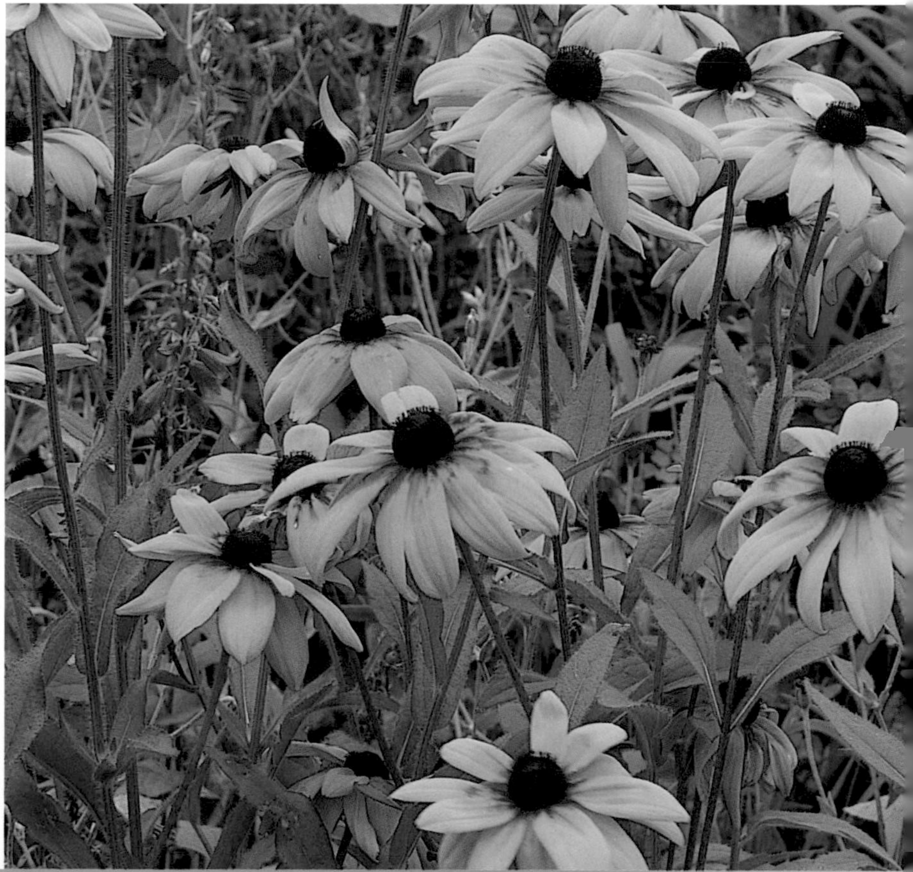

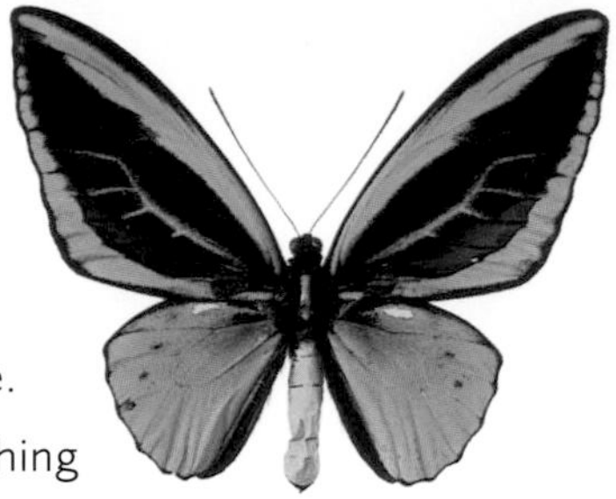

# Healing

We all give healing every day whether it is in the form of a hug or a gentle rub of someone's back, thinking of someone who has a tough time ahead of them, empathising with somebody's problems, or rocking a crying baby. Just being held by someone can be really soothing.

You might visit a healer for help with any sort of mental, physical or spiritual problem – grief or anger can be the cause of low energy just as much as any physical complaint. The main type of healing is hands-on, either where the hands literally touch you or hover above the body. In Reiki, a Japanese form of healing, certain positions are adopted and various symbols used. In distant healing people can heal by thinking of the person in question when they are not there or through a picture. Some healers believe that they are channelling a higher energy from gods or religious or spiritual sources, while others believe they are balancing the person's own energy system. I believe that healers do not actually heal but open up the body so it can heal itself.

Healers work in so many different ways that it is really only possible to say in very general terms what might happen when you go and see one.

A session with a healer can last anything from half an hour to two hours. Some healers talk to you first to establish how you need help, others prefer to let their spirit guides lead them to where help is needed. Some like to heal in silence with the lights turned down. Others feel that they can talk to you without disrupting the healing process and they also believe if you talk you are helping to release the problems from your physical body. Some will let their hands hover above your body, working in your aura and others will lay their hands on different parts of your body. You might feel their hands are very hot or you might find the area they touch feels cold or strange. Many healers will report to you what they pick up – for example, that an area feels hot or cold to them. Some might even yawn or burp during the treatment which shows they are expelling whatever they have drawn out of you. Some healers use clairvoyant skills as well and will tell you if they see or hear a spirit or advice from the spirit world, which many people find quite reassuring. Others might use crystals as well. After a treatment you will feel relaxed, spaced out, otherworldly and re-energised

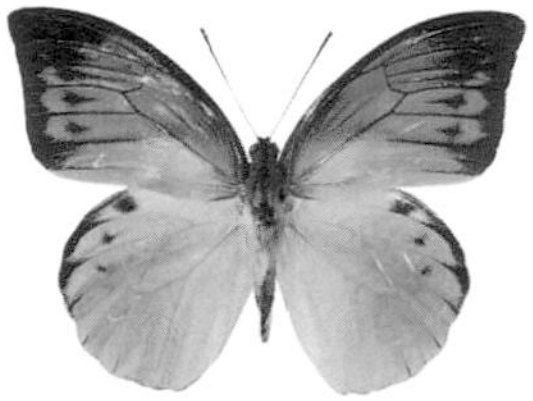

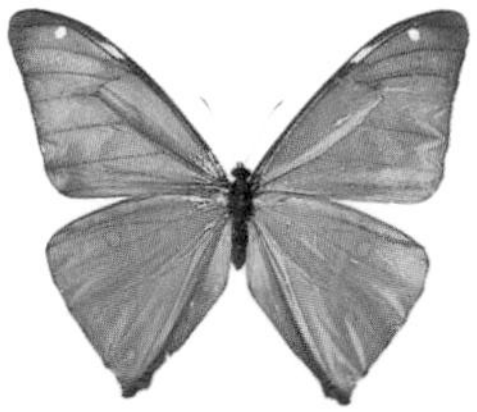

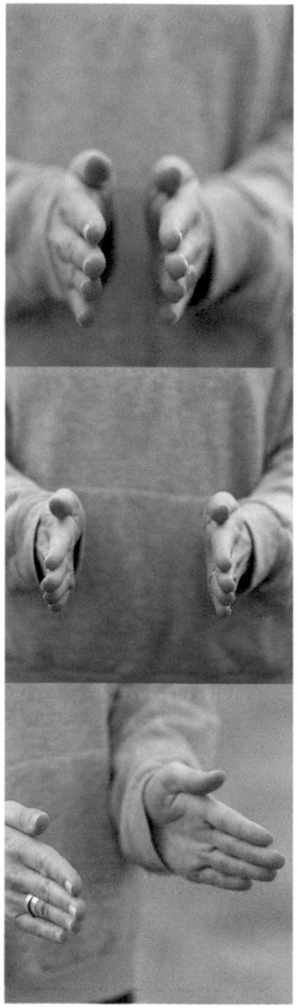

In order to practice healing on yourself or someone else you need to understand what it feels like to feel energy. The following exercise below should help you to do this.

## Feel the energy

In order to sense the energy put your hands a couple of inches apart, with palms facing each other, move your hands slightly like wheels on a train with one hand slightly behind the other in a circular motion. As you do this you should notice the magnetic pressure between your hands; you can then bounce off the energy by moving your palms slightly towards each other, and then slowly making the distance between them bigger again, ensuring you can still feel the energy between them. Your palms may tingle and feel warm. Imagine that energy is coming from the centre of your hands. A good device to help you focus is to close your eyes and imagine something opening like a butterfly's wings; as they open feel the energy coming from your palms. If you prefer you can ask for spiritual or religious guidance.

You can also practise feeling the energy with someone else. Stand facing each other and hold your palms out in front of you at shoulder height. Don't let your palms touch the other person's, close your eyes and focus on the energy between your own palms and your partner's. Practise moving slightly farther away and coming in closer. Always shake out your hands or wash them with water when you have finished healing.

## Giving/receiving healing

1 Close your eyes and either ask for guidance or imagine something opening up (see above).

2 Ask the person you are healing (or tell the person who is healing you) if there is any area that is bothering you, and if so concentrate on that area. Otherwise, go through the chakras or where your intuition takes you (see page 145 for more about chakras and their locations).

3 If you feel like touching the body then do so, or, if you feel more comfortable hovering a few inches above the body that is fine too. Again, let your intuition guide you.

4 Your hands might feel stiff, uncomfortable, hot or itchy; if so, just quietly shake them out.

5 Remember at the end of the treatment to either imagine the ritual closing (for example, the butterfly's wings) or thank your guides for their help and then wash your hands.Always shake out your hands or wash them with water when you have finished healing.

# Homeopathy

*Homeopathy is a safe and effective form of treatment, which has become more popular in recent years.*

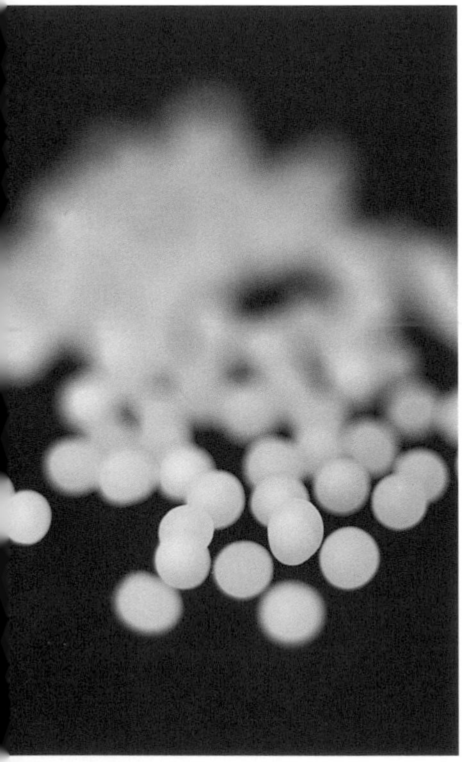

Its name, derived from the Greek words homoios, meaning similar and pathos, meaning suffering, reflects its basic premise which is one of similarity. In practice, this means that a substance that can cause a particular reaction in a healthy person can be used in the right dosage to treat similar symptoms or reactions in disease.

The idea is not a new one, and has been around for thousands of years – Socrates wrote of curing a disease with the substance that caused it. It wasn't until the late eighteenth and early nineteenth centuries, however, that it was developed into a formal discipline. Samuel Hahnemann, who founded homeopathy, believed that it worked along the same lines as classic immunisation: by administering an artificial illness to a patient that has similar characteristics to the illness that the doctor is trying to cure. This then stimulates the immune system, the body's natural defence system, to fight the original ailment or illness. Homeopathic remedies produce vibrational reactions rather than physical ones (everything, even illness, medicines and treatments, vibrates to a certain frequency). They produce a vibrational illness to stimulate the body to heal at a vibrational level.

Many people use homeopathy on themselves, for first aid, on children, or on animals. While it is possible to do this using over-the-counter remedies, it is always best to seek the advice of a qualified homeopath if you are pregnant or if you have a serious medical condition. Always ensure that you consult a fully qualified homeopath who is registered with the relevant body or council and fully insured.

A homeopath will take a detailed medical history of any illnesses and accidents. They will also ask you how you respond to certain situations and weather conditions, what you are like emotionally and what foods you like. The remedy or remedies they prescribe will be chosen specifically for you based on the information you have given. Remedies consist of a small white pill that is easy to take and may taste slightly sweet, or a tincture that is preserved in alcohol. The first treatment lasts an hour and a half and subsequent treatments normally last about three quarters of an hour. The remedies should be taken half an hour before or after food. Homeopathy can also be used alongside conventional medicine or other forms of treatment.

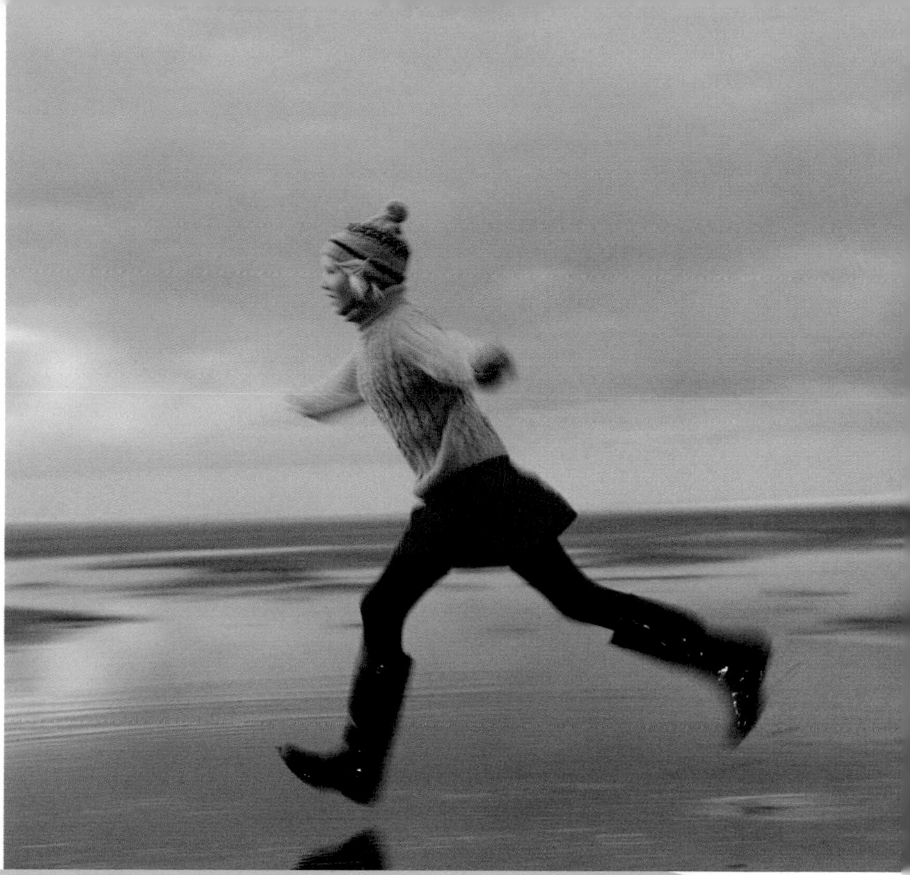

**HOMEOPATHIC REMEDIES RECOMMENDED FOR LACK OF ENERGY**

Kali phos (for nervous exhaustion causing loss of control)

Sepia (for feelings of being mentally, physically and emotionally static)

China (for lack of energy due to loss of fluids e.g. haemorrhage, diarrhoea, excessive perspiration)

Phosphorus (for feelings of exhaustion following a quick burst of energy, as in hypoglycaemia)

Carbo veg (for total inertia and low vitality, possibly as a result of illness)

Gelsemium (for mental, physical and emotional weakness)

Nux vomica (for lack of energy having done too much)

Ipeccac (for jetlag)

# Massage

*Massage mobilises and relaxes aching muscles but it can also help to reduce stress levels, lower blood pressure, relieve pain, strengthen the immune system, improve circulation, unblock repressed emotions and increase energy.*

Many of us are in a permanent state of stress and tension which prevents our energy from flowing and a daily massage would go a long way to relieving this, but if you can't afford that (and most of us can't) ask your partner or a friend to assist you. You can even self-massage, using your own hands or a machine.

If you visit a masseur it is important to ensure that it is someone who is qualified and registered with a relevant body or council and that they are fully insured. A practitioner may ask you a few questions about your medical history, before leaving the room to allow you to undress to your underwear (they will leave you some towels with which to cover yourself). You will then lie on the couch and the massage will begin. Massage is very relaxing and if you allow yourself you might even drift off to sleep. Once the massage is finished the practitioner will leave the room to allow you to dress.

## Giving/receiving a massage

- Allow between half an hour and an hour for your massage.
- Make the room warm and lie on a firm bed or mattress or on the floor. Your head and knees may be cushioned with a small folded towel and your arms should be bent loosely by your side. Make sure that you are covered with towels and warm, and that the 'masseur's hands are warm.
- Be careful not to massage injured areas, breasts or varicose veins . Tell the person if the massage is too painful and that they should go lighter.
- Massage strokes should always work towards the heart.
- Use oil to help massage; almond oil is good, and you might like to add in a few drops of clary

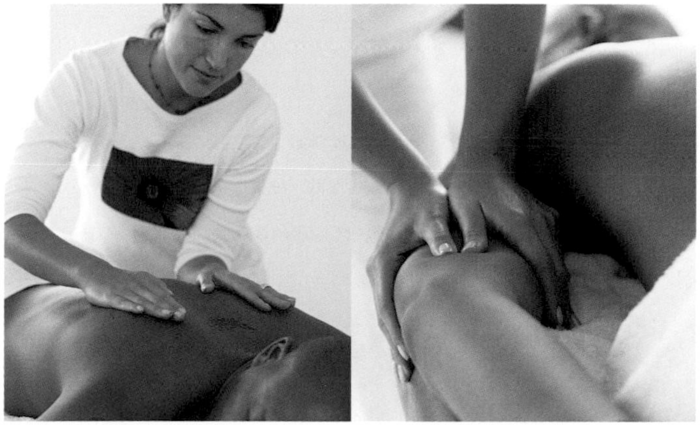

**1** Start by stroking up and down the back either side of the spine and across the shoulders and down the arms and down the bottom and legs.

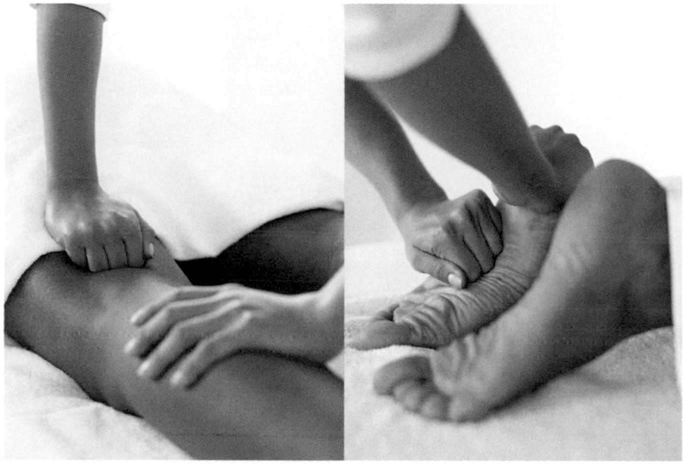

**2** Stroke down to the feet and knuckle the soles of the feet and massage the toes between your fingers and thumbs one foot at a time.

**3** Do the same again, this time more firmly, kneading and knuckling areas of tension and knots.

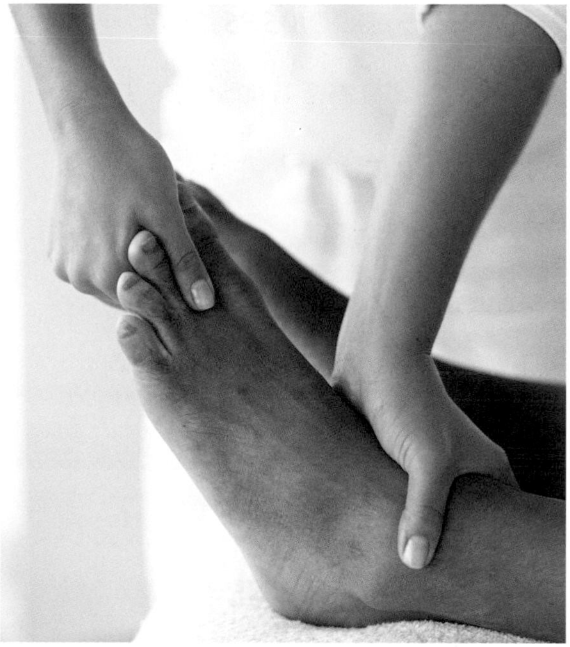

**4** Cover the person and let them rest until they are ready.

sage or lavender to make it more relaxing.

- There are various different techniques and strokes. Here are some basic technical strokes you can try (see pictures left to right):

– kneading: gather an area of skin, for example, in between the shoulder and the neck and knead, pull, squeeze and stretch the skin and muscle, making sure you check the pressure as this can sometimes be tender

– knuckling: with a light fist, knead the area with your knuckles; this is especially good for doing on palms and feet.

– stroking: speed and pressure can vary

There are a number of extra things that can be done on their own or as part of a massage:

- head and neck massage using circular pressure with the thumb and forefingers
- face massage: using your fingertips perform circular movements with light pressure on the forehead; then go round the eyebrows from the nose out to the temples. Exert a little pressure on the temples and then down through the cheekbones till you reach the nose, then make small circular movements just in front of the ears (it might be tender here). Finish by leaving your hands over the eyes for a few minutes.
- neck and shoulder massage with pressure and kneading. (Remove any jewellery.) Using the fingers of each hand stroke either side of the spine in the neck. Start with light strokes and get more firm if you feel you can. Stroke up towards the skull and then back down again.

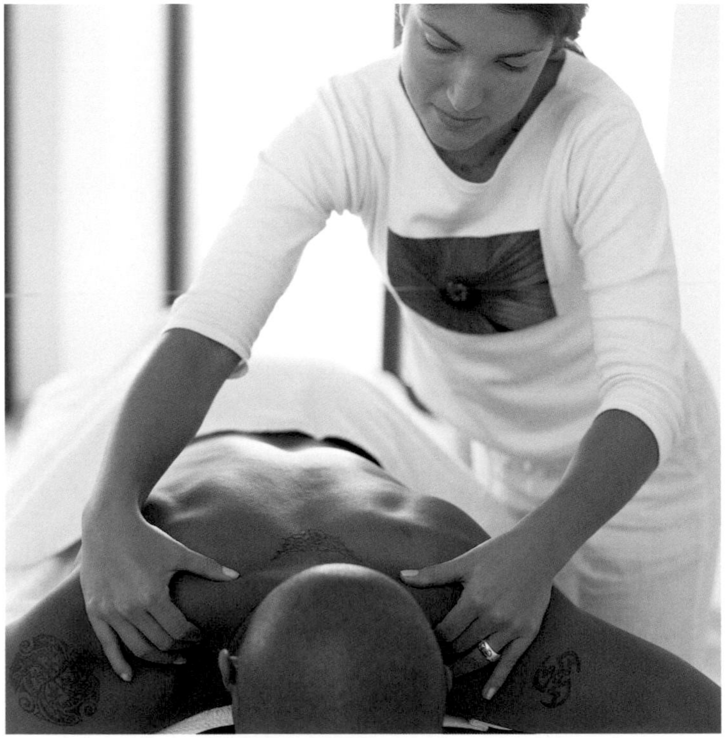

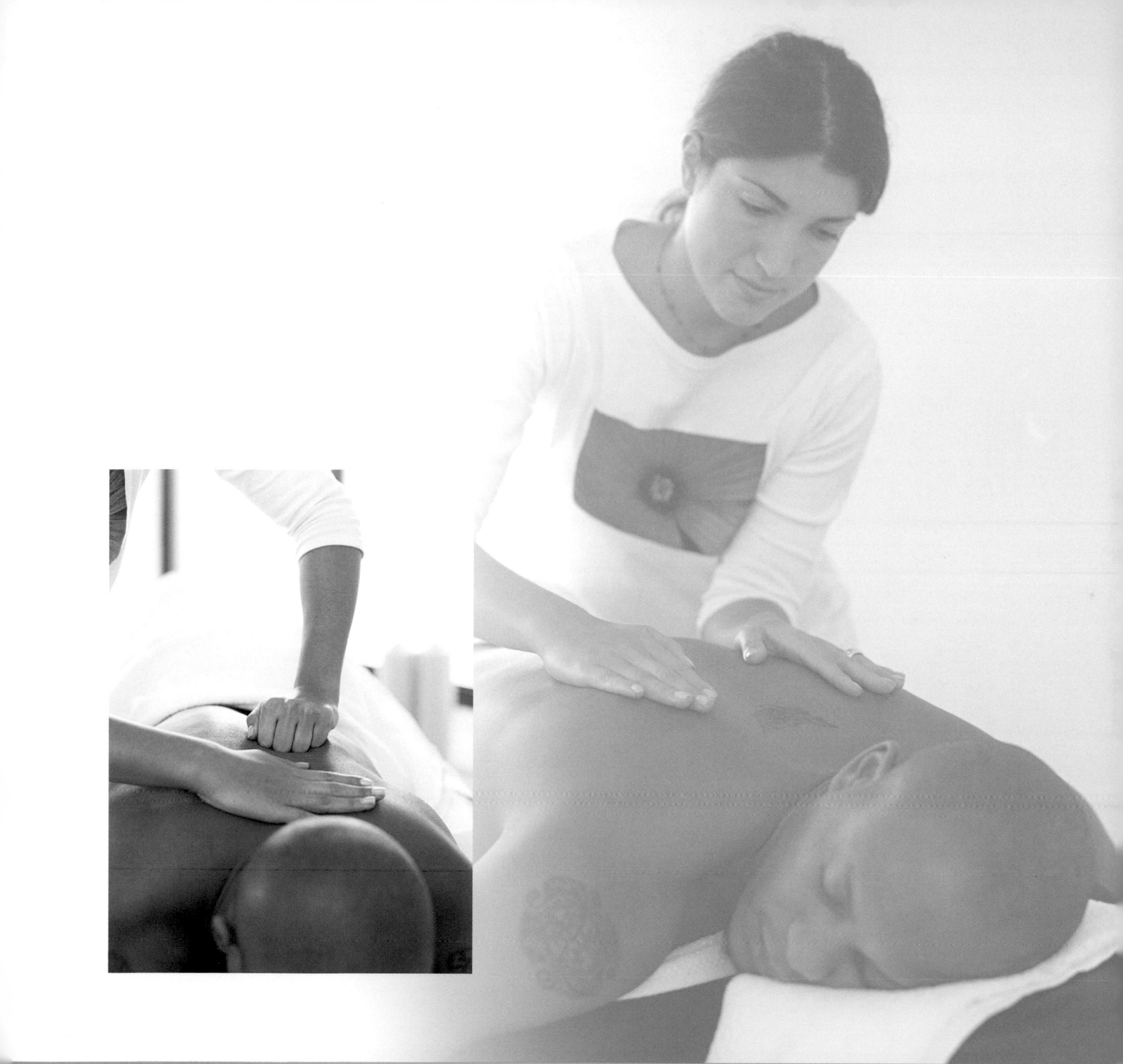

**Self-massage** is very helpful for reducing muscle tension, stress and for helping to increase energy. A face massage helps to reduce the amount of tension that builds up around the face, eyes, neck and scalp. Try and do the face massage twice a day for two to three minutes.

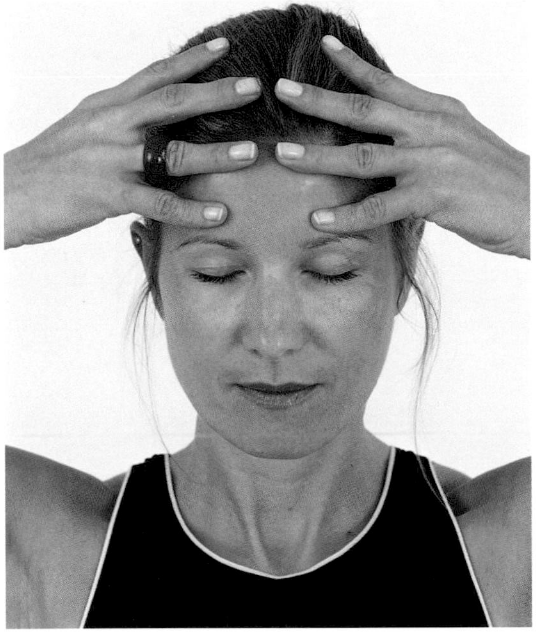

● Head massage: if you are tense the skin on the scalp will not move easily. Use small circular movements with your fingertips from the forehead to the back of the neck. Then work firmly and methodically all over the head, really moving the scalp as if you were shampooing your hair. This invigorating action helps to release tension and stimulates the circulation.

● Face massage: face and eye massages are good for easing eyestrain and headaches. Be gentle on the face especially around the eyes, where the pressure should be very light. Use vitamin E oil or almond oil, and if possible lie relaxed on your back or else in a bath or comfortable chair. Close your eyes and start massaging from under the jaw, moving slowly over the jaw and around the mouth, up the cheeks and around the temples and then across

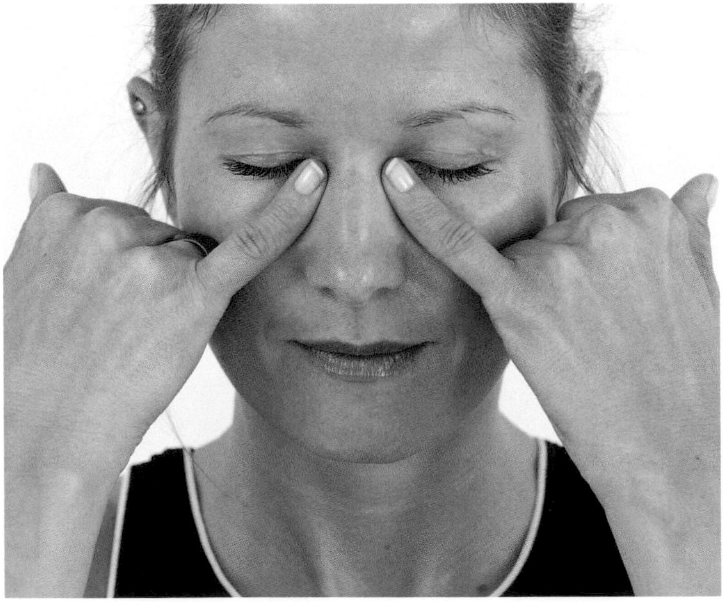

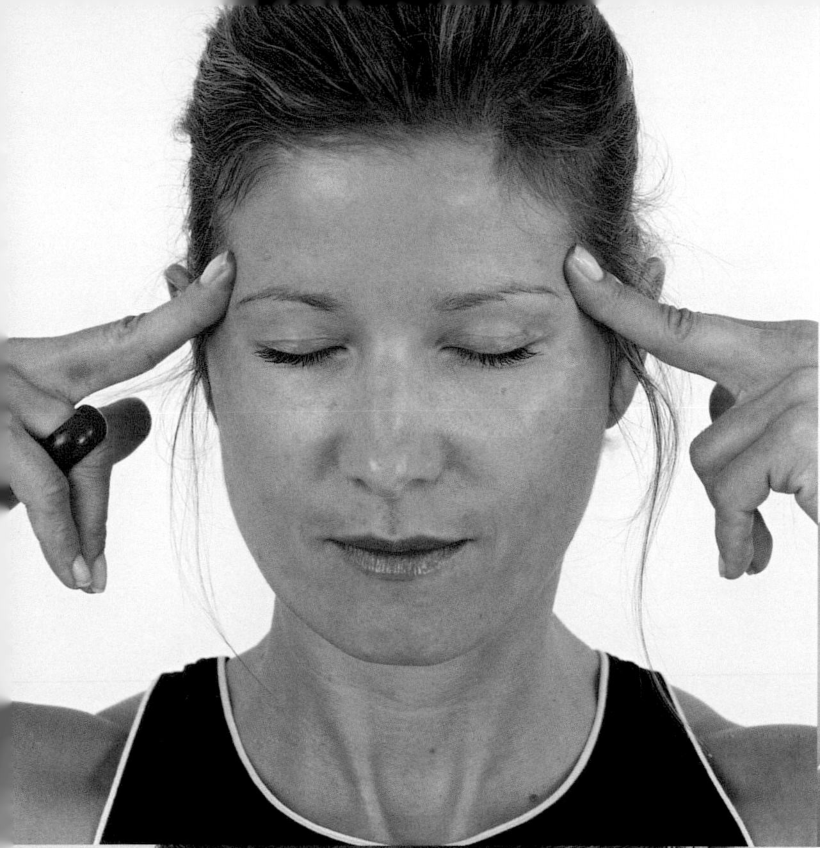
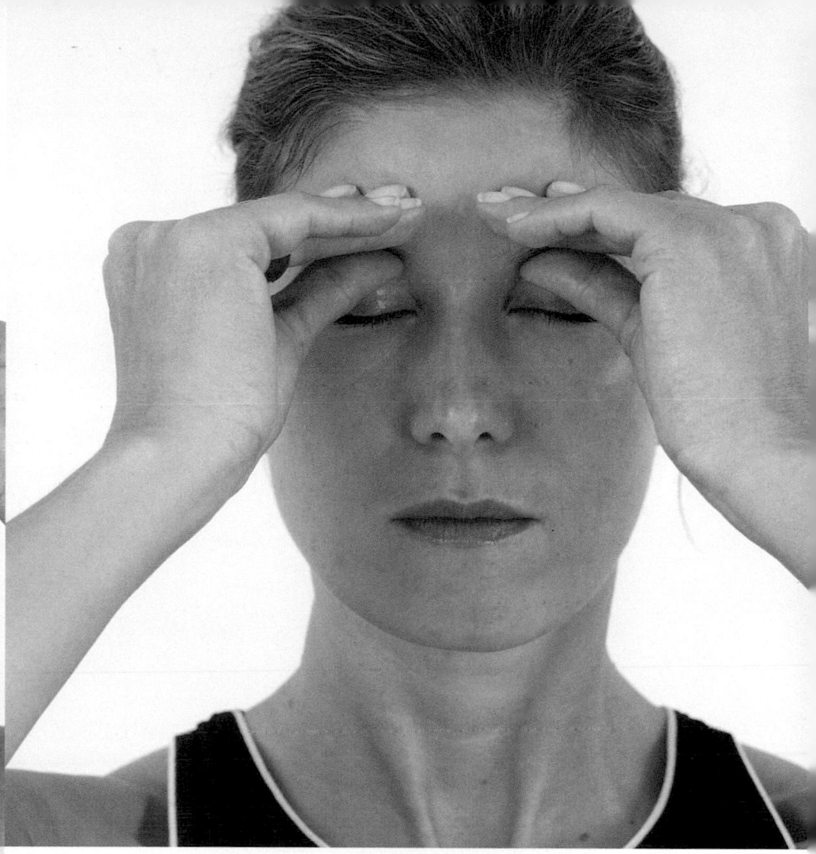
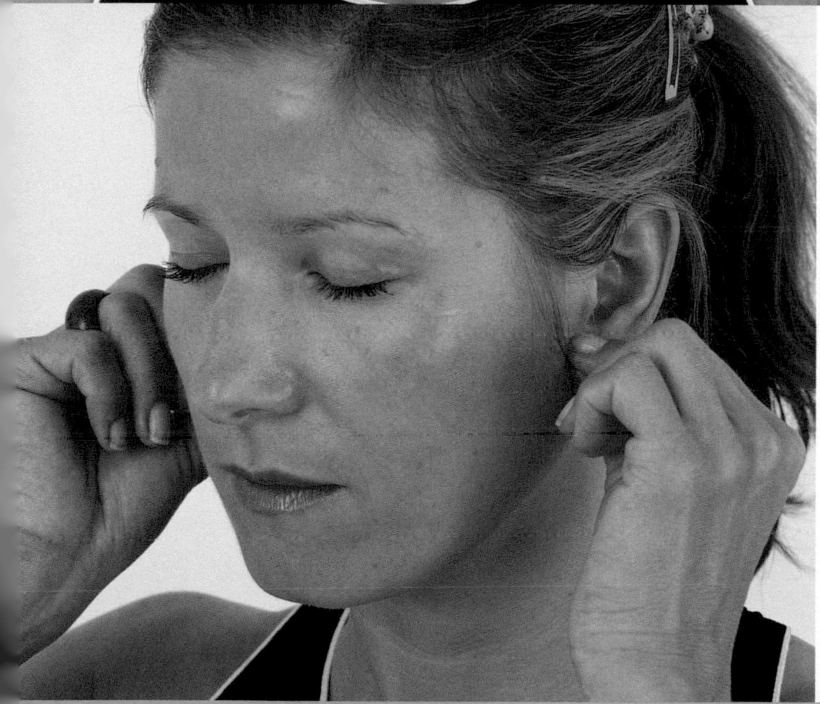
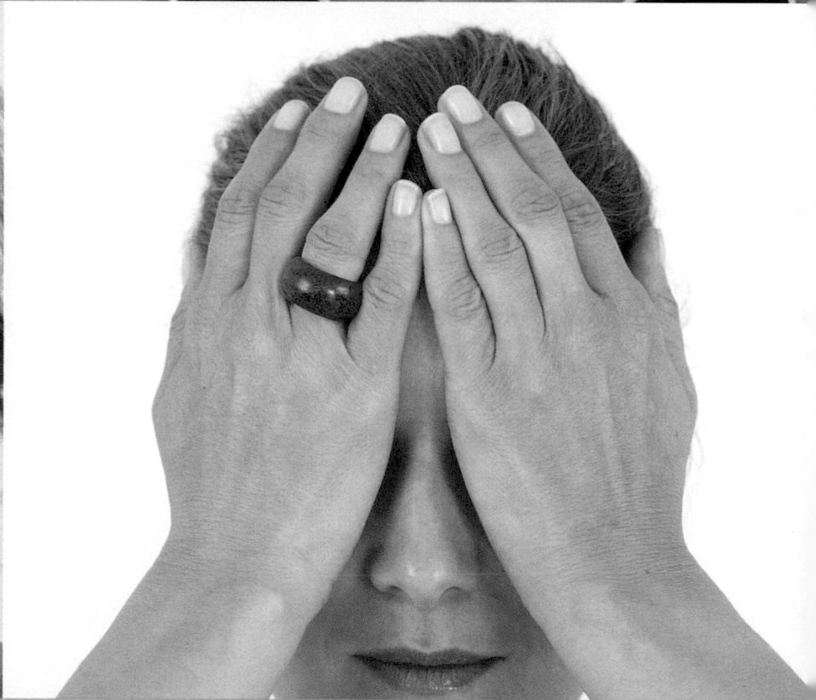

the forehead. Move along the forehead from the middle and out to the sides exerting pressure with your fingertips for a count of three and then moving down until you come down along the eyebrows out to the temples, and down the cheek bones. Use the little finger of both hands and slide up either side of the nose and round the eyebrows. Put your thumbs under your chin, slide the thumbs along the jaw until you reach the ear lobes. Repeat a few times. Pull your ear lobes. Lastly use your forefinger to do circular movements in the tender area under the cheek bones and in front of the ear, moving towards the ear. Place both palms over your eyes and relax.

- Neck massage: stroke either side of the spine and then up the back of the neck and then down. Use your thumbs to exert pressure on the points where your skull meets your neck (GB20).
- Shoulder massage: using the opposite hand for the opposite shoulder, exert pressure with all the pads of all the fingers.

Move from the back of the shoulder to the front. Use constant pressure on the tender points until it is relieved. Repeat for the other side.

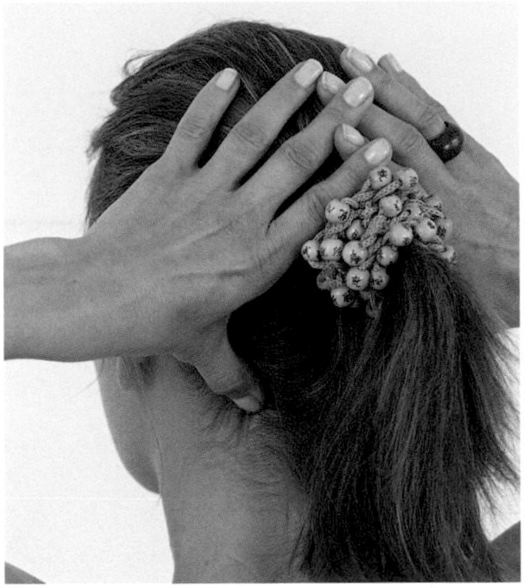

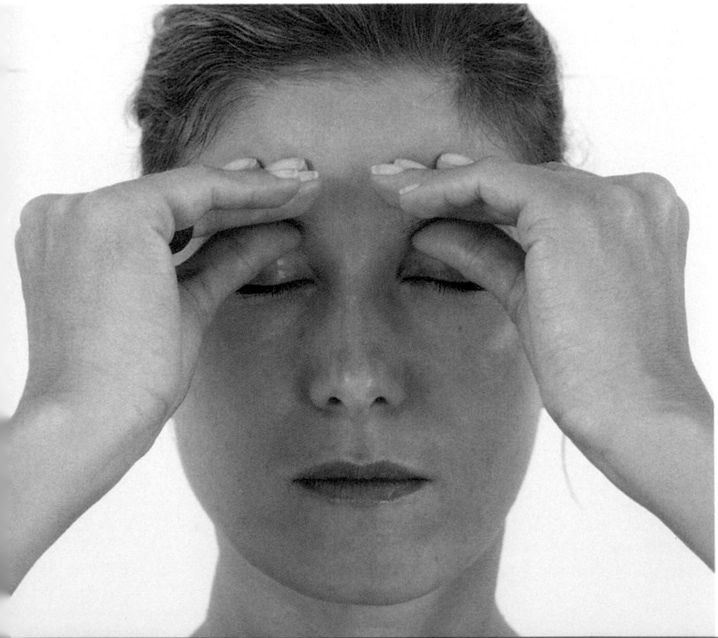

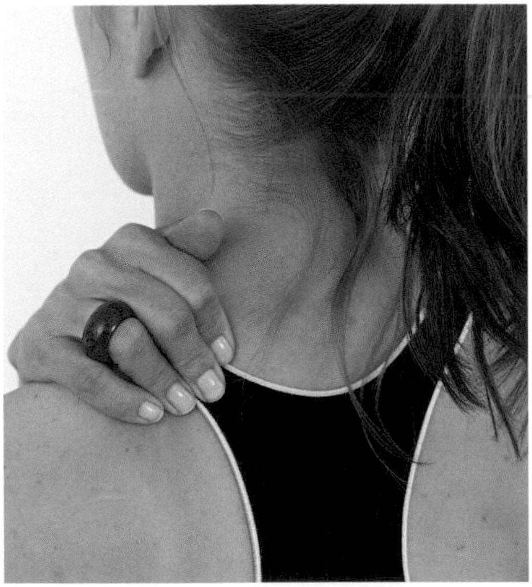

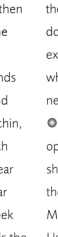

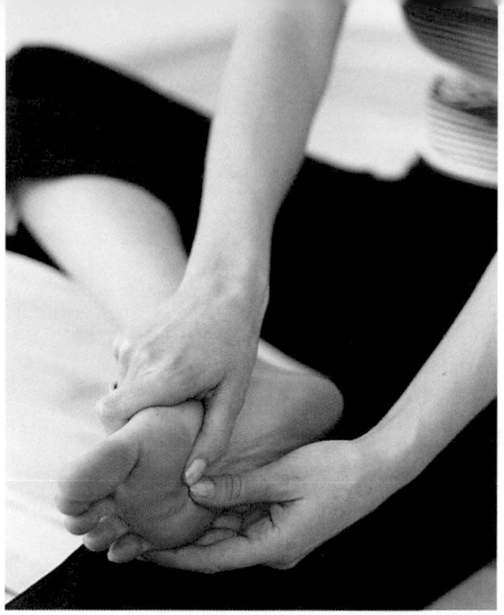

● Foot massage: this can be done at any time but should be done sitting in a comfortable chair with bare feet. Put your right foot on top of the your left knee so that you can see the sole of your right foot. Massage the sole using your thumbs from bottom to top, then massage each toe and give them a little pull. Massage between the toes in the web too, and work around the ankle bones and the heel and the top of the foot too. Repeat for the left foot.

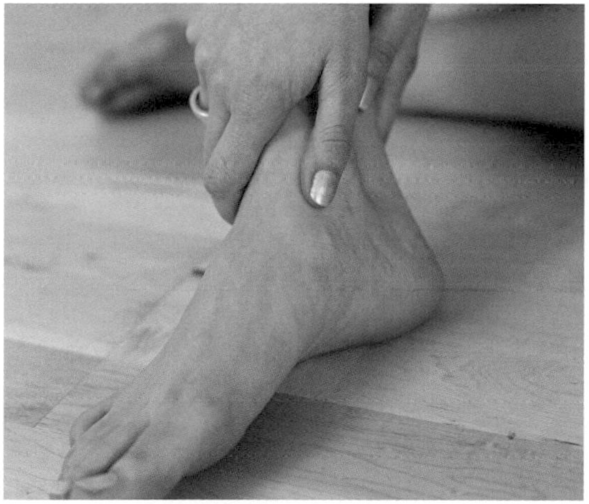

● Abdominal/tummy massage: for the abdominal massage use light strokes as the abdomen can be quite tender. Make small circular movements all over with the palm of your hand.

Note: do not try any of the above techniques if you are pregnant or suffering from a serious medical condition. You should, instead, consult a qualified masseur.

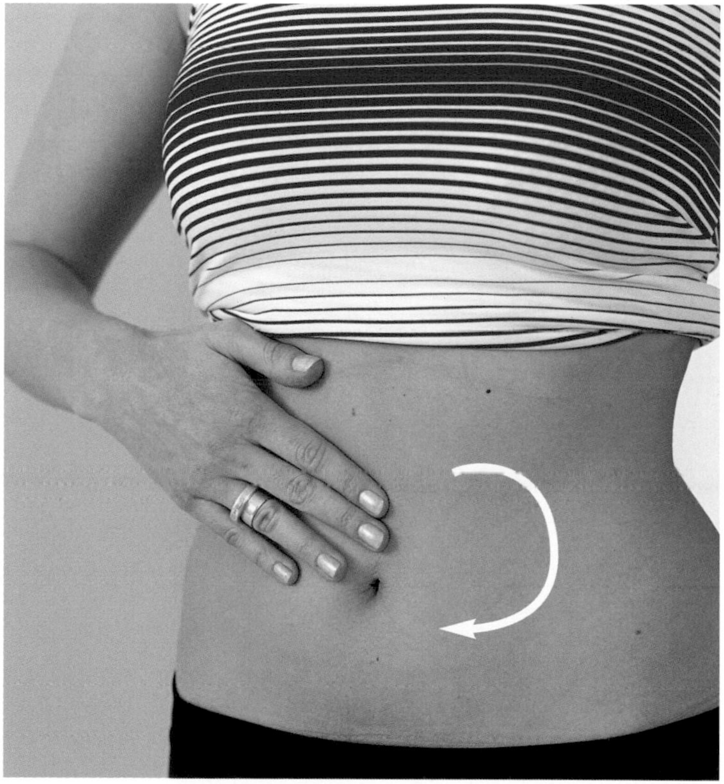

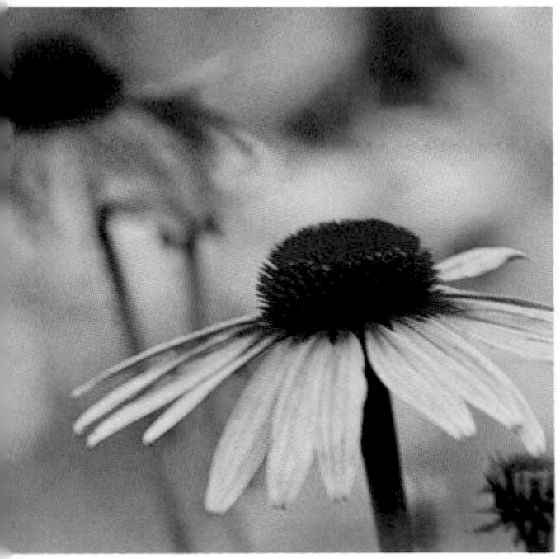

# Naturopathy

Naturopathy is a multi-disciplinary system of holistic medicine that incorporates diet and nutrition, fasting, hydrotherapy, iridology, herbs, massage and is based on the premise that nature heals. Naturopaths believe in using natural resources to get the body to heal itself using its vital curative force to fight illness and disease, eventually returning to a state of harmony known as homeostasis. The naturopath's aim is to help you to achieve homeostasis and to preserve it.

Naturopaths see illness as natural. They help to identify the cause of an illness, then assist the vital force in eliminating it. A naturopath looks at many factors when someone feels tired all the time, including: diet, stress factors, exposure to heavy metals, chemical and electromagnetic pollution, adrenal exhaustion, gut problems such as candida, underlying infections (often viral), imbalances in blood sugar levels and hormones, depression, anaemia and so on. Naturopaths believe that emotions play a big part in our health and energy. In other words, fear, hatred and resentment can adversely affect the digestive or hormonal systems or blood circulation, for example.

Most of the time a combination of many factors is responsible for tiredness. However, stress and poor diet are particularly harmful. Stress depletes the body of vital nutrients leaving it unable to function to its optimum level. Constant stress also leaves our body little time for relaxation, rest and repair. The adrenals work overtime producing hormones like adrenaline and noradrenaline to help us cope, but without sufficient nutrients and time to recover they reach burnout. Eventually when we require energy it is simply not available.

The balance between the nutrients and fuel that we put into our body and the rate at which they are processed has a huge impact on our health and energy. Sugary foods, and stimulants are toxic and deplete the nutrients required for adrenal support. Tobacco and smoke exposure should also be eliminated as it too is toxic.

A session with a naturopath will usually involve them taking a detailed medical history and questions about your emotional state and lifestyle. They will also look at your body type (if you are soft and round, muscular and stocky, long and lean) which will point toward certain constitutions and illnesses, and may use any of the tools/therapies mentioned above.

# Reflexology

Reflexology, or zone therapy, dates back at least five thousand years and stems from the Chinese use of acupressure. The ancient Egyptians also used similar methods and tomb drawings show their feet being held and massaged in a particular way. There is also evidence of American Indian and primitive African tribes using reflexology.

Many people are sceptical as to how reflexology, the application of pressure to points on the feet, or massaging the feet can be beneficial to their health, but it can be used successfully to treat a variety of illnesses, as well as being both relaxing and energising.

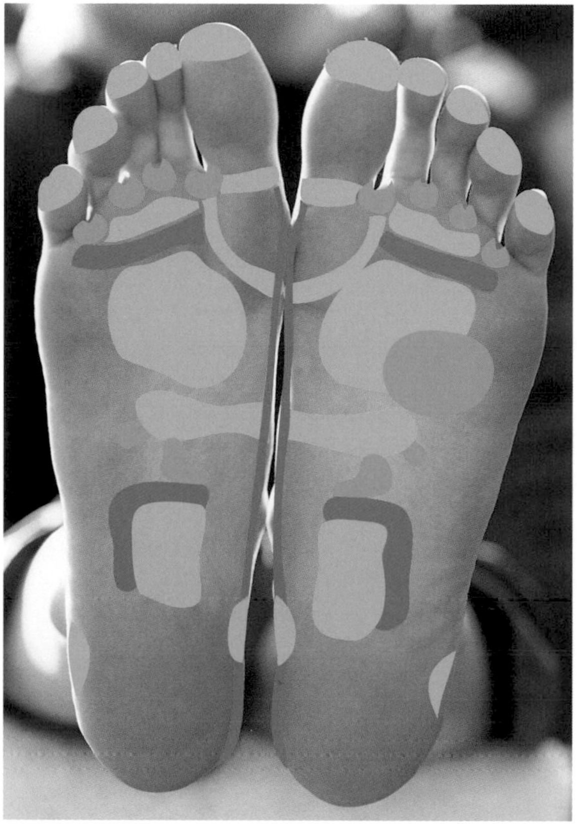

Each part of the body is reflected in particular areas of the feet, and on this basis, the whole body can be treated through the feet. Reflex points are found on the soles, sides and top of the feet (see diagram), and there are also reflex points on the palms and backs of the hands. The reflex points are organised through a system of ten longitudinal zones that extend through the body, as described by Dr Fitzgerald in 1913. The zones are divided into five, either side of the central line. Each zone has a corresponding reflex point in the foot which the reflexologist manipulates so as to diagnose and treat different parts of the body. As well as these longitudinal zones there are also three transverse zones. It is not yet fully understood how massaging a particular area of the foot has an effect on a corresponding organ, but we do know that it at least helps the circulation and helps to reduce tension.

Reflexologists work with the flow of energy in a similar way to acupuncturists. Because the flow of energy naturally strives for health and balance, it needs help when it becomes blocked in order to clear, release and balance the system. By applying pressure to the relevant points on the feet in a subtle yet effective way, reflexologists help to open energy pathways and release blockages.

The first session with a reflexologist usually lasts between an hour and an hour and a half. The practitioner will take a detailed medical history, and will then ask you to sit or lie at an angle on a couch. You only need to remove your shoes and socks. First the reflexologist examines your feet, looking at texture, colour and temperature; and your ankles to see whether there is swollen or puffiness in that area. They will then apply talcum powder to the feet to allow ease of movement, and using the tip of their thumbs, apply pressure and perform small circular movements on the various points, starting from the toes and making their way down the foot to the heel. The reflexologist will then gently rotate the toes and feet and massage the soles of the feet. The treatment ends with a breathing exercise, where pressure is placed on the reflex point for the solar plexus. You must tell the practitioner if the pressure is too hard as sometimes the points might be tender.

*A reflexology treatment is very enjoyable and relaxing, and even if your feet are ticklish, you will be able to cope with it because the pressure is hard enough.*

Though reflexology can be done at home, using the map of the reflex points to relieve, for example, a sinus problem, I have chosen to use a basic foot massage (see page 57) as a tool for increasing energy as it helps to relax and circulate the blood, and therefore enhance energy.

Note: if you are pregnant or suffering from a medical condition, consult a health practitioner before practising reflexology on yourself.

# Shiatsu

Shiatsu is a Japanese word (*shi* meaning finger, *atsu* meaning pressure) for a therapy similar to acupressure. It is an oriental massage where fingers are pressed on specific points (known as tsubo) of the body to help relieve tiredness, tension and the symptoms of disease. These points tend to be areas where the pressure feels uncomfortable because the flow of energy or ki is blocked. (Ki is the Japanese word for qi or energy.) Shiatsu works on the same points as acupuncture (see page 33), along the meridians through which the body's energy flows. However, shiatsu uses pressure not only from the fingers, but also the palms, knees, forearms, elbows and feet.

When you have a shiatsu treatment you can often feel the energy moving along the meridians, which is why it is often called acupuncture without needles. Like acupuncture, shiatsu can relieve many chronic problems and disabling aches and pains, and like all alternative therapies it is a great preventative discipline, helping to maintain health, vitality and stamina. It also strengthens the internal organs and prevents energy from becoming blocked in the channels.

To enjoy an all-over shiatsu you need to find a qualified practitioner who has had at least three years of training (see page 216 for contacts). You need to wear loose clothing because you will remain fully clothed throughout the treatment and the practitioner needs to be able to move and manipulate your body easily. The treatment is usually carried out on the floor on a futon mattress. The first treatment usually lasts for an hour and a half and includes questions on your health, lifestyle, diet and medical history. Sometimes the pressure points can be sore and you should communicate with your practitioner to establish the correct pressure for you. Shiatsu is most effective after a full course of treatments. You will also be given dietary and lifestyle advice.

Shiatsu is best from a qualified practitioner, but there are things that you can do at home or which you can get a friend or partner to do. Instinctively we all practise self-shiatsu when we an ache or pain using pressure or by rubbing an area that is cold. A mother rubs and caresses her baby when it cries and animals soothe each other and themselves with their tongues. Shiatsu is simply a more thorough and complex method of this sort of healing (without the tongues of course!).

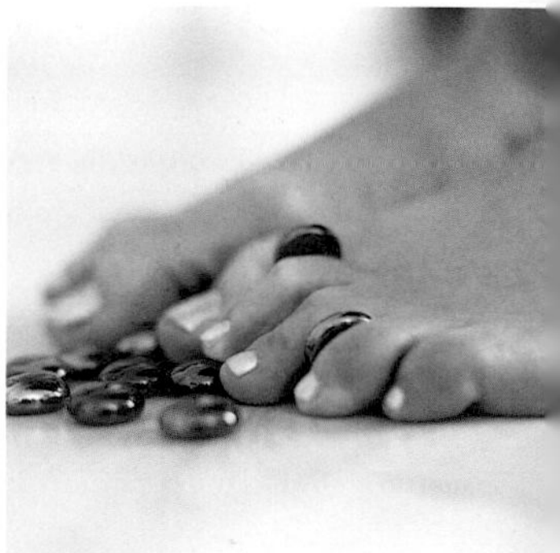

When you do shiatsu on yourself or others it is best to apply pressure slowly and evenly, this way it should not hurt. When you push on a pressure point use the pads of your thumbs, press down for a count of five, then slowly release. You do not need to move your finger while pushing down. If you practise on someone else ask them how much pressure they like; some people prefer a light pressure and others like it very deep. When you press the pressure points you are stimulating or releasing ki.For insomnia the points or tsubo to concentrate on are SP6, KID1, DU20, and, for fatigue, LI10, REN4, ST36 (see page 33).

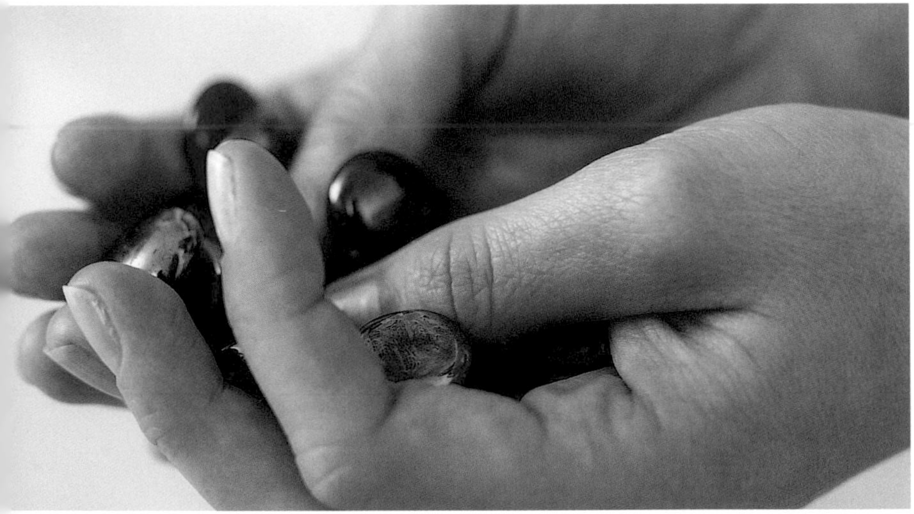

## Beating Fatigue

1 Lie on your back and put your hands behind your neck.

2 Starting at the top where the back of the head meets the neck apply gentle pressure with your fingertips (GB20) then make your way down to in between your neck and the tip of your shoulder and apply pressure (GB21).

3 Breathe deeply.

4 Tighten your whole body and release each part, bit by bit.

**No More Blues** This helps to beat the blues as well as increasing your energy. It's also good for stiff joints and bad circulation.

1 Hold some pebbles in your hand and roll and squeeze them in your palms.

2 Open and close your hands many times and then squeeze the pebbles between your fingers.

3 Put the pebbles on the floor and with bare feet roll the pebbles under your feet. Squeeze the pebbles if you can and try to pick them up between your toes.

Note: before working on any pressure points on yourself or anyone else, ensure that they are not pregnant or suffering from any illness; if they are they should consult a qualified shiatsu practitioner.

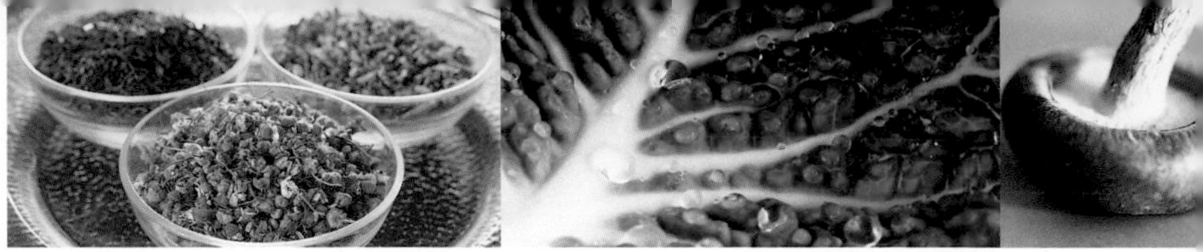

# Traditional Chinese Medicine (TCM)

## *TCM teaches the importance of eating well for optimum energy.*

Practitioners can help to relieve some illnesses using food alone, or in the case of a more complicated illness they might go on to use herbs, acupuncture and massage. In Chinese medicine good food is considered to be a good medicine.

As in Ayurvedic medicine, the Chinese believe that food contains a vital energy, qi, that is ingested when you eat. Chinese philosophy breaks food down into three main categories:

1 Hot foods (yang): warming and stimulating, for example, cooked fruits and vegetables, dried or stewed fruit, carrots, leeks, onions, watercress, lentils, oats, red meat and some cooked fish, pumpkin, sesame and sunflower seeds, chestnuts and walnuts, curries, garlic ginger, black pepper and cloves, basil, oregano, bay leaf, caraway seeds, ginger, cinnamon, mustard, chocolate, coffee, alcohol.

2 Cold foods (yin): calming and cooling, for example, raw fruits and vegetables, salads, broccoli, cauliflower, courgettes, sweet corn, asparagus, button mushrooms, lettuce, cucumber, celery, aubergine, spinach, squash, cabbage, watermelon, apples, melon, rice, barley, millet, wheat, soya, tofu, mung bean sprouts, alfalfa sprouts, salt, peppermint, nettle and dandelion tea, marjoram, tarragon, turmeric, seaweed.

3 Damp foods: create damp in the body (i.e. if you have a cold they will make more phlegm), for example, bananas, cheese, dairy and fried foods. Damp foods should not be eaten when it is damp and raining outside.

So, in essence, if you are feeling tired, lethargic, lacking in motivation, slow, sluggish and depressed you should eat yang foods to heat and speed you up. However, if you are feeling stressed, uptight, angry, anxious, overheated and with too much energy (this might be nervous energy), you should eat more yin foods to calm and cool you down. TCM also recommends that you avoid leftovers and processed foods.

TCM also looks at the thermal nature of people as well as food. Depending on whether you are a cold or hot person you should eat accordingly i.e. if you are a hot person you should eat more cooling foods and vice versa. A qualified TCM practitioner will be able to establish which type you are, but here are some general guidelines:

- Hot person: feels hot all the time; has a red face; is restless, impatient, excitable, hyperactive; walks and talks fast; can have problems sleeping; is always thirsty especially for cold drinks; fidgets a lot; likes to sleep with the covers thrown off and spread out on the bed; feels hot to the touch; has a loud voice and likes to talk; has dark urine.
- Cold person: feels cold all the time; is quiet and introverted; walks and talks slowly; is often tired, sleepy and lethargic; likes to be covered and curled up in bed; wears lots of clothes or layers; prefers hot drinks and foods; has a quiet or weak voice; does not like talking; is relaxed and easygoing; is vulnerable to the cold; is susceptible to colds; does not like to be active.
- Damp person: is lethargic or tired; lacks energy; has a muzzy head; has heavy, aching limbs; has a lot of phlegm, mucus or pus; has oozing skin conditions; has loose stools; may suffer with conditions that are worse in damp weather, e.g. arthritis; is depressed and listless; has difficulty making decisions; can feel nauseous.

If you are suffer from a damp condition it is best to see a qualified TCM practitioner but just cutting down on damp foods should help.

A consultation with a TCM practitioner will be very similar to one with an acupuncturist. Treatment will be with herbs together with advice on diet and lifestyle.

Note: if you suffer from a serious illness or are pregnant it is advisable to consult a TCM practitioner rather than trying to treat yourself.

## Western Herbalism

Plants give us materials for shelter, transport, clothing and tools, they provide us with food and clean our air and most importantly they have a vast array of healing properties.

Herbalism recognises the existence of a vital life-giving force or energy flowing through nature. It also believes that in order to maintain vitality and good health we need to be able to maintain our inner balance (of, for example, body fluids, sugar levels, temperature and breathing rates) regardless of what is going on around us and to heal ourselves when we become out of balance.

When we experience a physical symptom it is simply the vital force of the body trying to re-establish balance. For example, a high fever is a sign that the body is trying to fight an invading pathogen more efficiently, and by suppressing this symptom you are fighting against the body's own vital force. And so it is with energy: if you feel tired all the time it is a sign that the body needs to reinstate the vital force that has been depleted; trying to suppress this with stimulants will further deplete the body's vital force.

The herbalist's job is to recognise the body's attempt to heal itself and to support and enhance this using herbs. A herbalist will ask you in detail about your medical history, as well as your emotions, mental attitude, diet, work, relationships and lifestyle. The herbalist can help to relieve symptoms but will, more importantly, address the underlying problems that are causing the symptoms, for example tiredness. After forming a diagnosis they will formulate a herbal prescription, and offer advice on diet and exercise. Herbs can be taken as a tea, tincture (based in alcohol), syrup, inhalation, gargle, poultice, herbal bath or balm/ointment or compress. Ensure that your herbalist is fully qualified, insured and registered with the relevant body or council.

## Herbs for energy

- For stress: wild oats, vervain, liquorice and skullcap
- If you are run down or recovering from an illness: dandelion, burdock, echinacea, red clover and nettles
- To boost the immune system and fortify the nerves: garlic and sage
- For energy and nervous exhaustion: avena sativa (oats)
- For insomnia and nerves: camomile
- For low mood: hypericum
- If you or people around you are sick or to increase mental energy by clearing the mind: mint (be careful if you are breastfeeding as it can reduce milk flow)
- For vitality: saffron

Note: if you are pregnant or suffer any serious medical condition do not take any herbs without consulting a professional medical practitioner.

**SLEEP AND RELAXATION**

# Sleep

*We all need to sleep, and in fact, tiredness at the end of a fulfilling day is a signal that prepares us for a good night's sleep in order to re-energise ourselves for the next day.*

Even when our energy is in plentiful supply sleep is still very important as without it the body cannot function properly.An indication of just how important a part sleep plays is the way we feel and function when we are sleep-deprived. We feel ratty, groggy, unable to concentrate, lacking in energy, edgy, stressed and oversensitive.

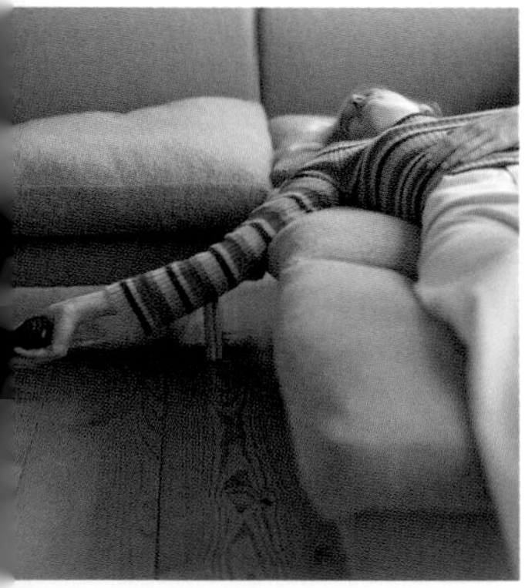

**How much sleep do we need?** Most adults need on average seven to eight hours' sleep, but many get by with six or even fewer, while others need more. As long as you are going to bed and sleeping through the night and waking refreshed and energised then you are getting enough sleep. If, however, you wake up every morning to an alarm clock feeling tired and resentful it would be best to try and get to sleep earlier as it is most likely that your alarm disturbs you during your deep sleep stage.

Research has estimated that about 5 million people in the UK suffer from TATT (Tired All The Time) syndrome. These people feel that no matter how much sleep and rest they get, they still feel exhausted, weary, lethargic, fatigued and unable to live life to the full. If you are a TATT syndrome sufferer you may find that one of the following is the cause of your problem:

- Illness: diabetes, under-active thyroid, flu and many other illnesses can cause tiredness. Check with your doctor that there is no underlying physical problem at the root of your tiredness.
- Depression: this can cause tiredness and lethargy regardless of how much sleep you get, indeed if you are depressed you probably feel that you want to sleep all the time. Your doctor or health practitioner should be able to help you.

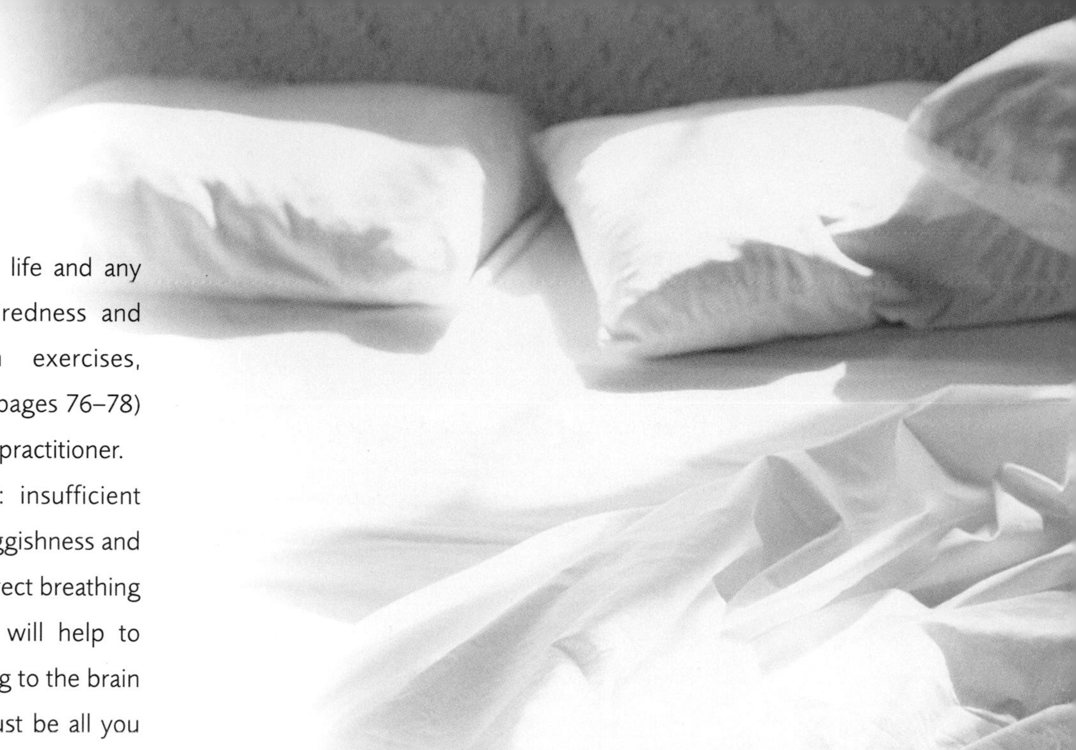

- Stress: dissatisfaction with your life and any negative emotions can lead to tiredness and lethargy. Try some relaxation exercises, meditations and visualisations (see pages 76–78) and/or seek the help of your health practitioner.
- Lack of exercise and oxygen: insufficient oxygen can cause tiredness and sluggishness and a whole host of minor illnesses. Correct breathing and posture, stretches and yoga will help to increase the amount of oxygen going to the brain and around the body. This might just be all you need to help you recover from tiredness.
- Holding on to emotions: regular body massages can help to increase your energy and stop you feeling tired all the time, by releasing stored emotions such as anger, resentment and so on. Some people actually cry during a massage as they experience this release, and afterwards they report having lots more energy as a result. Massage also helps with circulation, making the blood and oxygen circulate around the body better. This makes you feel and look refreshed, rejuvenated and re-energised (see page 54 for some simple self-massage techniques).
- Lack of fresh air: if you live/work in a centrally heated environment and spend a lot of time in cars and trains, it is important that you spend more time outdoors. Pure fresh air contains negative ions which energise you, whereas indoor and polluted atmospheres contain more positive ions which make you feel tired. Try and find places full of trees and plants and little traffic to walk in, and keep lots of plants at work. If you cycle in cities wear a good anti-pollutant mask. Keep your home and work cool and fresh. An ioniser or a salt crystal at work/home will help to clean the air and take away the positive ions.
- Poor diet: make sure that you are eating well (see pages 84–99) otherwise you will be lacking in essential vitamins and minerals/nutrients which will eventually lead to tiredness and ill health.

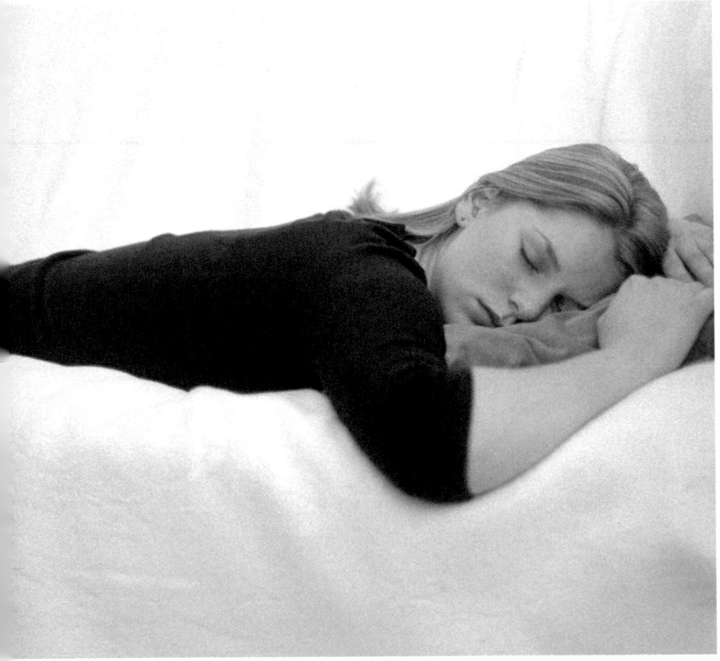

**Body clocks** The body has its own natural rhythm, monthly cycle (even men) and a heartbeat rhythm. Added to these are the earth's rhythm and the cycles of the seasons, moon and day and night. The cycle of day following night really affects us as we secrete hormones depending on whether it is dark or light outside. But features of modern living such as late-night parties, the contraceptive pill and flying across time zones, have made us lose touch with some of these rhythms.

Living life in tune with your body clock allows you to conserve and create more energy. The twenty-four hour circadian cycle dominates our body clock, encouraging us to sleep when it is dark and wake when it is light. These and all the other body clock rhythms are controlled by suprachiasmatic nuclei in the hypothalamus area of the brain.

When we are asleep these nuclei lower our heart rate, lung function, urine production, temperature and blood pressure by balancing the hormones and chemicals of the body. When we wake up the same nuclei stimulate everything again ready for the daytime rhythms to begin (so the heart rate increases, the lungs function faster, more urine is produced, our temperature rises and so does our blood pressure). There are also many mini cycles in the day which is why you might notice your energy fluctuating with dips and dives at certain times.

In order to function with optimum energy it is important to recognise these cycles: don't try and fight what your body is telling you at times when you have less energy, and do more energetic things at a point in the day when you have lots of energy.

## How a typical body clock might function

- 12–4 a.m. This is the time for deep, restful sleep. The body is repairing and refreshing itself ready for the day ahead, so this sleep is important.
- 4–6 a.m. Blood pressure and body temperature are low, so it is difficult to work during this period.
- 6–8 a.m. The brain starts to become more active again as REM (rapid eye movement, see below) sleep occurs (it also occurs during the night), so it is fine to get up at this time if that's what feels right. Melatonin, a hormone that helps to promote sleep is starting to dip, while cortisol which wakes us up, is being released at this time.
- 8 a.m.–2 p.m. Adrenaline is rising so this is when the brain is most alert. This is a good time to get a lot of work done especially mental work
- 2–5 p.m. Energy levels can start to dip now so it is a good time to eat lunch and do jobs that require less energy or concentration.
- 5–6 p.m. The muscles are warm and the heart and circulation are working at their best, so this is a very good time to exercise.
- 6–8 p.m. The sleep hormone starts to be released around now, so you will begin to feel more relaxed and tired. In the summer this will be slightly later as it gets dark later.
- 10–12 p.m. This is the best time to go to sleep as melatonin levels are high; this means you will be asleep in time for the deep sleep around midnight in preparation to wake up refreshed the next day.

The above is a very average body clock and not everybody does or should work in this way. There

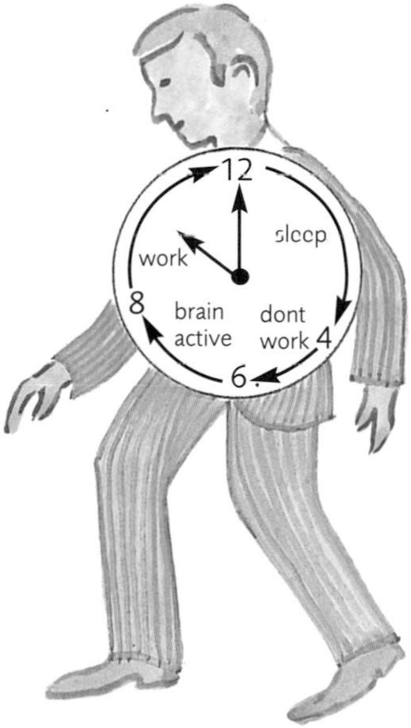


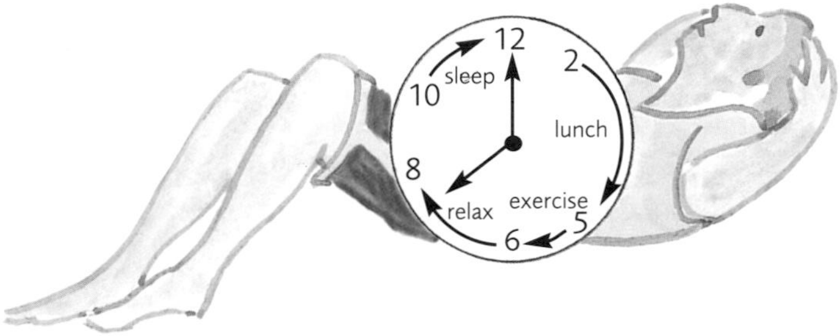

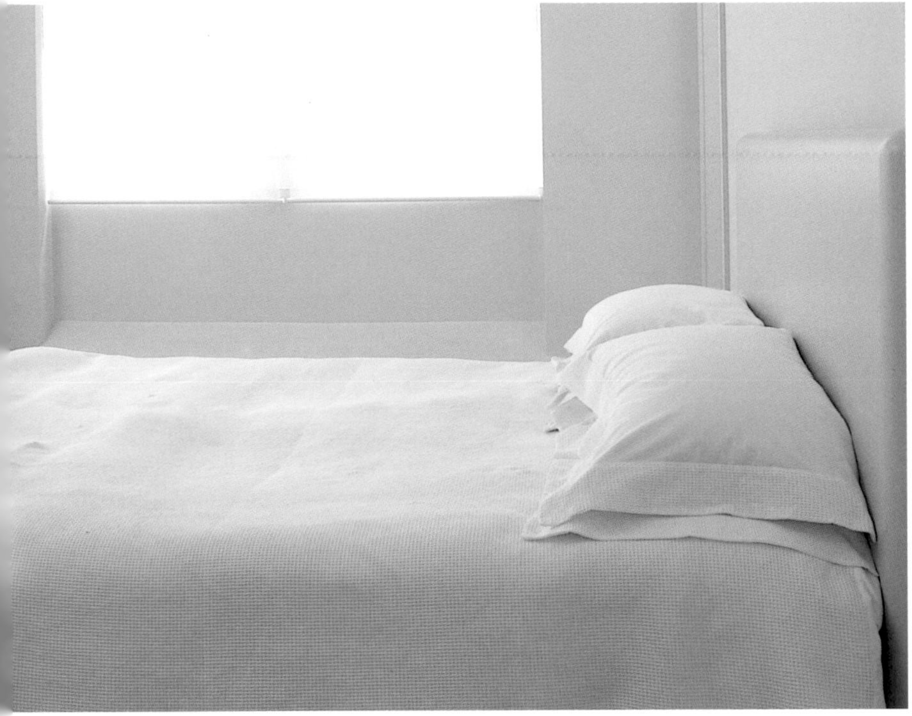

are many reasons why one person's body clock may not fit into the typical pattern, for example, frequent travel to different time zones, but the important thing is that your body clock suits your lifestyle and works for you. If, however, you feel that you would like to re-establish your body clock to maximise your energy levels, it is possible to re-programme it.

To re-programme your body clock to fit the standard pattern, simply set an alarm to go off at the same time, early every morning until you are waking up before it goes off. You must get out of bed as soon as you wake up. Do this for another week and your new clock should be set.

## JETLAG-BUSTERS

- To help regulate sleep patterns when travelling try clary sage, lavender, geranium or rose essential oils.
- To awaken the body and mind try bergamot, melissa, orange, peppermint, rosemary or ginger.
- The Australian Bush flower remedy, travel essence, may be taken before and during travel and on arrival. It really does help.
- A homeopathic remedy that is good for jet lag is ipeccac.

**Getting to sleep** Some people find that no matter when they go to bed, they still have difficulty in getting off to sleep. Here are some tips to help:

- Avoid caffeine after five p.m. and, if possible, cut down on the amount you have during the day. Ideally you should cut it out completely.
- Drink a cup of camomile or valerian tea instead before bed.
- If you can't sleep, get out of bed and do something else; don't stay in bed as your body needs to relearn that your bed is for sleeping.
- Don't read in bed or watch television as that will stimulate you.
- Have a hot bath before bed with a few drops of lavender, juniper and marjoram oils.
- Try some relaxation exercises (see page 79–80) either in bed or in the bath.
- Try playing some soothing background music.
- Eat a couple of hours before going to bed so you don't go to bed hungry.
- If you can't sleep because you are worrying over things that need to be done the next day, write down all the things you need to do; that way you should feel more relaxed knowing that everything is on a list and won't be forgotten.

And here are a few more tips to ensure that you have a good-quality sleep once you've managed to fall asleep:

- Try going for a walk every day.
- Write a list of things to do the next day before going to bed.
- Avoid sleeping medication; they do not address the root cause of your problem and they also suppress REM sleep (see page 73) which is essential for good health. Try a natural alternative such as valerian which is non-addictive and helps promote sleep.
- Ensure that your bed is comfortable and that the room has a soothing, relaxing atmosphere.
- Never leave the heating on overnight as this will make you wake up tired and sluggish in the morning.
- Avoid big meals before bed. A light, meal of calcium-rich foods around two to three hours before you go to bed is recommended. (These foods are known as nature's tranquillisers.)

**Sleep and stress** When when we are under a lot of pressure we experience stress. This can leave us feeling quite exhausted by the end of the day and if the stress continues over a period of time we can really be drained of energy. When we de-stress we allow the body time to recharge: just think back to your last holiday and how much energy you had when you first got back. However, before you realise it the stresses pile back on and slow you down, making you tired again all too quickly.

Regular relaxation exercises and activities (see pages 100–109) can help enormously to counteract the effects of stress, but just being aware of when your body is under stress is a vital key to stress-busting. Stress factors need not only be negative things such as bereavement, divorce or losing a job; many positive things like getting married, moving house or even going on holiday can induce huge amounts of stress. So many people in today's busy world are unaware as to just how stressed they really are. Try answering the stress questionnaire below to find out how much stress you are carrying:

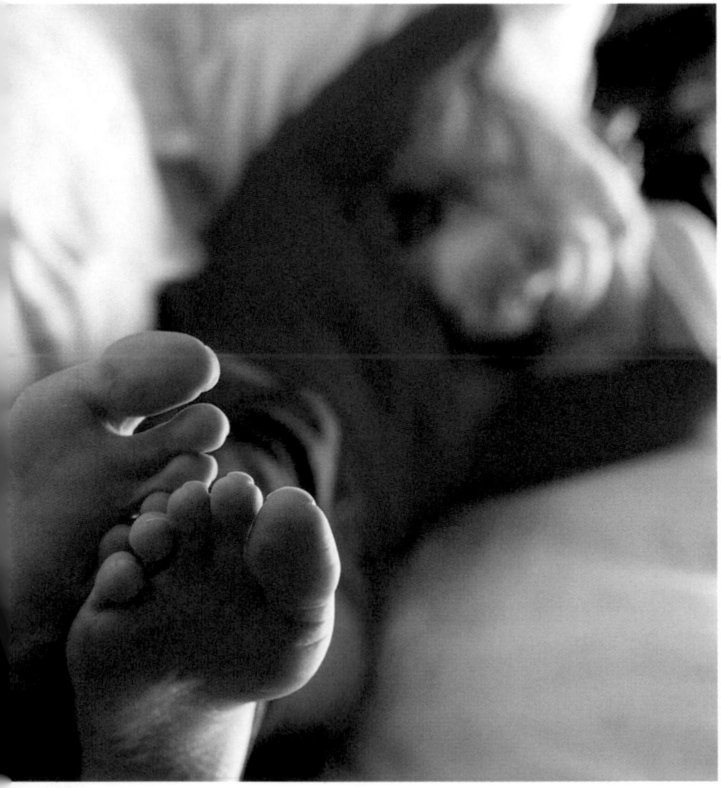

**1** Do you have difficulty sleeping or trouble staying asleep?

**2** Do you feel anxious a lot of the time?

**3** Do you often have a stiff necks and shoulders?

**4** Do you grind your teeth at night?

**5** Is your jaw clenched tight even now?

**6** Are you constantly going over and over things in your mind?

**7** Do you find it difficult to stop relax/switch off?

**8** Do you find that you need alcohol, cigarettes or social drugs to help you to relax?

**9** Do you have problems with your skin or digestion?

**10** Do you take offence very easily and have mood swings for no apparent reason?

**11** Do you eat and talk quickly and want people to tell you things quickly so you can carry on?

**12** Does your leg shake under the table when you are working or sitting down to a meal?

**13** Do you feel that there is not enough time in the day for everything?

**14** Do you long for a holiday/break/change of life?

If you answer 'yes' to most of the above questions then you are carrying a lot of stress.

When you are stressed the quality of your sleep is diminished. Quality sleep contains adequate REM and deep non-REM sleep. REM sleep is light dream sleep, when the brain sorts through all of your daily activities and thoughts. Deep sleep is when the body repairs itself and growth and sex hormones are released. With sufficient amounts of both types of sleep you will wake up feeling refreshed and raring to go. It is therefore essential to try and de-stress before bed.

## RELAXING THE TENSION BEFORE BED

Regular relaxation exercises and/or alternative therapies will help you to get a good night's sleep. Massage, deep breathing, stretching and yoga will all help to relax your brain and calm your body especially if you do them before going to sleep

Try the following exercise every night when you get into bed. It's great if you are feeling stressed and/or can't sleep:

1 Lie down with the lights off. Close your eyes and observe your breathing.

2 When you are ready begin, tense each part of your body individually starting with your toes, then your feet, calves, knees right up to your eyes, nose cheeks, top of your head.

3 Starting with your toes, hold the tension and then release, exhale and move on to the next part of your body. Notice the difference between holding the tension and relaxing.

4 When you have done your whole body front and back top and bottom you should (if you're not asleep already!) feel very relaxed.

# Relaxation Techniques

*Learning to relax both physically and mentally is a very important skill.*

It is important to find the relaxation technique that works for you: if you are an impatient person, for example, you should try a short relaxation technique. When a relaxation method works you will feel physical benefits: your heart rate slows down, your blood pressure falls and your breathing becomes slower and more rhythmic. Your saliva and bile are also stimulated to aid proper digestion allowing your bodily functions to work properly. You will also feel calm.

When you feel calm your mind works at its best, concentration is better and so is memory. You see problems in perspective and you feel lighter, stronger and more centred. You are able to let go of emotions such as anger and frustration, allowing your body to recharge and create new energy.

Learning to unwind at the beginning, middle and end of each day gives you a simple tool with which to help your body to cope better and to give you more real energy throughout the day.

During a meditation or visualisation your heart rate and breathing slow down, the bronchi of the lungs dilate, blood pressure drops and the production of stomach acid is reduced. Most importantly, no stress hormones are released into the bloodstream. Relaxation exercises (including visualisations and meditations) are not the same as sleeping, as during a meditation and/or visualisation the brain emits alpha waves showing the brain to be mentally alert but physically relaxed.

**Meditation** Being in a meditative state is actually very similar to what we might call 'daydreaming'; we all switch in and out of simple meditative states throughout the day without even realising it. I have included the walking meditation on page 77 to show how a 'normal' meditative activity can be enhanced simply by increasing awareness, and to take away many people's fear of meditation.

When you meditate (as with visualisations or relaxation exercises) you turn your attention inward. Even though you are aware of where you are it is no longer at the centre of your mind. Meditation helps you to find inner peace by calming the mind and helping it to focus. It provides a rare opportunity to find a little space in a hectic world and often a hectic mind.

Meditation requires practice and discipline. When you meditate you let go of your thoughts just for the time of the meditation in the knowledge that you can think about them all again when the meditation is over. The mind loves to be active and it is very easy to get swept along on a daily basis by your thoughts and emotions but this can be very tiring. The first step of meditation then, is to become aware of how busy your mind is and then learn to let it go.

During everyday activities the brain operates on fast theta waves but when you meditate the brainwaves change to the slower alpha waves that occur with relaxation. Experienced meditators can even experience delta waves similar to those activated during sleep.

There are many activities that we do on a daily basis that are quite meditative, such as cycling, cleaning, painting or anything where the mind is used in a disciplined way so that it can't wander off into a whole chain of thoughts.

It can take weeks or even months to really see the benefit of meditation so don't give up too soon, and once you have found the meditation that works well for you, try to stick to it and use the same method every day. The walking meditation on page 77 is a good example of a simple activity that has a meditative quality.

**Rules for doing any relaxation technique:**

1 Find a quiet space in which to relax (this can even be the toilet if you are at work), preferably first thing in the morning, at noon or when it gets dark, and not straight after a meal.
2 Turn off all phones.
3 Ask your family/colleagues not to disturb you.
4 Make yourself comfortable (for example sit on a chair with your feet resting on the floor).
5 Try to use the same place at the same time every day so that your body gets into a routine.
6 Tell yourself to let go of your worries for just ten to twenty minutes; you can think about them all again when the exercise is finished.

**Simple meditations** Try to do one of the following simple meditations every day.

**Breath meditation**

**1** Sit comfortably on a chair or lie down.

**2** Close your eyes and slowly focus your attention on your breathing. Don't judge your breathing by thinking it's too fast or too slow, just observe it objectively.

**3** Every time your mind wanders, which it most certainly will do with thoughts like, 'I wonder what I will have for tea?', just let the thought go (you can always think about it later) and go back to observing your breathing.

At first you might find it difficult to stop your mind wandering especially if you are stressed and/or very busy, but with practice you will find that you might have just one second or minute when your mind is clear, and this will feel like bliss. You can do this breath meditation anywhere, anytime – on a train or a bus, in a waiting room, just anywhere.

**Mantra meditation:**

**1** Pick a word or phrase that you like like – 'peace', 'love', 'health', 'energy' – and repeat it over and over either in your head or aloud. This word is your mantra. The traditional Hindu mantra is 'om', said to be the sound of the whole universe,

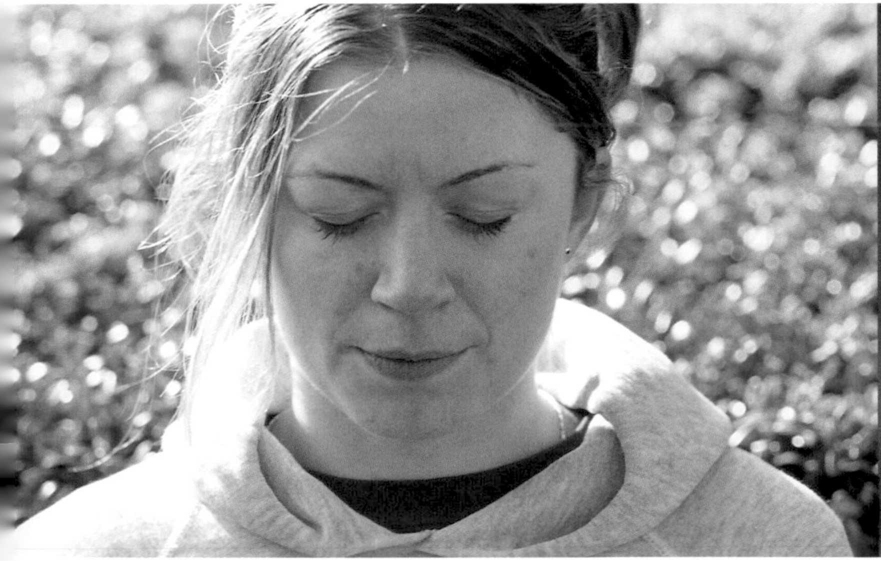

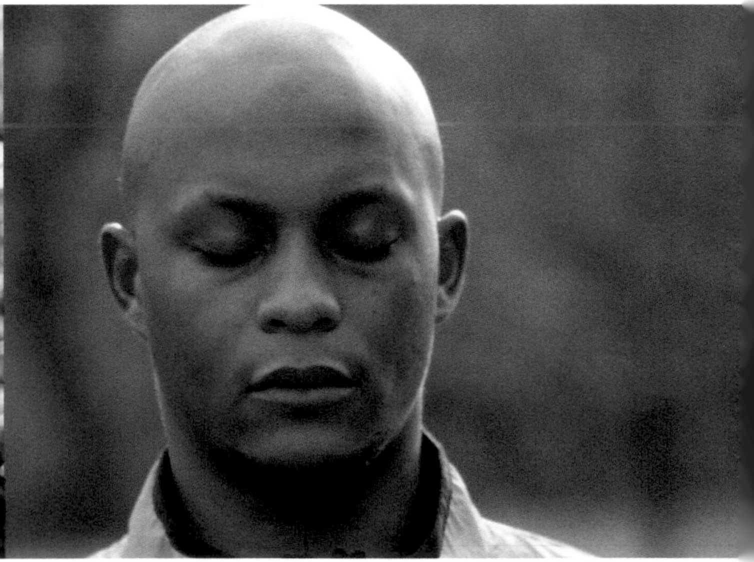

and it will help you to bring about changes in your real self. It is also very balancing and massages the internal organs, increases blood flow, stimulates the nervous system and relaxes the respiratory system.

**2** Close your eyes and take a few deep breaths when you are ready start.

**3** Concentrate and focus on your chosen word or phrase. Try to still your mind and turn your attention inward. By doing this you will focus your mind on your inner world and find a state of peace.

This type of meditation is particularly good if you find it difficult to stop the constant internal dialogue, as it helps you to focus the mind.

**Walking meditation**

**1** As you walk become aware of your feet.

**2** Begin by saying in your head, 'left right left right', then just let the rhythm take you into a meditative state. If any problems are bothering you try and put them aside until after the walk.

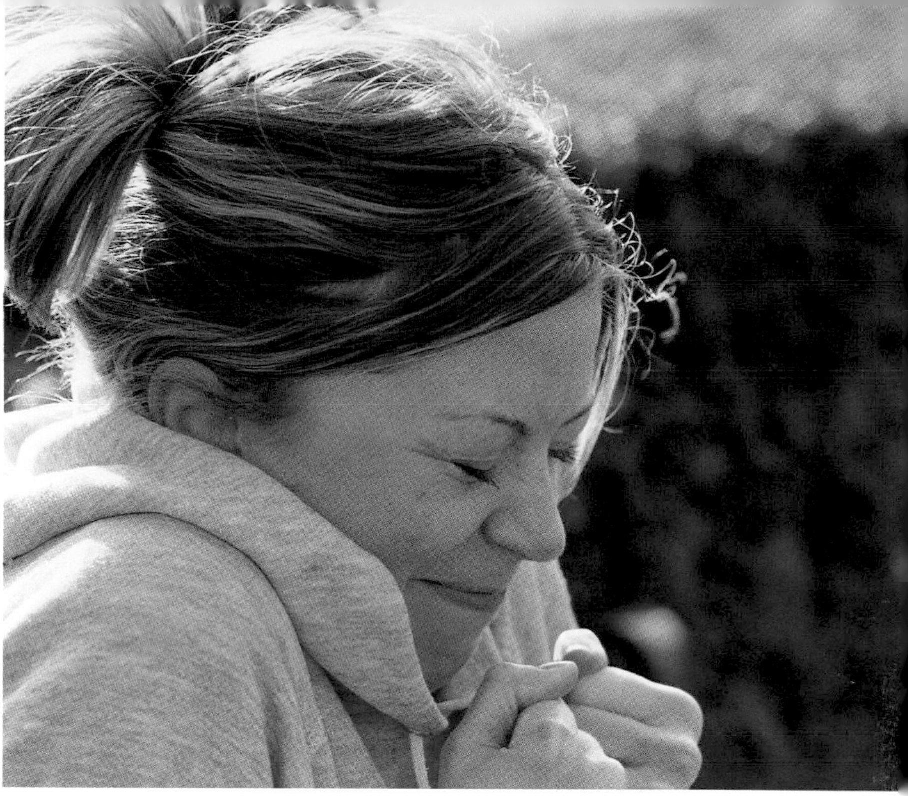

**Visualisations** To visualise simply means to see something in your mind's eye, something which we all do instinctively every day. If someone stops to ask you for directions you will automatically visualise the route in your mind; if you are thinking about what you did last night you visualise the events of the previous evening in your mind. When you listen to the radio, or hear someone describing something, or even when you read a book you will automatically produce pictures in your mind. In fact when you see a film based on a book that you have read, you are often disappointed because the characters in the film do not look as you'd visualised them. So if you feel that you have 'no imagination' and worry that you will not be able to visualise, fear not. Everyone can visualise, and everyone does!

A good friend of mine, Pete Cohen, who does NLP (neuro-linguistic programming) and also wrote the foreword to this book, once told me that the key to visualisation is not to concentrate too hard with your mind. This really helped me to relax and stopped me from constantly trying to force my mind to think of the image I wanted to see.

**Earth's energy visualisation** Allow yourself fifteen to twenty minutes for this visualisation:

**1** Close your eyes and innocently observe your breathing objectively (see page 76). Don't judge it.

**2** Imagine yourself sitting under a big old tree. Feel your back supported by its firm trunk as you lean against it. Keep observing your breathing.

**3** With your feet on the ground feel the earth's energy pull your stress out through your feet. Observe your breathing again.

**4** When you are beginning to feel relaxed, allow the energy of the earth and tree to fill your body starting with your feet and working its way up your body through your back right up into the top of your head. Your feet will probably tingle and you may feel like you have butterflies in your stomach.

**5** Whenever you are ready and feel recharged, slowly come back to the room and open your eyes.

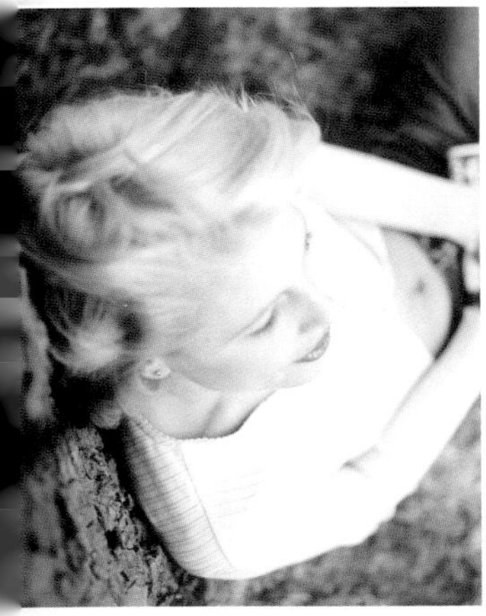

**Ten-minute sun visualisation** This is designed to be a ten-minute visualisation but if you can find twenty minutes, so much the better:

**1** Find a comfortable chair to sit on, (although a toilet will do if necessary.) Close your eyes and begin to observe your breathing (see page 76).

**2** Empty your mind. If you find this difficult then when and if a thought comes into your mind, tell yourself to let it go, and you can think about it in ten/twenty minutes' time.

**3** Once you have started to relax, revisit a beautiful beach, park, waterfall. Allow the energy of nature to recharge you. Remember how good it feels to bask in the sun. Feel the sun warming your face and tickling the rest of your body from your head right down to your toes. Let it calm and re-energise you. Keep observing your breathing. Stay basking in the sun for as long as you want.

**4** When you are ready slowly open your eyes.

When you get used to doing this you will find that you can even meditate on a busy train or bus or just about anywhere. But to begin with, try and do the sun meditation in the morning when you wake up, at midday or when you get back from work. If your day is particularly stressful try to take ten minutes out just to recharge.

## Relaxation Exercises

Relaxation exercises are simply exercises that make you relax the muscles in a particular way, or make you conscious of how you are holding stressed muscles.

### Relax any time, anywhere

**1** Take a deep breath and clench all your muscles.

**2** Make a fist with your hands, tighten your jaw, scrunch up your face, lift your shoulders up to your neck (that is if they are not there already!), tighten your bottom, curl your toes.

**3** Hold all these positions for a few minutes and then breathe out fully and relax every muscle letting every bit of tension out with your breath.

**4** Breathe normally, then repeat a couple of times.

### Stressbuster

**1** Lift your shoulders up and down a couple of times, then rotate them forward and backward a few times.

**2** Close your eyes and concentrate on your breathing.

**3** When you are breathing deeply look up and stretch your arms above your head. Stretch higher with one hand first and then the other.

**4** Rub your head and tap it with your fingertips, tug your hair and then release your hands.

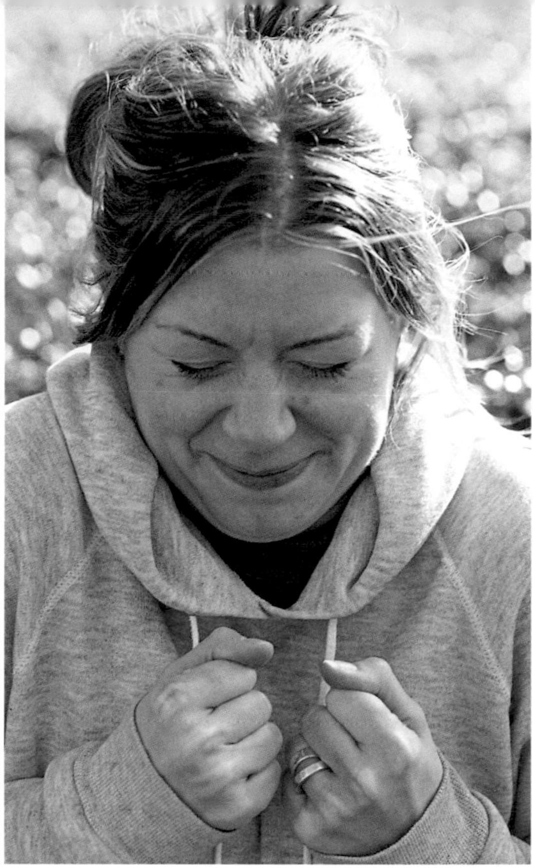

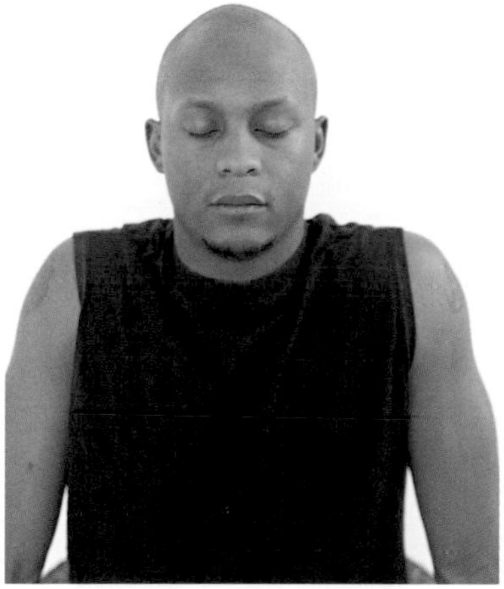

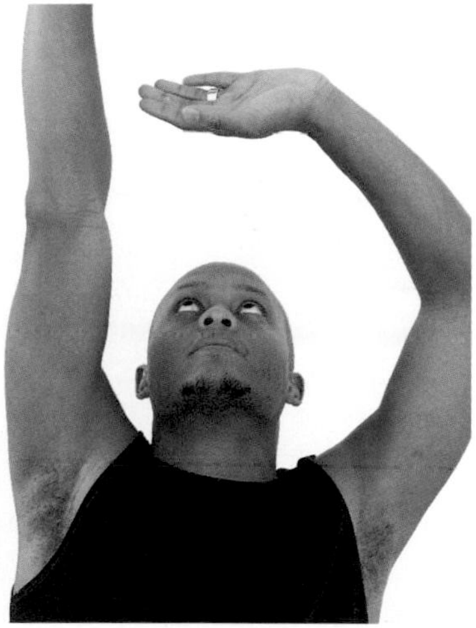

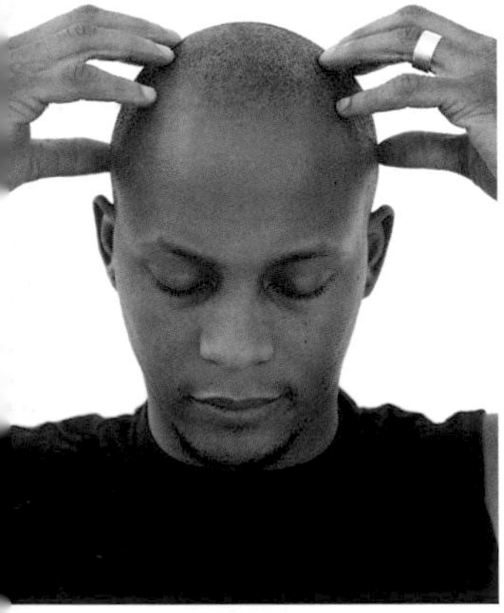

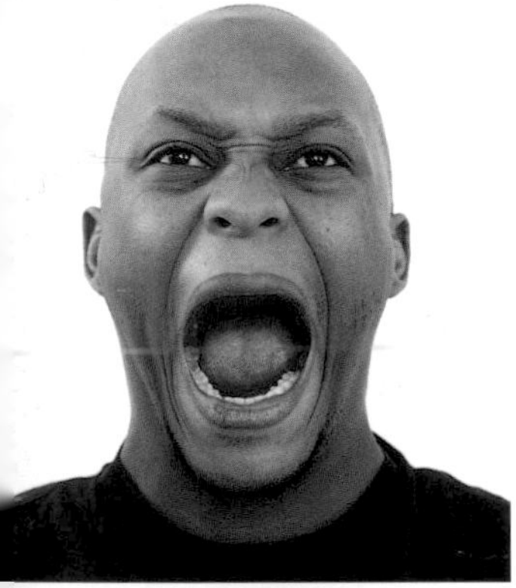

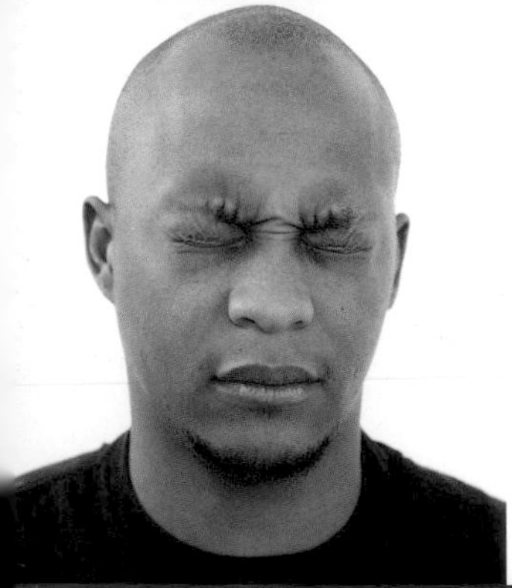

**5** Squeeze around your jaw and then tap it to release the tension often held there, especially if you grind your teeth.

**6** Clench your jaw and then open wide and say, 'Aaaahhhhh'.

**7** Squeeze your eyes shut and then open them wide.

**8** Close your eyes and breathe through your nose while imagining something very peaceful.

### Ease the tension

This exercise can be done anywhere, at any time.

**1** Close your eyes.

**2** Place your thumb and first finger on your eyebrow and squeeze it between them, starting at the nose and moving outward.

**3** With your thumbs push down for a count of five and then move along the bone, under your eyebrow, again starting at the nose.

### Private release of tension

**1** Stand with your feet hip width apart.

**2** With your arms at your sides shake out your hands and then your arms.

**3** Roll your shoulders forwards six times and then backwards six times.

**4** Roll your neck from side to middle to side one way and then the other.

**5** Shake your head, as if saying 'No', and while letting your face relax completely, allow a strange warbling sound to come from your relaxed mouth and cheeks.

**6** Lift up one foot and shake it, then shake out your leg; repeat with the other leg.

**7** Put your hands on your hips and move your hips in a circle one way and then the other. Move your pelvis backwards and forwards.

**8** Making sure that your feet are still hip width apart and your knees bent, clasp your hands together.

**9** Lift your arms above your head and breathe in. Exhale and shout 'Ha', while swinging your arms down as if you are chopping wood, and swing between your legs.

**10** Swing your arms back up again until you are standing upright.

Repeat as many times as you feel necessary.

# Mental Attitude

When looking at energy we have to realise that we are more than just our physical bodies. What happens to us emotionally and psychologically is reflected in physiological changes. Taking this into account it is obvious that our energy levels will also be affected by our mental attitude, the way in which we relate to others and whether we are enjoying life or finding it a struggle.

Just as negative emotions can zap your energy, learning to love and feel positive emotions can boost it. Liking yourself is also very important. A poor, negative self-image can drain your energy and by constantly criticising yourself you use up energy that could be used on other things.

**Here are a few tips to help you achieve a more positive mental attitude:**

- Try to see a positive outcome to every situation.
- If something doesn't happen that you wanted, for example you don't get a job that you were hoping to get, remember the phrase, 'It obviously wasn't meant to be, something better will be waiting around the corner'.
- Give yourself compliments and confidence-boosts: 'I am a nice person', 'I am talented and good at art/self-expression/poetry writing', 'I am a good listener' etc. Make a list of these things so that you can look at it whenever you feel yourself starting to be negative or self-critical.
- Every time you catch yourself being negative turn the situation or sentence round to a positive one.
- Make choices for your own life; don't just accept what comes to you because you believe you don't deserve any better.
- Start the day with an activity that you like, for example reading with a cup of herbal tea.
- Do something that you have never done before and thought that you could never do, like parachute-jumping, roller-blading, acting classes, surfing etc.
- Surround yourself with people who are very positive.
- Repeat positive mantras to yourself whenever you catch yourself being negative, e.g. 'I have loads of energy and can do anything that I choose to do in life'; 'I know that every day and in every way I am getting better and better'; 'Throw it away, throw it away, let it go, let it go'; 'If I will it, it is no dream'; 'I can do anything'.
- Always remember, you are unique and only you can do the things you do.

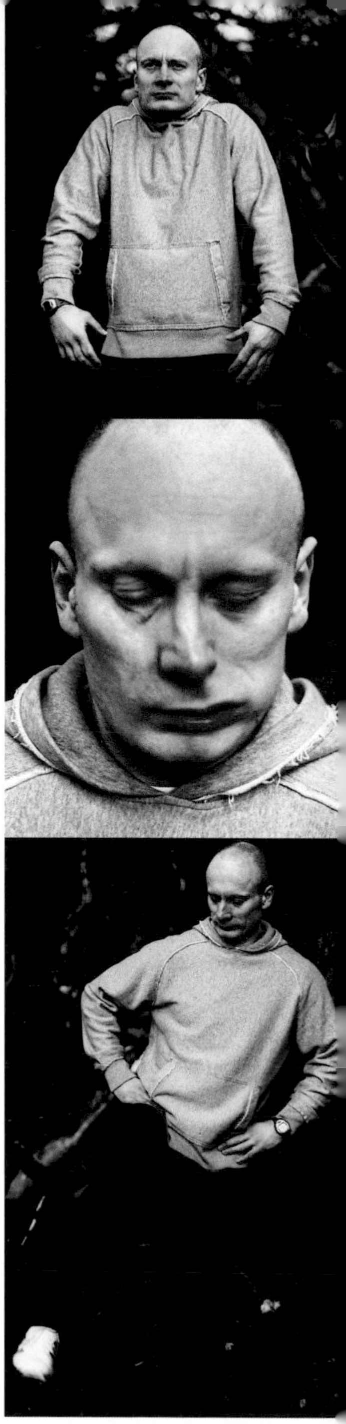

# Structured time

Many people take their work home with them either literally, when they do not have enough hours in the working day to get through it all, or figuratively, by worrying about it after hours. When working on energy levels it is very important to set structured times for work so that there is always time to unwind.

In order to structure your time, a 'To-do' list is a must, otherwise before you know it a firm intention becomes yet another thing you wanted to do but work and other things got in the way.

**To-do lists** We all spend a lot of energy trying to remember things that we have to do and worrying about doing them. Writing a to-do list helps us to stop worrying; it allows us to stop carrying around lots of jobs and worries in our head so that we can spend that energy either on getting those jobs done, or elsewhere.

Try to write your lists either every morning or every afternoon, whichever works best for you. You may find that you don't need to do it daily and that a weekly list that you can add to on a daily basis works better. Some people like to include sections such as work, home and personal. Try to prioritise the various jobs and write in your diary when you plan to do them. It is best to do the jobs you don't like or those that are particularly difficult first, otherwise they won't get done, or you will waste a lot of energy worrying about doing them which will make you irritable and even depressed, draining you of energy still further.

To-do lists mean that you can enjoy your relaxation time more as you are not trying to relax while your brain is still worrying over that day's chores. It will also help you to sleep better which, in turn, will give you more energy.

Don't be afraid to reshuffle your lists: if you don't manage to get something done move it to another day; the lists are there to take the stress off not, to add more.

## QUICK ENERGY BOOSTERS

E*mergency*C made by Alacer increases energy levels quickly due to its rapid assimilation into the body. Use between meals as a drink.

## *A typical to-do list*

*Week starting Monday 18 February 2002*

***Work:***

*All week – Start in-house magazine, decide topics and structure*

*Monday – call suppliers and see if they want to advertise in magazine*

*Tuesday – work out price of printing and mailout*

*Wednesday – organise open day*

*Thursday and Friday – open*

***Home:***

*Monday – Organise baby sitting for anniversary*

*Tuesday – Buy nappies*

*Tuesday – Buy light bulb for hallway*

*Friday – Get money for cleaner and childminder*

*Saturday – Go through baby clothes and put away clothes that are too small*

*Saturday – Do washing*

***Personal:***

*Monday and Friday – Exercise at gym*

*Tuesday – Dance class*

*Thursday – Anniversary dinner*

*Friday – Brother arriving from California*

*Sunday – Wedding*

## CONSERVE YOUR ENERGY

- Get your partner and kids if you have any to help with chores around the house. If you can afford it get some home help from a weekly cleaner.
- If you are always running around doing things for other people but find at the end of the day that you are exhausted with no time left to do anything for yourself, you should try to learn to say 'No' when you are asked to do yet another favour.
- Cut down on going to places or events that you really don't want to go to; only go if you really want to and if you have the energy.
- At work and at home learn to delegate especially at very busy times. This will help to get the job done and will allow you to conserve your energy so that whatever you do yourself is done efficiently. Don't fall into the trap of thinking that the job isn't done properly unless you do it yourself; eventually you will collapse with exhaustion and nothing at all will get done.

# Nutrition and Diet

*Food is like fuel or petrol for the body. If you put poor quality or no food into your body, then like a car with the wrong or poor quality petrol, it won't function as it should, and eventually it won't run at all*

Poor diet and tiredness can very easily become a vicious cycle: a poor diet makes you feel more tired, when you are tired shopping for food and cooking become yet another chore that has to be done which means that snack meals and stimulants become more appealing (chocolate, cakes, coffee and tea) and more vitamin deficiencies occur, with the end result that you are more tired than ever.

If you are lacking in energy, ask yourself if you are over- or under-eating, missing meals, eating enough protein and fibre, drinking enough water, drinking too much alcohol, eating lots of sugary foods, and getting enough vitamins and minerals.

A good diet for making sure you have enough energy is one that includes:

- fish (especially oily fish such as sardines and herring)
- freshly made soups
- chicken
- free-range eggs three times per week
- lots of vegetables especially green leafy ones
- salads
- fresh fruit
- lots of pulses
- nuts and seeds,
- muesli and porridge
- soya, tofu, miso paste (in soups)
- vegetable oils (such as olive and grapeseed)
- only a few dairy products (and none if you are a damp person – see page 63–4 – or have a cold)
- no sugar
- plenty of yang foods (e.g. brown rice, whole-grain cereals, root vegetables, fish, pulses and lentils) – see page 64
- lots of water, filtered if possible

All foods should be organic wherever possible, and alcohol should be avoided altogether as it is a depressant (it makes your blood sugar levels fluctuate which can make you feel tired). Avoid coffee (even decaffeinated) and be careful with tea as both coffee and tea over-stimulate the adrenals. Herbal teas are the best choice, and chamomile, peppermint, verbena and lemon teas are all great for relaxing the nervous system. Dandelion, nettle, sage and rosehip teas all help support the liver and help with detoxing.

If you are under-eating or missing meals because you don't have enough time to prepare them, you can always fall back on eggs, pulses, nuts, seeds, salads, avocado or soups, all of which are quick and easy to prepare, yet still supply you with the right vitamins and minerals to fill your energy requirements.

## HOW TO EAT FOR ENERGY

Sometimes it is not what you are eating that is the problem but how you are eating it.

Here is a list of things to help you get the most from your food:

- Do not sit down to eat if you are upset or angry as this will prevent you from digesting your food properly.
- Try to give yourself time to relax after work before eating.
- Don't eat quickly and try not to overeat.
- Don't eat a heavy meal before going to sleep.
- It is better not to drink while eating as this dilutes the digestive enzymes.
- Always sit down to eat and try to concentrate on enjoying your food – its taste, smell and colours.
- Eat three small to medium meals a day and two to three snacks.
- Don't go more than two and a half hours without food.
- Eat a big breakfast as you won't have eaten anything for about twelve hours and your blood sugar levels will be low.
- Between-meal snacks should be rich in vitamins and minerals, EFAs and antioxidants. Fruits, either fresh or dried, and nuts and seeds make great snacks.

**Cooking** The way you cook your food is also important; some cooking methods can help to preserve nutrients, while others have exactly the opposite effect. Here are some simple guidelines for cooking for health:

- Remember that vitamins and minerals can be lost in the cooking process especially vitamins B and C which are soluble in water, so when you cook vegetables it is best to steam them rather than boil them (if you boil them you lose all the vitamins into the water). If you must boil them at least save the water for stocks or drink it as it is rich in nutrients.
- Fry as little as possible (although stir-frying is fine).
- Brush vegetables clean and scrape them rather than peeling them as the skin is full of goodness.
- Vitamin C is killed when exposed to the air, so eat your fruit and vegetables fresh and only prepare them just before cooking.

## CAFFEINE

Caffeine is found in coffee, tea, cocoa, chocolate, cola and other fizzy drinks. It has effects on the nervous system, the heart and circulation which give us a fake energy boost. It also acts like a drug: the more you have the more you need to be able to feel its effects until eventually you will have to have huge amounts of caffeine just to get a slight energy boost.

Tea is not as bad as coffee but cutting them both out is preferable. Soft drinks with caffeine in them are even worse than coffee and tea as they also contain lots of sugar or artificial sweeteners. Too much of these can give you 'the sugar blues', making you feel low and depressed: the body responds to a sudden influx of sugar into the bloodstream by producing insulin which lowers the blood sugar level too much leaving you drowsy, irritable and unable to concentrate.

Note: caffeine can cancel the effects of homeopathic medication for up to sixty days afterwards.

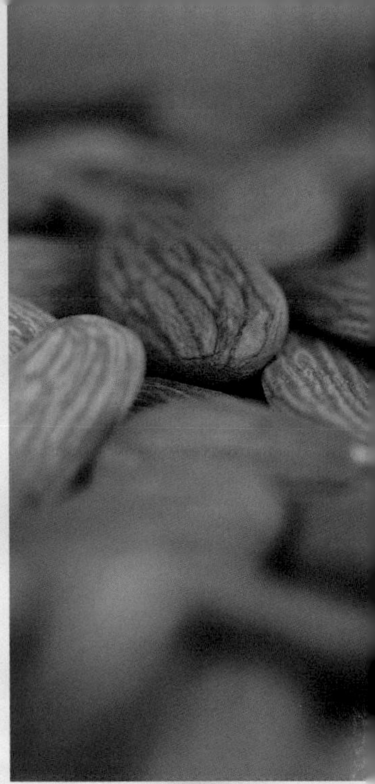

**Balancing your diet** In order to maintain your health, have enough energy and to be able to fight off disease you need a balanced diet that includes all five of the main nutrient groups (carbohydrate, protein, fat, fibre and vitamins and minerals), in the correct proportions, along with plenty of water.

**Carbohydrates** are made up of carbon, hydrogen and oxygen, and produce energy when their carbon molecules bind with oxygen in the bloodstream. They supply the body with instant energy and should therefore make up about 50–60 per cent of our diet.

Carbohydrates are either starches or sugars, but we should mainly eat those that are starches such as plant-based foods (cereals, bread, pulses and root vegetables). As with all foods it is better to eat them in their natural form (or as natural as possible) rather than refined. Fruits contain sugary carbohydrates as do vegetables but in much smaller quantities than fruit. Refined carbohydrates like cake, biscuits and desserts, provide instant energy which is fine in an emergency, or when playing sports, but it won't sustain us over long periods of time. Starchy carbohydrates, on the other hand take two hours to be absorbed, providing you with energy throughout the day. So for constant energy it is best to eat starchy carbohydrates at the majority of your meals, with only a small intake of sugary carbohydrates for short bursts of energy. Beware of eating too much carbohydrate, however, as if you eat more than you need for energy it will be converted into fat and stored.

**Protein** The body needs protein in order to be able to build muscle, repair tissue, maintain cells and regulate bodily functions. We also need protein for energy and if we don't eat enough of it we feel tired, irritable, and unable to concentrate. Between 10 and 15 per cent of your food intake should be made up of protein depending upon how much exercise you do and how much muscle you have.

There are twenty-two amino acids in proteins. Different foods contain different combinations of these, so you need to eat a variety of proteins to get all of them.

Protein foods are meats, pulses, dairy produce, cheese, eggs, fish, poultry, nuts, seeds, wholemeal bread, beans, lentils, tofu, soya beans. Some starchy foods like potatoes, bread and pasta also contain proteins.

If you eat more protein than you need for building muscle your body will use it for energy by converting it to glucose. However, if you don't use this energy it will be converted to fat and stored. Because protein takes longer than carbohydrate to be used by the body it is good for giving you energy over long periods of time and for helping to control blood sugar levels.

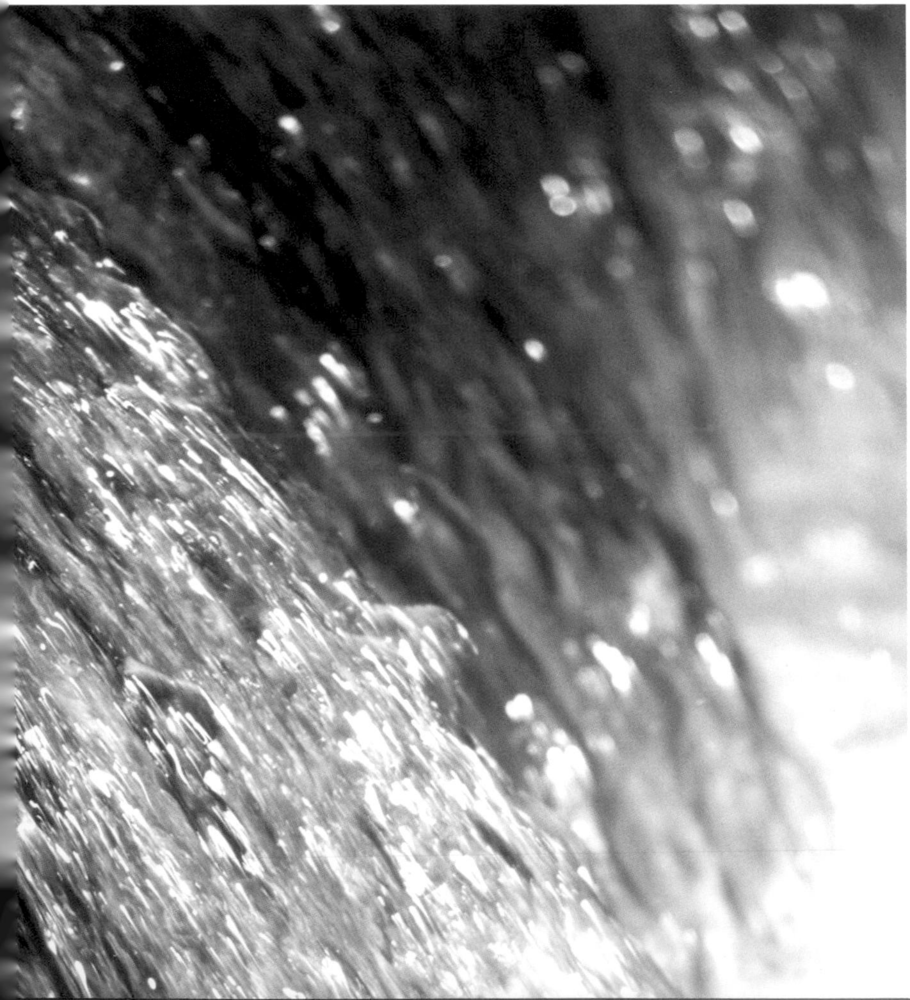

**Fat** The food industry promotes low-fat food because people who are conscious of putting on weight are prepared to pay more for them even though many of them are full of sugars and additives. But not all fats are bad for you, it is just important to eat the right kinds.

There are three types of fat: polyunsaturated, monosaturated and saturated. Fat is found in lots of foods and is the slowest food group to be converted to glucose and used as energy, so it is good for providing longer-term energy. Be careful though, because just as with proteins and carbohydrates, the energy that is not used is stored as body fat. Fat also helps vitamins A and D to be carried into the bloodstream and absorbed as they are fat-soluble vitamins. A mixture of all three fats should make up 30 per cent of your diet.

Saturated fat is found mainly in dairy foods, eggs, meats and processed foods like pies, cakes, biscuits and pastries.

Polyunsaturated fat is found mainly in plant oils including corn, safflower, sunflower, and nut and seed oils. They contain essential fatty acids (EFAs), linoleic acid and alpha linolenic acid all of which are important for a healthy immune system, for energy conversion and for keeping you well. If you are low in EFAs, as most people are, you will suffer from low levels of energy. Fatty acids, EPA and DHA are found in oily fish.

Monosaturated fat is found mainly in olives, olive oil, rapeseed oil, groundnut oil, plant oils, nuts, seeds and avocados. They are high in vitamin E which is an antioxidant.

**Fibre** Lack of fibre in the diet can be a cause of sluggishness and low energy, as well as headaches and constipation. There are two types of fibre: insoluble and soluble. Insoluble fibre is found mainly in whole wheat, corn, brown rice, vegetables and pulses. They help to speed up the elimination of waste which is good for your energy levels as it prevents constipation and the bloated sluggish feeling that can accompany it. Soluble fibre is found mainly in pulses, oats, rye, apples and citrus and other fruits. All types of fibre help to regulate blood sugar levels, keep a constant flow of energy and help to prevent hunger.

**Alcohol** Excess alcohol is damaging to many bodily functions and can reduce energy levels by disrupting sleep and also blood sugar levels.

**Water** is vital for life and energy; if you don't drink enough you can become dehydrated making you feel weak, faint, and eventually very unwell. It plays a part in almost all bodily functions, transports nutrients to and from cells and is important for the circulation, digestion and excretion. Water also helps regulate body temperature.

### CLEANSING DIET

Cleansing your body will make you feel more energised, especially if you have been eating too much of the wrong foods. You should eat lots of fresh fruit and vegetables, and drink lots of water to aid detoxification. You can also drink herbal teas.

Most of us don't drink nearly enough water. Drinking about eight glasses a day should help to improve energy and give a healthy glow to the skin. Filtered water is preferable, and a glass in the morning with lemon helps to balance your energy.

**Macrobiotics** The theory of macrobiotics holds that the more 'living' foods we put into our bodies the more alive we will actually feel. Living foods are fresh foods that still have life in them and do not have colours, additives, emulsifiers, preservatives and stabilisers added to them. Vegetables, fruit, nuts, seeds and pulses are all living foods. They are also easy to digest and provide vitamins, minerals and fibre.

Macrobiotics looks at the energy of food in terms of yin and yang (see page 32). If we eat too many yang or heating foods we will feel restless, over-reactive and have difficulty relaxing and sleeping, as if we have too much energy. This is especially true if we are already a 'hot' person, i.e. someone who feels hot, has a red complexion, is often restless and walks and talks quickly.

On the other hand too many yin or cooling foods will make us feel listless, lacking in energy, even depressed. Again this is especially true if we are already a 'cold' person, i.e. someone who feels the cold, is quiet, walks and talks slowly and is often tired. See p. 64 for 'warming' and 'cooling' foods.

**Food, culture and religion** Some cultures believe that food is not just fuel to fill our bodies but that many food-related illnesses are due to a lack of spiritual connection with the food we eat. Almost all religions and spiritual traditions regard food as sacred and the eating of

## ENERGY DIET FOR TRAVEL

When you are travelling your diet should comprise one kind of food as much as possible. This diet has proved to be very successful for many politicians who need to be fully alert on arrival at their destination in order to participate in important international conferences:

- Eat one kind of food, preferably protein, throughout the twenty-four hours, from when you wake up on the day of travel (eggs, fish, low-fat cheese, meat, poultry, fish, nuts, seeds), plus three to five portions of fruit throughout the day. Add more fruit if desired.
- Drink a minimum of eight glasses of water (mug-sized) throughout the twenty-four hours and no alcohol until arrival. If jetlag is to be avoided, no alcohol should be drunk even on arrival. The following morning your regular diet of complex carbohydrates, fat, protein (see page 87) should be resumed as usual.

## POWERFOODS

Make sure you that you eat at least one power food every day. Some examples of powerfoods are:

- Avocado: a great food for helping to increase your energy because it is a good source of B vitamins, contains monosaturated fat which protects against heart disease, and because it also contains vitamin E which is an antioxidant and great for your skin and circulation. Avocado is also a good source of copper which helps red blood cell development and the absorption of iron from other foods. It also contains fibre.
- Bananas: a good source of fibre that beneficial bacteria crave, full of vitamin B6, good for digestion and rich in potassium which helps with high blood pressure. Because bananas are naturally high in carbohydrate they give you piles of energy.
- Citrus fruits: help with energy levels because they are a powerful antioxidant and good for the immune system. They are also vital for the formation of collagen and connective tissue in the skin and blood vessels which is important if you are training or doing vigorous activities. They are a good source of folic acid which helps to produce red blood cells to carry oxygen around the body which, in turn, is vital for your energy.

it a sacred act (including native Americans, Jews, Christians, Hindus and Muslims).

Ayurvedic medicine teaches that food should not only taste good but it should also attract all the other senses as well. It is therefore necessary to ensure that you like the look of your plate and table before you eat and enjoy the smell of the food you choose to eat. Even finding foods that you like the sound of is encouraged, and ones

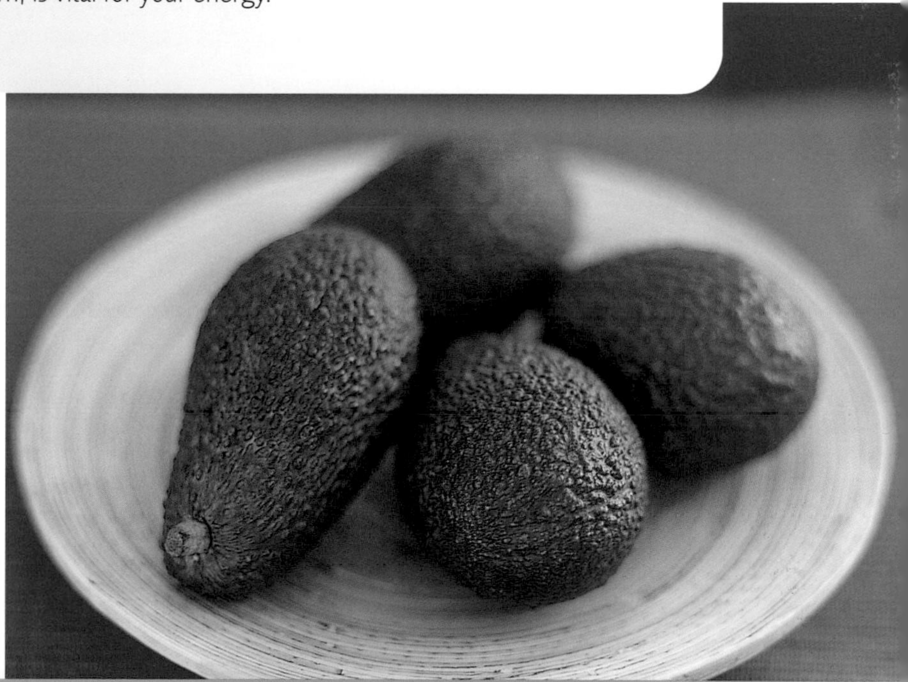

whose texture feels good to you. Many religions and New Age followers believe that food should be prepared with love. For example, if you are making soup, say a prayer for everyone who is going to eat it, imagining that you are making a magical broth with healing powers to increase everyone's energy.

**Foods for balancing blood sugar levels** Fluctuating blood sugar levels are a common cause of low energy. If your blood sugar is low (hypoglycaemia) you may feel tired, dizzy and unable to concentrate and have a craving for sweet foods. Low blood sugar can be caused by missing meals, taking prolonged exercise without any sustenance or by a diet that is high in sugar or alcohol. The body responds to these by releasing extra insulin which may make blood sugar levels dip too low. Many women experience low blood sugar before their periods. Chromium deficiency is said to be a cause of low blood sugar so it is a good idea to eat lots of foods containing chromium, such as shellfish, cheese, whole grains and pulses. Caffeine is best avoided.

Meals consisting of whole foods and a combination of carbohydrates, proteins and fat at each meal should be taken regularly. Also plenty of low glycemic foods in every meal will help to maintain blood glucose levels and give energy throughout the day. It will also help with hunger pangs. Fat and protein are low glycemic foods so a little of each should be included in every meal.

Other suitable foods are: pulses, lentils, chick peas, soy beans, baked beans, kidney beans, butter beans, barley, apples, dried apricots, peaches, plums, cherries, grapefuit, avocado, courgettes, spinach, peppers, onions, mushrooms, leafy greens, leeks, broad beans, green beans, sprouts, mange tout peas, cauliflower, broccoli, natural yogurt, milk and peanuts.

Note: the worst thing you can do if you suffer from low blood sugar is reach for a sugary snack.

**Allergies** If you suffer from allergies lots of whole, unprocessed and most importantly organic foods are best. If you have a wheat or gluten allergy try millet, rice and corn (polenta) buckwheat, and corn or rice pastas. Soya and rice milk are good alternatives to cow's milk for anyone who has a lactose intolerance.

**Vitamin and mineral supplements** Vitamin and mineral supplements help to increase your energy by treating deficiencies. For example,

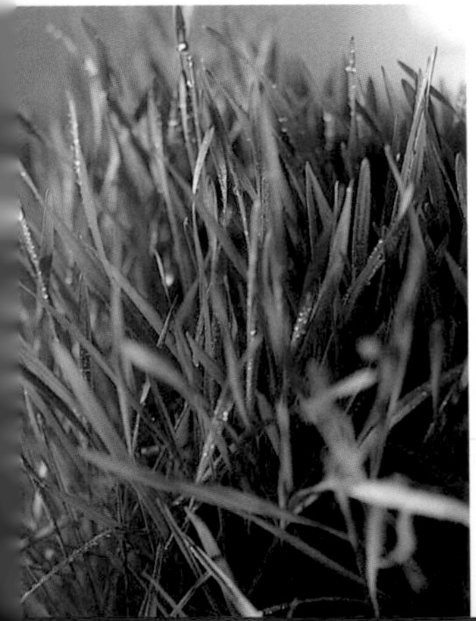

if you have blood deficiency, supplements of iron and blue green algae along with a good quality multivitamin and mineral supplement will help to build the blood, and hence your energy, more quickly than if you try to do it with food alone.

Some people know that their diet is poor and they like to take supplements for peace of mind, so that they feel they are getting the nutrients that they need in spite of their bad eating habits. This is better than nothing, but is not a substitute for a good healthy diet. Others believe that the quality of food and the soil in which it grows is so bad these days that no matter how healthy your diet is you cannot possibly get the full range and quantity of nutrients required.

Either way, you will certainly be short of energy if you neglect to ensure that you are getting enough vitamins and minerals either through your diet or with supplementation.

Below is a list of supplements that will help if you are feeling tired all the time or low in energy. You should be able to find most of them at good health food shops:

- **Bee pollen:** dramatically increases energy.

DOSE: a few granules daily for three days, then slowly increase to two teaspoons daily.

Note: some people can have an allergic reaction to it so discontinue use if you develop a rash, wheezing, discomfort or any other allergic symptoms.

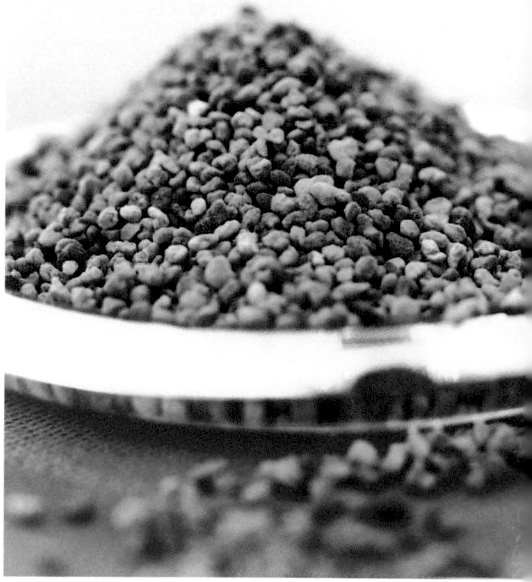

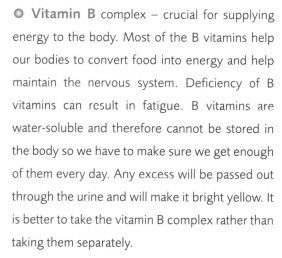

- **Brewer's yeast:** a good source of vitamin B which is very important for maintaining energy levels.

DOSE: one teaspoon daily, then work up to two teaspoons daily over a two-week period.

- **Vitamin B** complex – crucial for supplying energy to the body. Most of the B vitamins help our bodies to convert food into energy and help maintain the nervous system. Deficiency of B vitamins can result in fatigue. B vitamins are water-soluble and therefore cannot be stored in the body so we have to make sure we get enough of them every day. Any excess will be passed out through the urine and will make it bright yellow. It is better to take the vitamin B complex rather than taking them separately.

DOSE: 100 mg, three times daily with meals.

- **Vitamin B1 (thiamin):** essential for growth, health of muscles and nerves and the conversion of carbohydrates into energy. Signs of deficiency are irritability, depression, loss of appetite, poor digestion and dark shadows under the eyes. B1 is found in meat, fish, beans, nuts, seafood, whole grains, pulses, potatoes, wheatgerm and yeast.

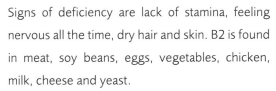

- **Vitamin B2 (riboflavin):** extracts energy from proteins and carbohydrates. It is essential for growth, health of skin, eyes and red blood cells.

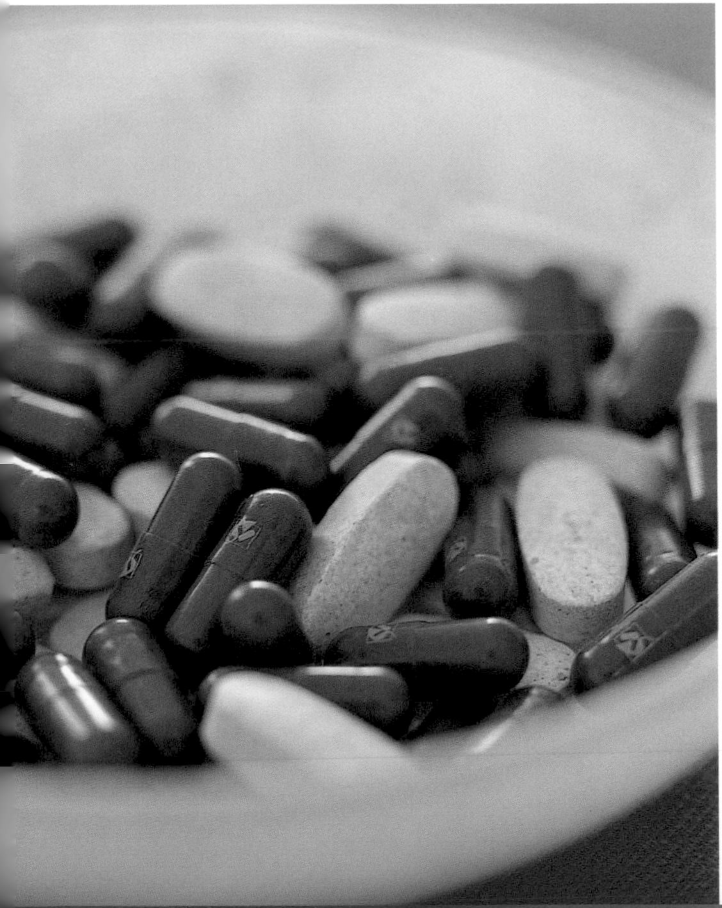

Signs of deficiency are lack of stamina, feeling nervous all the time, dry hair and skin. B2 is found in meat, soy beans, eggs, vegetables, chicken, milk, cheese and yeast.

- **Vitamins B3 (niacin) and B6 (pyridoxine):** important for growth, health of the nervous system, help to counteract stress (therefore help energy) and important for the health of the skin. Signs of deficiency are insomnia, irritability, anxiety, depression, headaches, and feeling shaky. They are found in lean meat, fish, whole grains, chicken, nuts, potatoes, dried fruit and green vegetables. B6 is also found in bananas.
- **Folic acid:** essential for growth, blood (therefore energy) and fertility. Signs of deficiency are fatigue, feeling weak, depression and anaemia. It is found in spinach, Brussels sprouts, broccoli, potatoes, whole-wheat flour and lentils.
- **Vitamin B5 (pantothenic acid):** converts energy from proteins, fats and carbohydrates. Signs of deficiency are dry skin and hair and fatigue. It is found in eggs, liver, meat, nuts, whole grains and yeast.
- **Vitamin B12:** fights fatigue and helps to prevent anaemia; important for the health of the nerves, blood and skin. Signs of deficiency are

fatigue and anaemia. It is found in liver, chicken, lean meat, eggs, yeast, milk and cheese.

Vitamin B12 is not found in vegetables so it is very important for vegans to take B12 supplements (2000 mg daily).

- **Vitamin C:** increases energy and helps to prevent disease and recovery from illness, essential for combating stress, helps in the body's absorption of iron. Signs of deficiency are regular colds, bleeding gums, susceptibility to bruising, fatigue and frequent infections. Found in fresh fruit, especially citrus, strawberries, rosehips and vegetables especially green, leafy ones.

DOSE: 3000–8000 mg daily.

- **Minerals:** present in the soil and absorbed by plants. We get our minerals either by eating plants or animals that have eaten plants. For optimum health, energy and vitality we need more than fifteen different minerals, including iron, calcium, phosphorus, sodium, magnesium, potassium and sulphur. Without them we develop symptoms of deficiency such as fatigue, depression, emotional tension and anaemia. Of all the minerals it is most commonly a lack of iron and calcium that is associated with energy loss.

- **Iron:** deficiency is very common, especially in women. Iron deficiency starves the cells of oxygen causing tiredness, irritability and depression.

It is found in meat, liver, kidneys, whole-grain cereals, spinach, lentils, dried apricots, prunes and peanut butter.

DOSE: as directed on the bottle.

NOTE: do not take iron if you have a bacterial infection as it can feed the bacteria.

- **Calcium:** deficiency upsets the function of the nerves and muscles causing excitability and inability to relax or sleep. It is found in dairy foods, fish, vegetables and eggs.

DOSE: as directed on the bottle.

- **Royal jelly:** the food supplied to the queen bee by the worker bees. It is taken from bee larvae and provides the queen with an amazing amount of energy and stamina enabling her to produce in twenty-four hours eggs that exceed her body weight by two thousand times. She also lives five times longer than her workers. Research on royal jelly suggests that it is a great energiser because it contains protein, B vitamins, amino acids and enzymes. Not only does it increase your energy, vitality and stamina but it also boosts the immune system and improves skin, nails and hair. The

Japanese believe that it helps old people to recover their zest for life.

DOSE: two capsules, three times a day.

- **Shiitake/reishi mushrooms:** help to build immunity and boost energy levels

DOSE: as directed on the label.

- **Spirulina:** an excellent protein source and full of all the essential vitamins and minerals.

DOSE: between one and four pills, three times a day (if you get loose stools start more slowly and build up).

- **Ginseng:** known as 'the root of life', Chinese doctors prescribe it for loss of vigour, anaemia, nervous disorders, insomnia and even as a sexual potency remedy. Even though it can help insomnia it should not be taken late in the day as it is such a potent energiser that it could actually prevent you from sleeping. The Russians give ginseng to their astronauts on space missions in order to heighten their alertness, endurance and energy. It is rich in nutrients, minerals and trace elements.

DOSE: consult a qualified herbalist for correct dose. Note: do not take at all during pregnancy.

- **CoQ10 (co-enzyme Q10, also known as ubiquinone):** a vitamin-like substance that helps the body to convert food into energy. It can

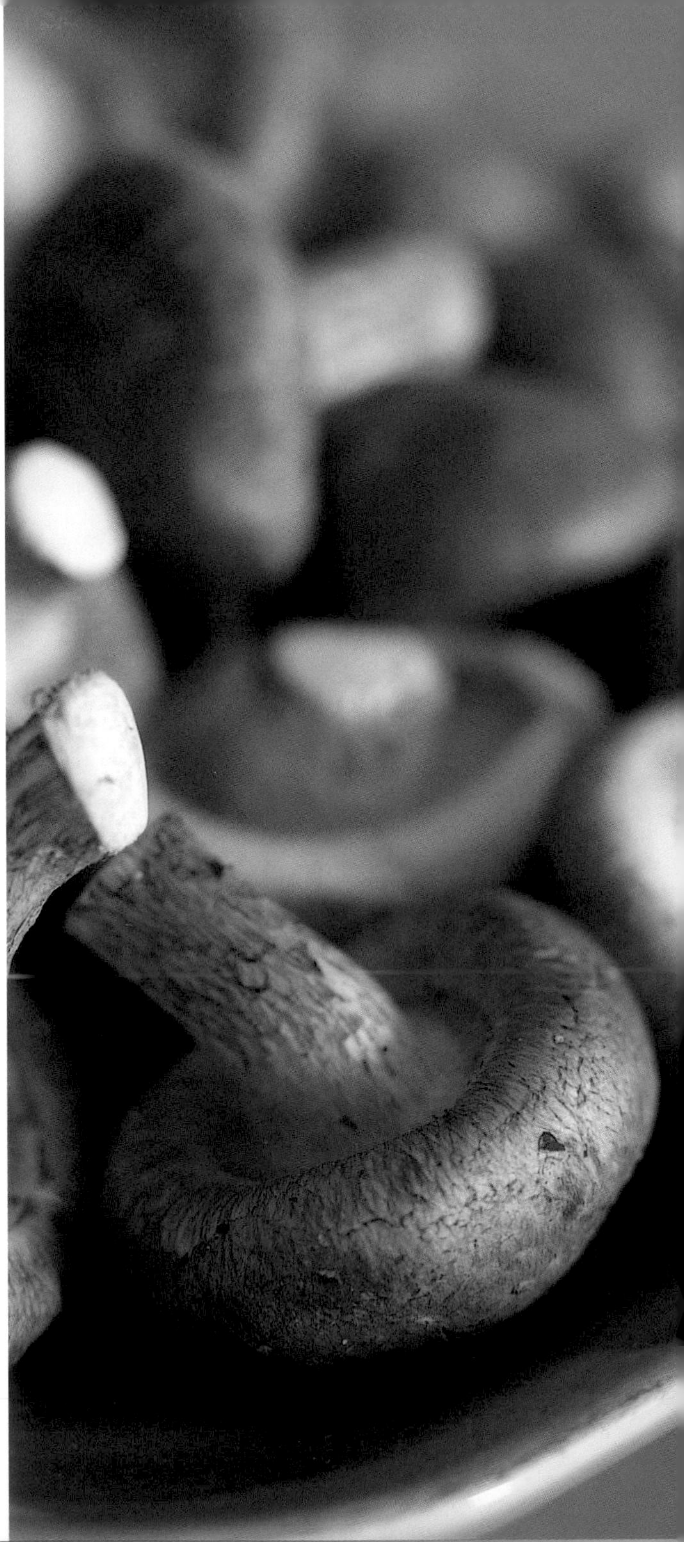

be found in food and the body can make its own, but as we get older or if we are sick we tend to make less of it.

DOSE: one to two 60 mg tablets with meals daily.

- **Blue-green algae:** a complete food source which contains all the vitamins and minerals we need to be healthy and full of vitality.

DOSE: one to four pills, three times daily (if you get loose stools or feel too speedy then take a lower dose and build up more slowly).

- Wheat grass: can be made into a drink or taken in capsule form. It is rich in vitamins, minerals and antioxidants.

DOSE: a half to one teaspoon daily.

Note: always seek advice from a fully qualified and insured naturopath or nutritionalist before taking any of the above if you are pregnant or suffering from any serious medical condition.

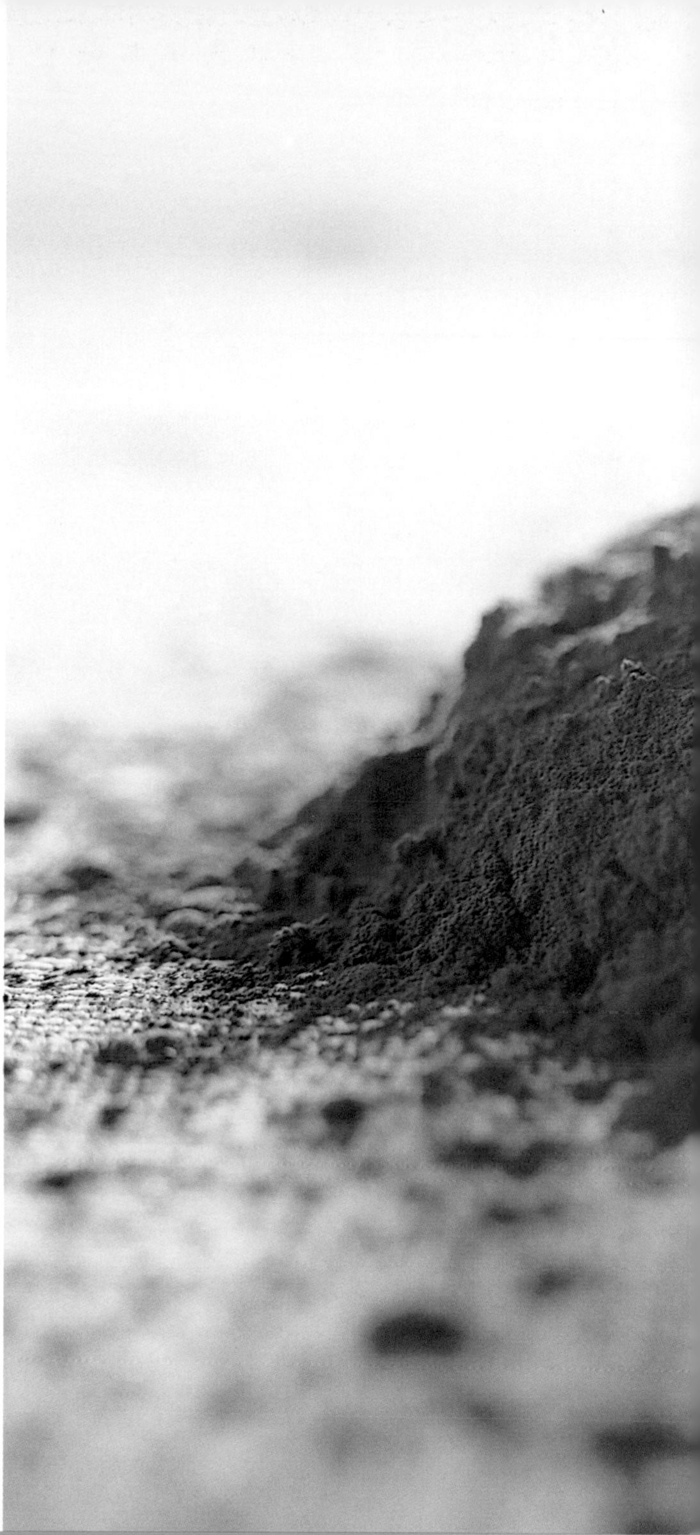

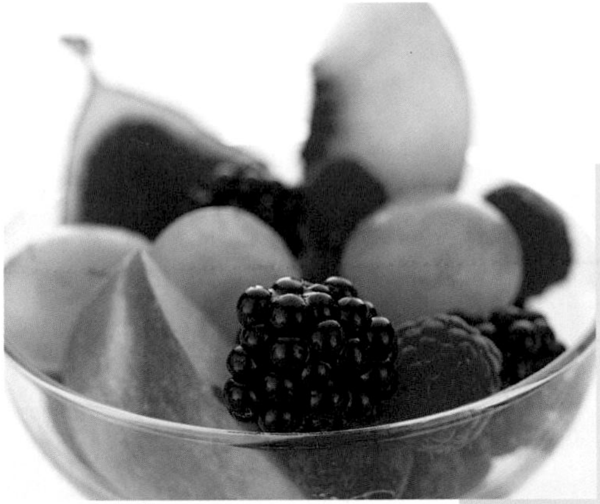

Your energy is your responsibility. What you choose to eat can determine how much or how little energy you have. If you choose to eat a high percentage of refined carbohydrates in your daily diet (i.e. white bread, pasta, pastries, snack bars etc.) then your energy levels will be low. However, if you choose more complex carbohydrates (i.e. whole-grain bread, fresh fruit and vegetables, pulses, nuts and seeds) then your energy levels will be much higher. Acquiring and sustaining your energy levels can be that simple. It's about getting back to basics – naturally.
*Helen Jones, Nutritionist at Bliss*

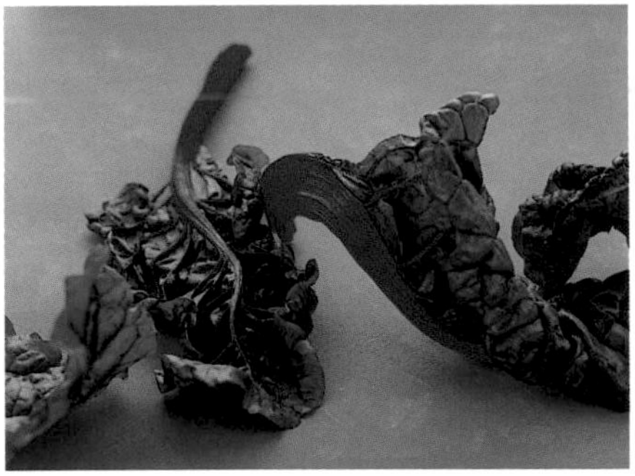

As the saying goes, 'you are what you eat', but more accurately speaking you are what you assimilate. Good digestion of food depends upon the quality of the food we eat. A varied and natural diet, preferably organic-based, provides the body with the nutrients it needs for optimum energy.
*Adrian Mercuri, Naturopath at Bliss and co-author of* The Detox Cook

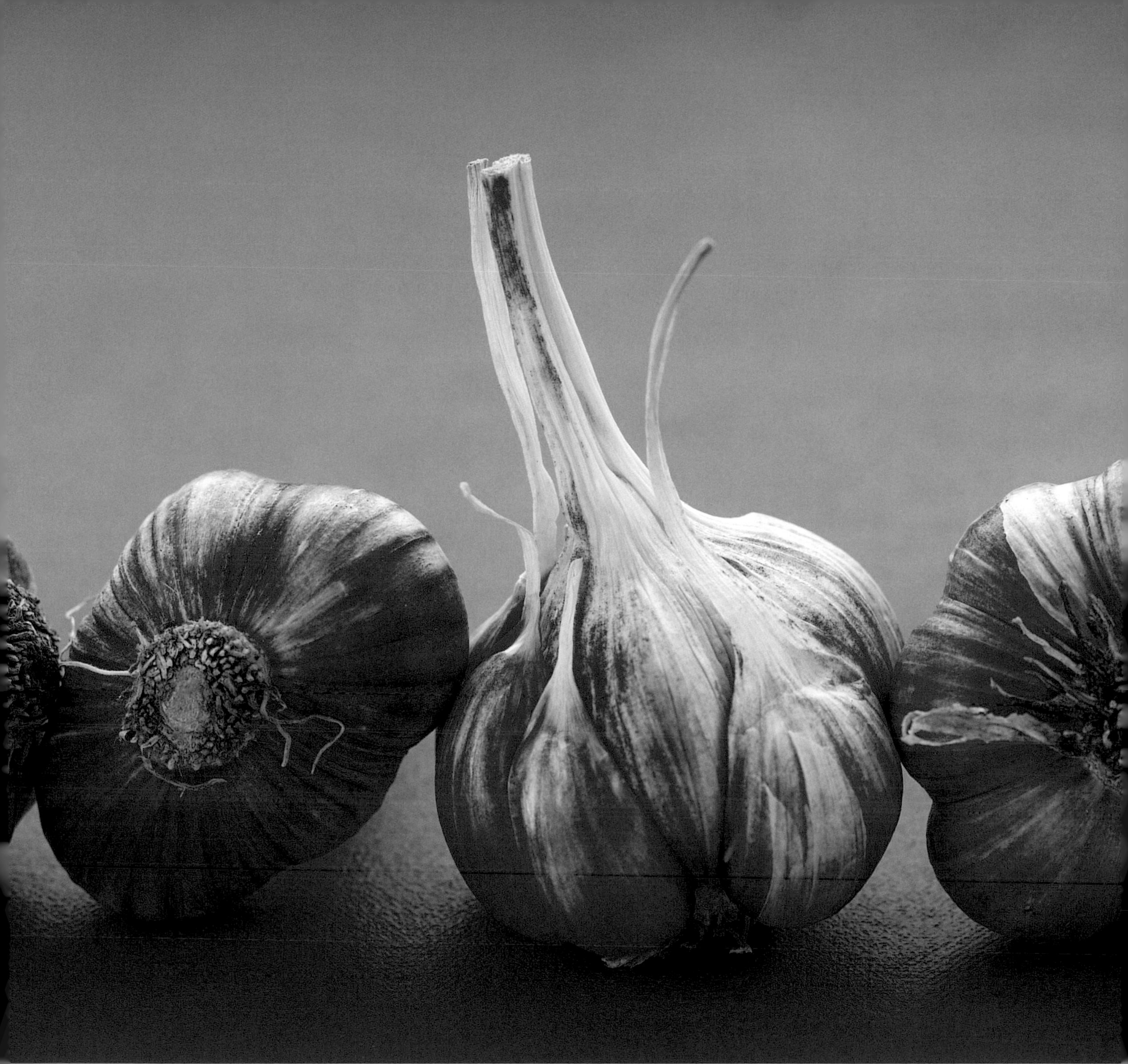

# Exercise

*One of the quickest ways to increase your energy levels is to move your body.*

Staying in one position for too long for whatever reason is not healthy: it slows the body down, impairs circulation, making the body hungry for oxygen and stops energy from flowing, leaving you tired and lifeless.

Aerobic exercise increases the amount of air that you breathe into your lungs giving the body

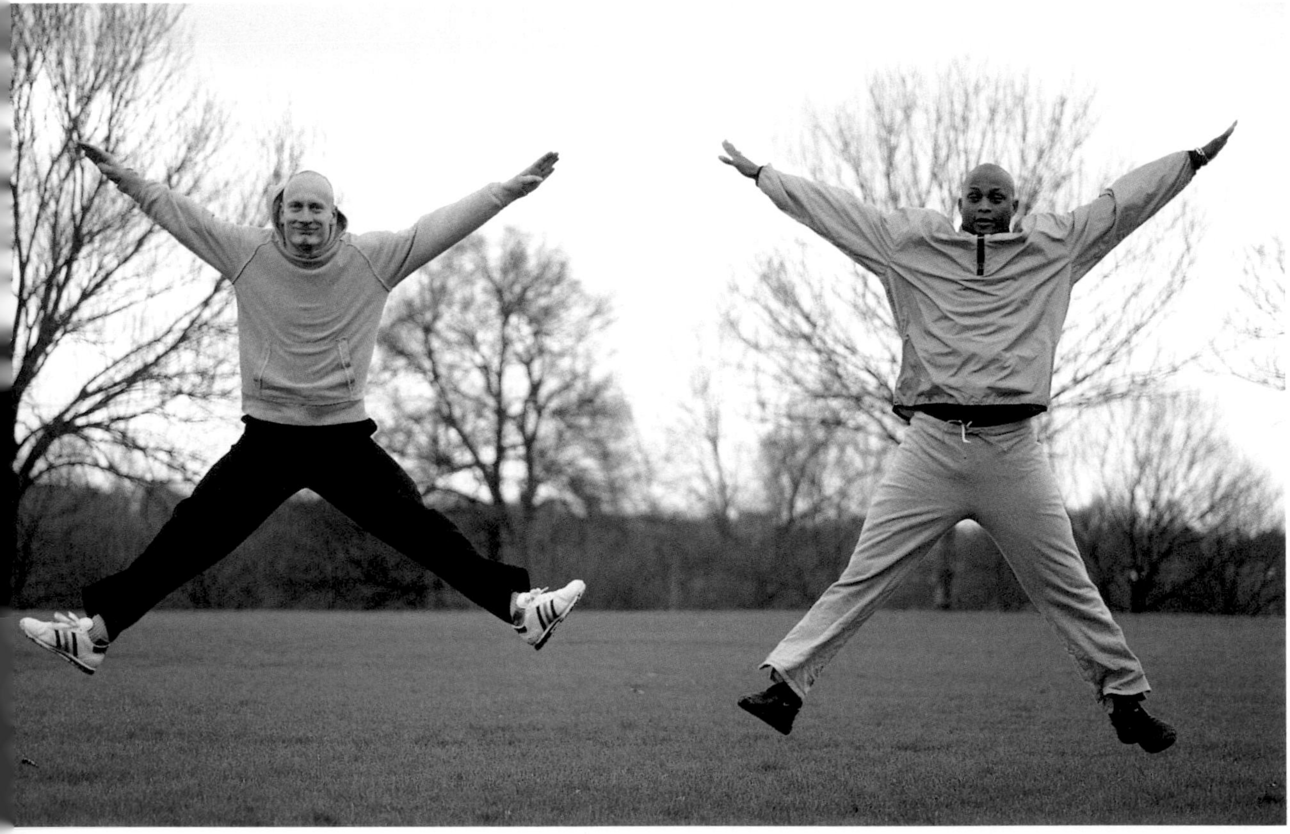

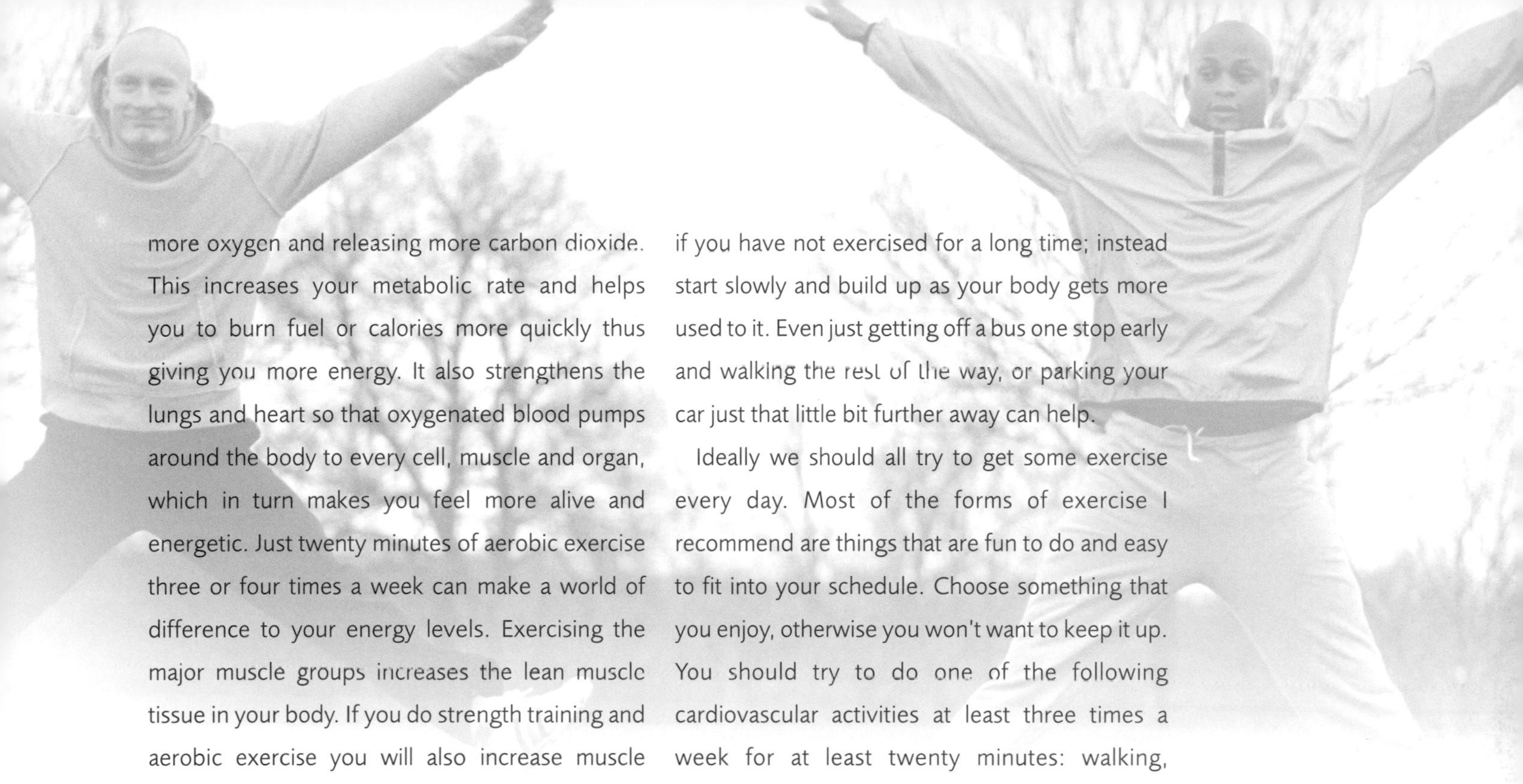

more oxygen and releasing more carbon dioxide. This increases your metabolic rate and helps you to burn fuel or calories more quickly thus giving you more energy. It also strengthens the lungs and heart so that oxygenated blood pumps around the body to every cell, muscle and organ, which in turn makes you feel more alive and energetic. Just twenty minutes of aerobic exercise three or four times a week can make a world of difference to your energy levels. Exercising the major muscle groups increases the lean muscle tissue in your body. If you do strength training and aerobic exercise you will also increase muscle strength so that you have a stronger and more energised body.

Exercise improves flexibility and helps to prevent osteoporosis. And as well as releasing tension in muscles, it also makes you feel happier because when you exercise you not only release endorphins, but you also stimulate the lymph system and increase blood circulation all of which help you to feel more energetic.

Exercising early in the morning leaves you raring to go for the rest of the day. How much exercise you do depends on your age and physical condition and it is very important not to overdo it if you have not exercised for a long time; instead start slowly and build up as your body gets more used to it. Even just getting off a bus one stop early and walking the rest of the way, or parking your car just that little bit further away can help.

Ideally we should all try to get some exercise every day. Most of the forms of exercise I recommend are things that are fun to do and easy to fit into your schedule. Choose something that you enjoy, otherwise you won't want to keep it up. You should try to do one of the following cardiovascular activities at least three times a week for at least twenty minutes: walking, swimming, roller-blading, cycling, squash, basketball, tennis, boxing, dancing or horse-riding. Try to fit in a session or two of an activity such as yoga, tai'chi, qi gong, martial arts, Pilates or stretching as well.

The exercises below include yoga and stretching and qi gong. They will help you to feel relaxed, become more flexible and energised. I have chosen them because I know that they are quite easy to do and will definitely start the ball rolling for increasing your energy. So, go for it; the more energy you use the more energy you will get!

Note: it is important to have at least a twenty-four hour break between tougher aerobic exercise sessions to give the body time to recover. Walk on the days in between and do gentle warm-up and cool down exercises (see opposite).

Consult your doctor before doing any of the exercises in this book if you have had an illness, are pregnant or overweight or you haven't exercised before or for a long time.

## Warming up and cooling down

It is always very important to warm up before and cool down after any exercise so as to avoid any muscle aches or injuries.

## BREATHING

### Breathing

How we breathe is very closely connected to how we feel. When we are relaxed or asleep our breathing becomes slower, deeper and more even, breathing from the diaphragm and stomach, not the chest. When we are frightened it is faster and more shallow, creating an imbalance of oxygen and carbon dioxide which can make us feel light-headed and panicky. If you are constantly feeling stressed you may develop a habit of breathing in this way so that even when you are relaxing you still feel stressed.

### Correct breathing

1 Sit and relax.

2 Breathe deeply through your nose and sigh.

3 Breathe in again, this time ensuring you breathe into your chest, diaphragm and stomach (until they expand) to the count of five.

4 Breathe out through your mouth from your stomach, diaphragm and chest to the count of five.

You might find that the diaphragm doesn't expand as it should due to stiffness but it will with eventually become easier with practice. Find a few minutes throughout the day to check on and practise your breathing.

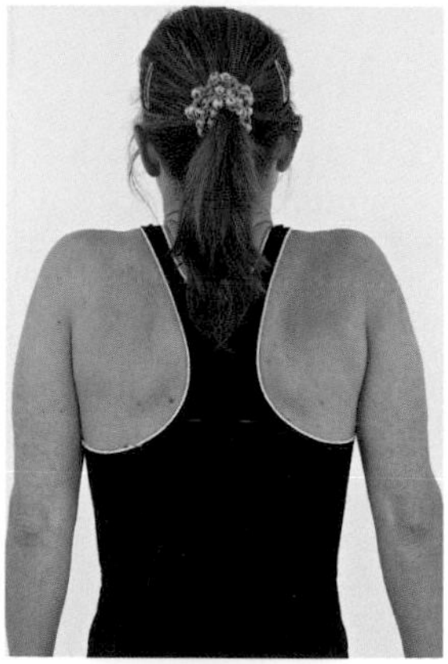

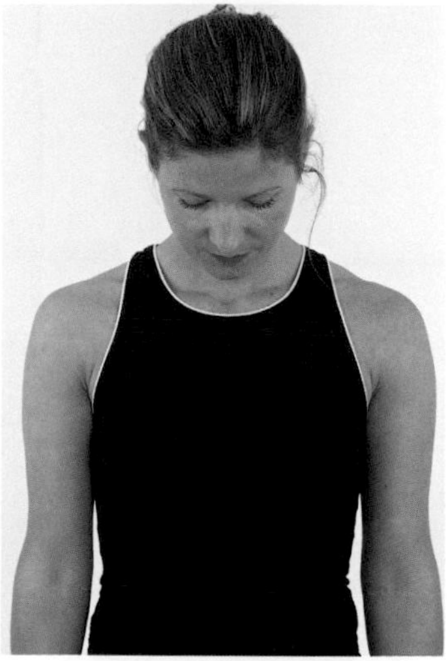

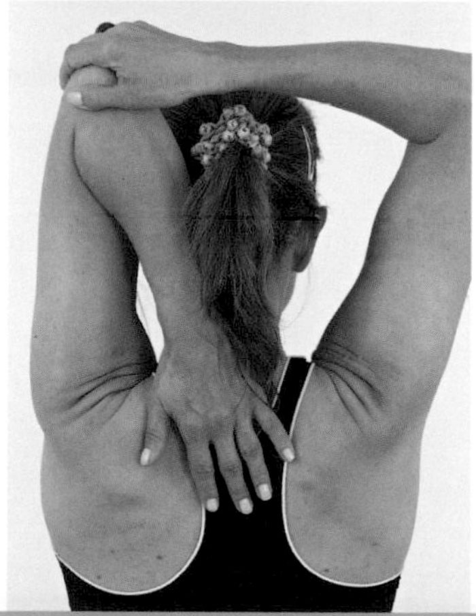

## Warm up and cool down exercises

(All warm-up exercises should be held for a count of ten.)

**1** Shrug your shoulders up and down a few times.

**2** Turn your head from side to side and up and down.

**3** Stretch your arms by lifting one arm up, bending it at the elbow, then letting your hand dangle behind your head. Repeat with the other arm.

**4** Hold one arm straight out in front of you parallel to the floor and with the other hand move the arm towards the other side of your body till you feel a stretch in your upper arm. Repeat on the other side.

**5** Now, step one foot forward and with your heel on the floor bend your knees slightly and bend slightly forward – you should feel a stretch up the back of your leg. Repeat with the other leg.

**6** With one hand holding on to a wall for balance bend your left leg backwards and hold your foot with your left hand. Repeat on the right. If you find this difficult, try it lying down on your side.

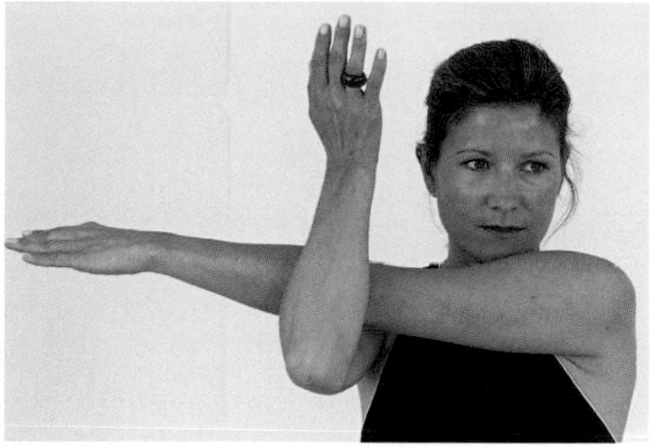

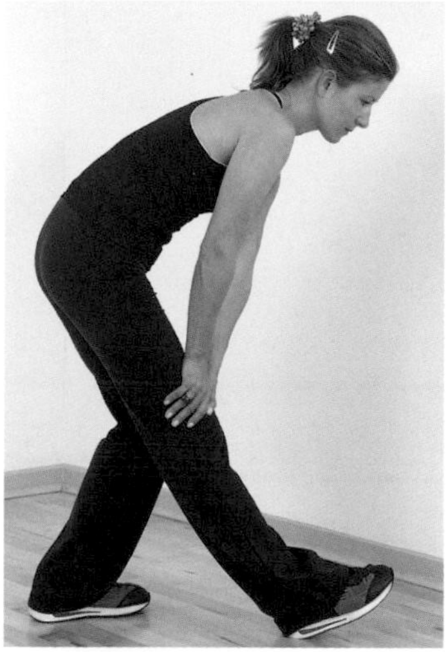

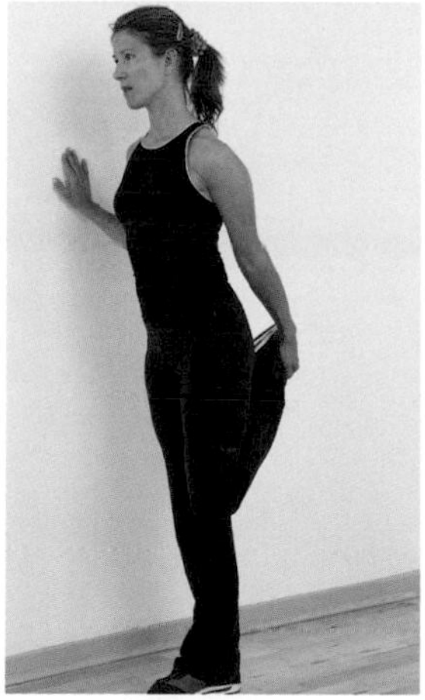

## Walking

Of all the different types of exercise, walking is one of the easiest, as well as being free of charge and very good for you.

In order to really benefit from walking you need to walk at a good pace without stopping for about twenty minutes. As you get fitter you need to increase the time and speed to reap the benefits. You should feel your lungs really working and breathe in more deeply than when at rest. However, you should be able to just about continue a conversation with someone who is walking beside you.

Always wear suitable clothing and comfortable, supportive walking shoes. You should warm up for three minutes before your twenty-minute walk by walking slowly and gradually build up your speed and do the same at the end for cooling down. Also stretch your legs before and after to prevent aches and pains (see previous page for warm-up and cool-down exercises).

## The windmill routine

My grandfather lived to the age of ninety-one, was vibrant, active and healthy right up until his last few months, and was an inspiration to all who knew him: he did the windmill exercise routine his whole life, wherever he went whatever the weather. If you do nothing else in terms of exercise, at least try to do the windmill daily.

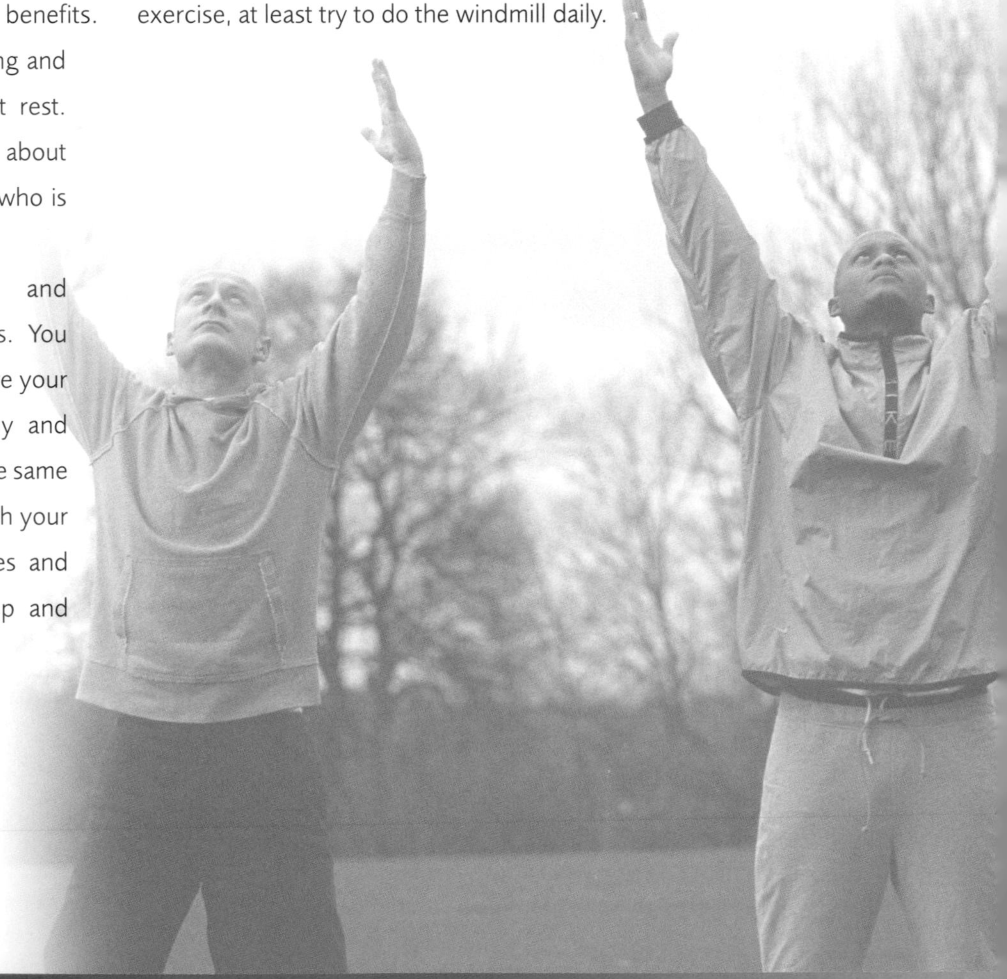

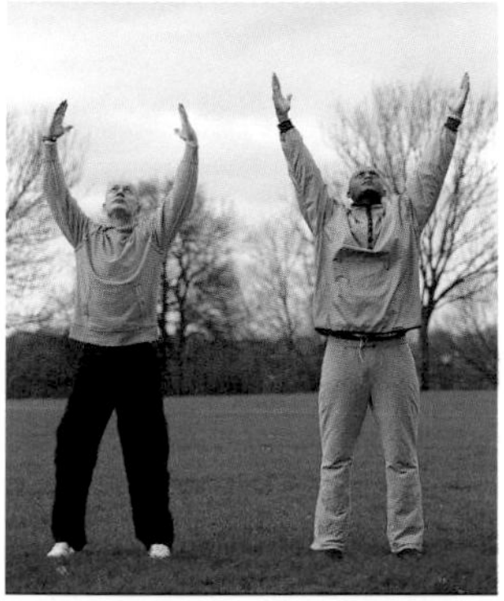

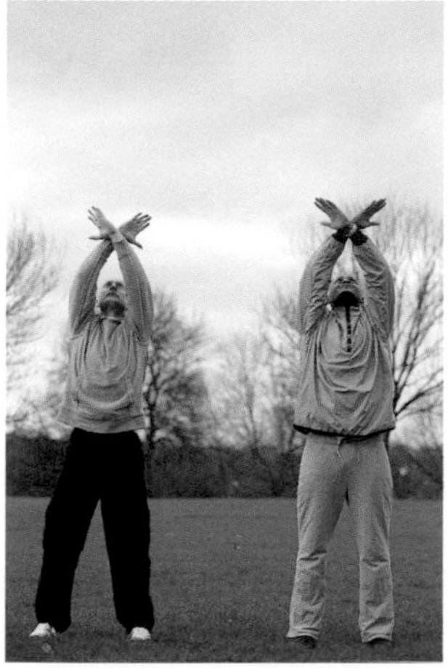

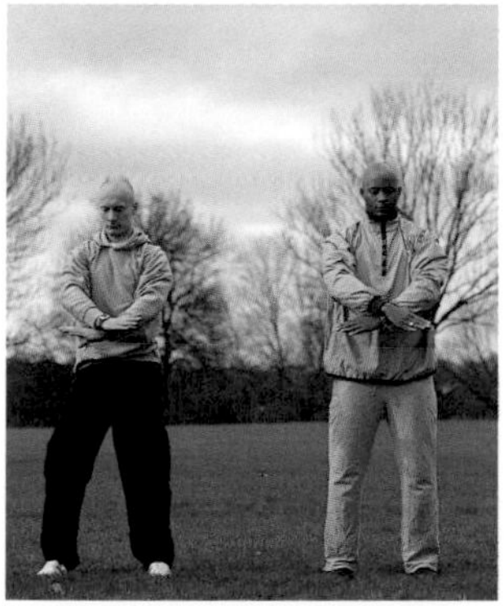

**1** When you wake up in the morning, open the window and, whatever the weather, stand by the open window.

**2** Take ten big, deep breaths of fresh air.

**3** Put your arms up to the ceiling, with elbows just slightly bent, cross your hands above your head and move them down to the side (like a windmill), still taking big, deep breaths.

**4** Now bring both arms up from the side, cross them in front of your face and up above your head, then down to the sides again, breathing deeply throughout. Repeat ten times.

**5** Lift your arms above your head and take a big breath in.

**6** Bend down with straight legs, reach for your toes, exhale slowly, come up to standing position. Repeat five times.

**7** Now do ten jumping jacks, breathing deeply all the time.

**8** Don't forget to close the window!

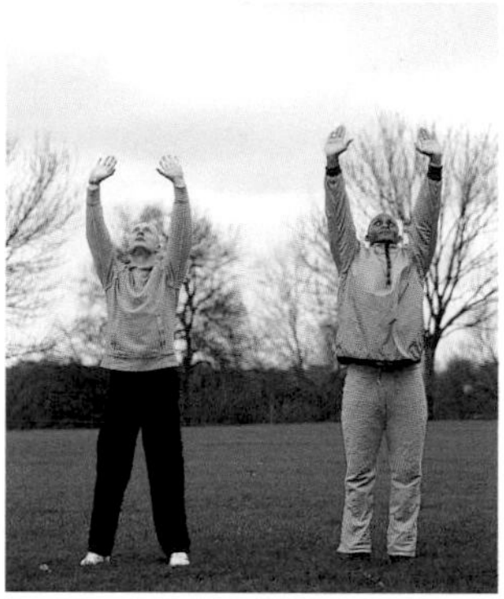

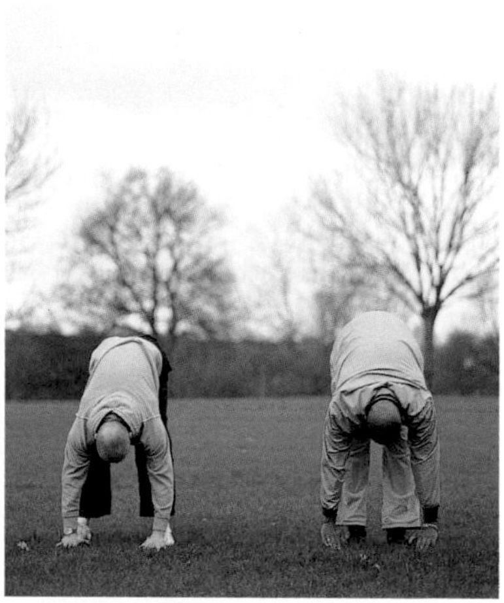

## Strengthening exercises

Strengthening exercises should be done three times a week for about twenty to thirty minutes. Repeat fifteen times (one set) and increase as you begin to build strength. Work until the muscle begins to feel tired or shake slightly.

You will need an exercise band or ball (see bottom right) or a free weight or tin of beans for some of the exercises (see page 216 for suppliers).

## Half press-ups for your chest (below)

**1** Kneel on all fours with your palms flat on the floor.

**2** Bring the knees slightly backwards.

**3** Bend your elbows and, keeping your back straight, allow your upper body to dip towards the floor.

**4** Try and go as low as possible and then slowly raise yourself back up again.

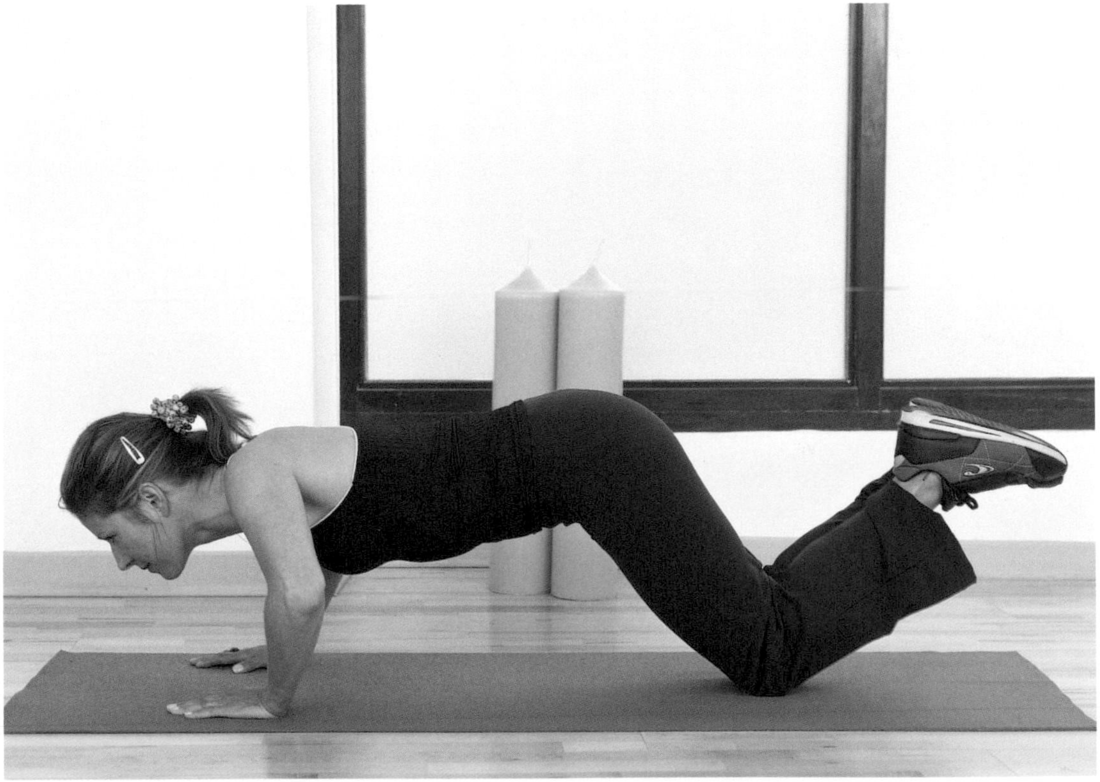

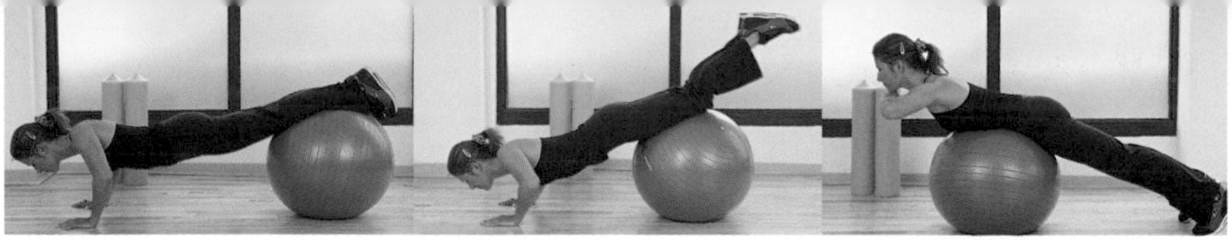

If you find the half press-up too difficult, try using an exercise ball (above):

**1.** Lie on the exercise ball and getit into position with your thighs resting on it and your feet raised

**2.** Put your hands on the floor and lower your body down between your hands, with a straight back. Slowly raise yourself back up again.

**3.** For a full push-up, rest your shins on the ball and continue as above.

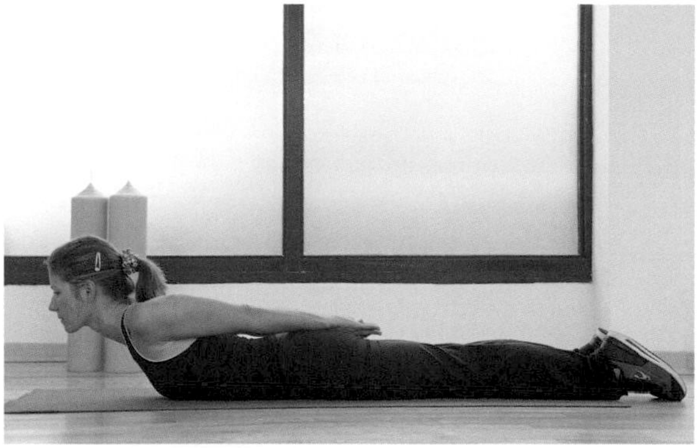

### For your back (above)

**1** Lie on your stomach with your hands behind your back or under your chin.

**2** Keep your legs and hips on the floor and raise your upper body a few inches from the floor or as far as you can go. Don't look up.

If you find this too difficult, try using an exercise ball (see top right).

### Bicep curl (right)

**1** Stand on a band with your feet hip width apart.

**2** With knees bent, tuck in your stomach and bottom.

**3** Hold the band in one hand and slowly bend your arm until your hand comes up to your shoulder.

**4** Gently lower back to your side again.

**5** Repeat for the other side.

### Lateral raise (below)

**1** Hold the band in your right hand, left arm by your side, feet hip width apart and knees slightly bent.

**2** Lift your arm with the band out to the side till your arm is parallel to the floor then slowly lower your arm to the floor.

**3** Repeat on the other side.

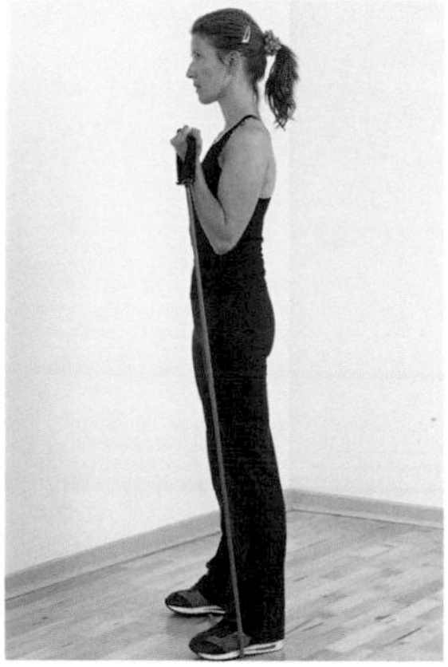

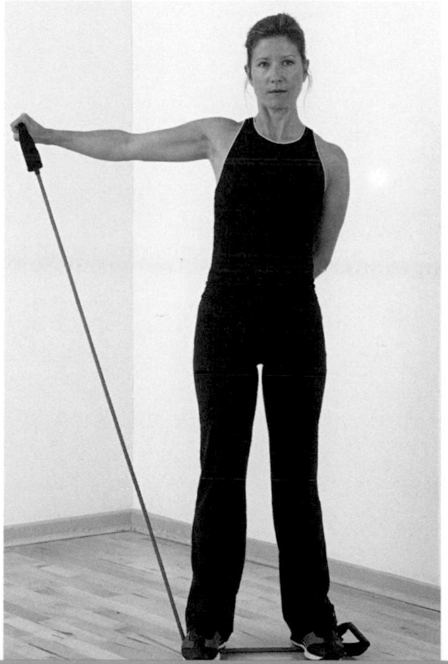

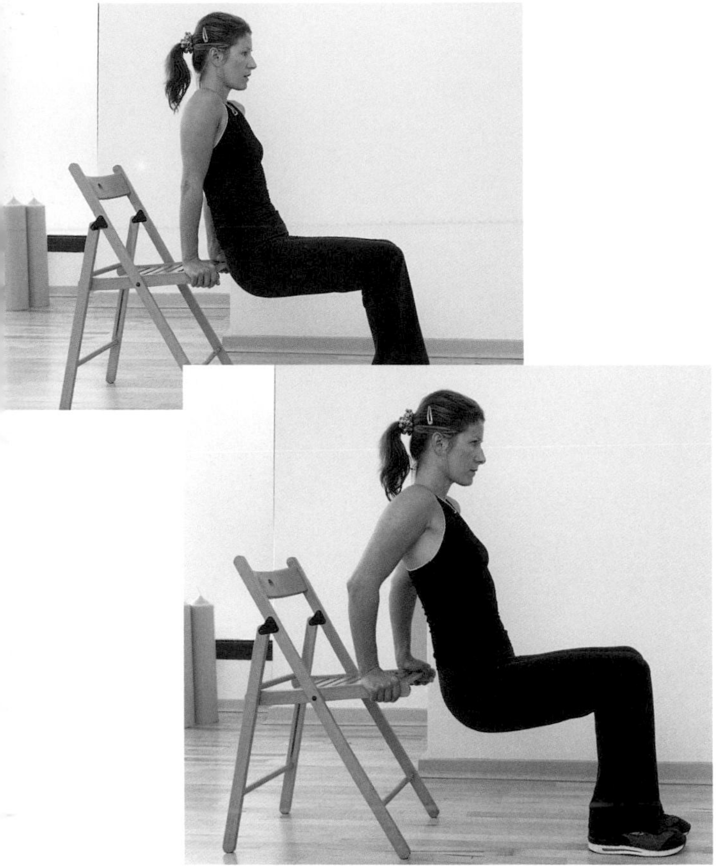

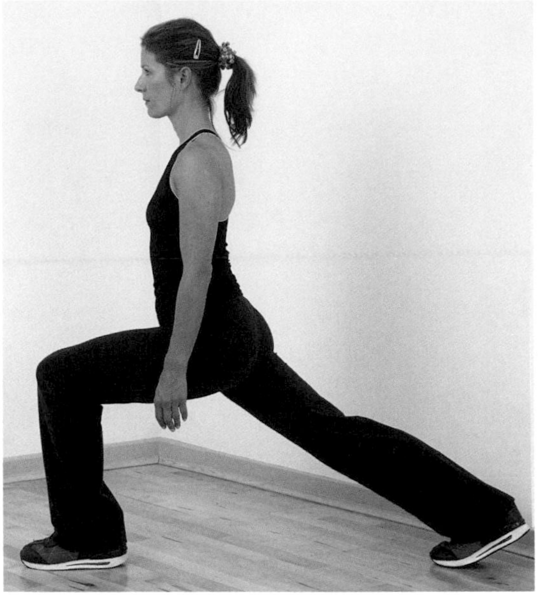

### Tricep dips (above)

**1** Sit on the edge of a sturdy chair.

**2** With your hands holding the edge of the chair lower yourself off the chair until your elbows are at right angles to the floor.

**3** Pull yourself back up without sitting on the chair.

**4** Repeat.

### Lunge (above)

**1** Stand with feet hip width apart and your arms by your side. Step forward with one leg and bend both legs till the front leg is at right angles to the floor.

**2** Come back to starting position and repeat with the other leg.

### Squat (right)

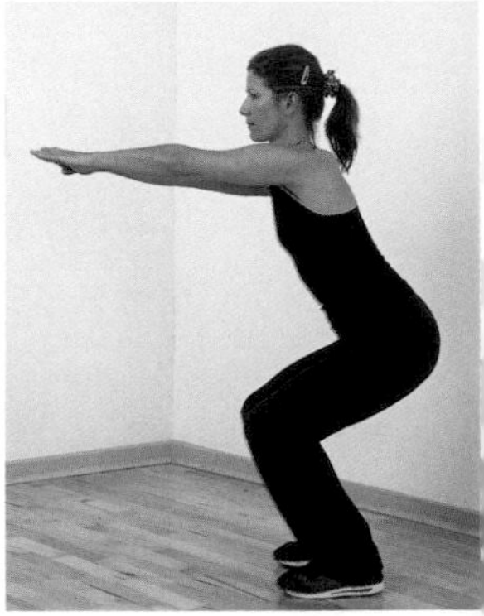

**1** Stand with feet hip width apart and arms parallel to the floor.

**2** Squat down keeping your back straight and your knees in line with your feet. Try and get your thighs parallel to the floor.

**3** Slowly return to starting position and repeat.

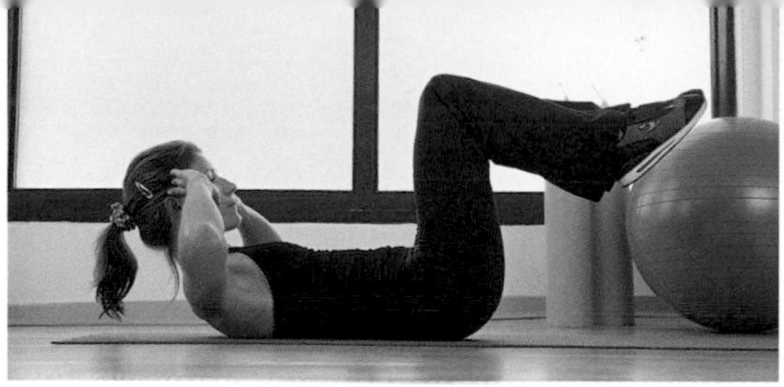

## Crunch (above)

**1** Lie on your back with your knees bent and your feet firmly on the floor.

**2** With your hands at your temples breathe out and raise your head and neck off the floor. Slowly go back but without touching the floor.

**3** Repeat. You should feel it burn in your abdominals.

## Side crunch (right)

**1** Like the crunch, but this time raise one knee in towards the head and neck.

**2** Put the knee back down and then raise the other knee in while raising your head and neck off the floor.

**3** Raise both knees. Repeat all three parts of the exercise each time.

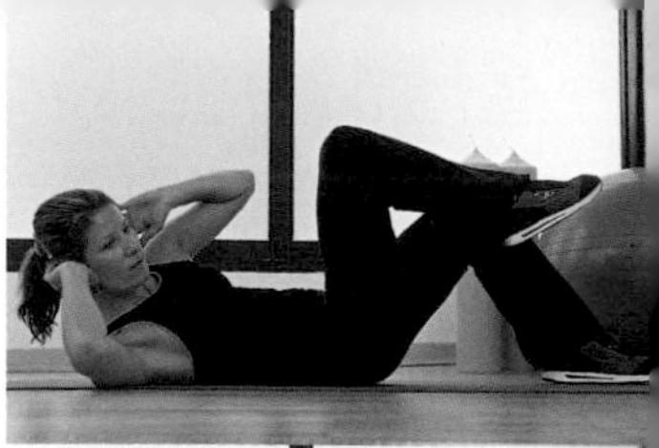

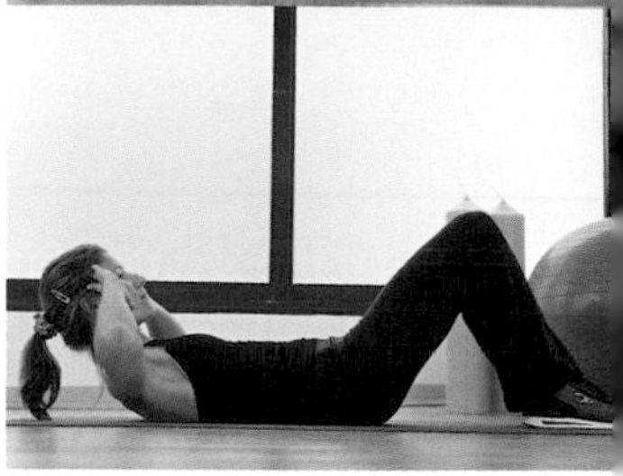

## EXERCISE WHEN YOU'RE TRAVELLING

After travelling it is important to do some form of exercise and activity to keep the blood and oxygen flowing to the muscles and brain and to help your body and mind to adjust to any differences in time, food, weather and culture.

Normal energy levels can plummet and may not return to normal as quickly as usual, even after rest. If this happens be patient and listen to your body and mind. If your metabolism has slowed down and become sluggish it might take more time than you would expect for your body and mind's co-ordination to return to its normal patterns, especially after crossing time zones.

Listen to what your body is telling you that it is willing to do. Try gentle exploratory stretching exercises to bring your mind–body connection together again in a quiet 'one-to-one' way and develop your routine slowly, possibly to include the following:

- simple rolling of shoulders backwards and forwards
- tilting neck toward one shoulder then the other, looking over one shoulder and then the other
- rotating ankles round in both directions and up and down with toes/also heels up and down
- shrugging shoulders up and down towards ears.

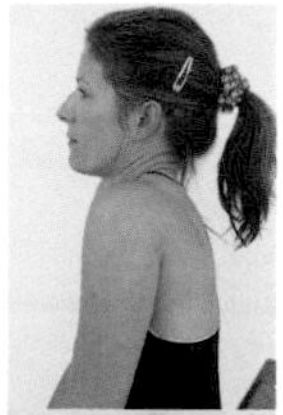

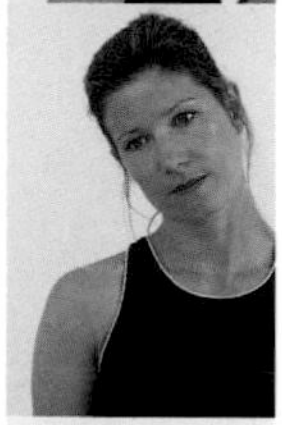

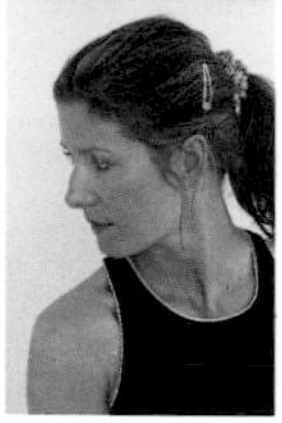

# Chinese wisdom

*The Chinese believe in balancing the flow of energy, or qi, around the body.*

They believe that the qi can become blocked due to many factors such as stress, shock, toxins and emotional problems such as anger or grief, thus causing disease and disharmony. The ancient Chinese mapped out channels (meridians) through which qi flows and used pressure and needles on precise points along these meridians to stimulate or regulate the qi's flow, thus increasing energy, lifting mood and helping to treat specific illnesses. As well as working on these specific points they also used medicines and exercises to remove blockages.

## Qi gong

One exercise practice that helps to move the qi and build it is known as qi gong which has been practised in China for thousands of years. The term qi gong means energy practice. It is a combination of breathing, posture and meditation, and like yoga, it focuses our energy inwards. It is often translated as 'working with life energy'. It is a precise exercise routine that finds energy imbalances and corrects them. It helps to increase energy flow and emotional stability, promotes clear thinking, physical fitness, good health, and spiritual wellbeing.

Everyone can do qi gong; you can even perform it sitting down. Ideally it should be practised every day and in doing so, you will notice a dramatic change in your energy levels.

Below are just a few qi gong exercises that are easy to do and will help to increase your energy and vitality.

### Holding the dantien

The dantien is about an inch below the navel and is where the qi is stored. It helps in lymphatic drainage and aids proper circulation.

**1** Men should place their left hand on the dantien and the right hand over the left. Women should place their right hand on the dantien and the left hand over their right (see picture right).

**2** Relax your whole body, straighten your legs (but don't lock them) and concentrate on and breathe into the dantien.

**3** Bend your knees and breathe out.

**4** Repeat for a few minutes.

You can do this exercise for longer when you get used to it and you have the time.

## Vital energy

Many people spend so much of their life running around chasing their tails that they forget what it feels like to be aware of their vital energy. Vital energy is always there but we often tend to be so busy that we ignore it. Here is an exercise to help you reconnect and feel your own energy again. Most people feel a tingling sensation throughout their body after doing this exercise.

**1** Stand with your shoes off, your feet hip width apart and your knees slightly bent.

**2** Let your hands fall by your sides.

**3** Imagine there is a rope from the middle of the top of your head to the sky holding you upright.

**4** Relax your shoulders and neck.

**5** Close your eyes and become aware of your breathing.

**6** Just stand and breathe for a few minutes.

**7** Become aware of the centre of your body, the area around your navel (your dantien). Breathe big, deep breaths into this area.

**8** Focus on the dantien being the centre of yourself and keep breathing slowly and steadily.

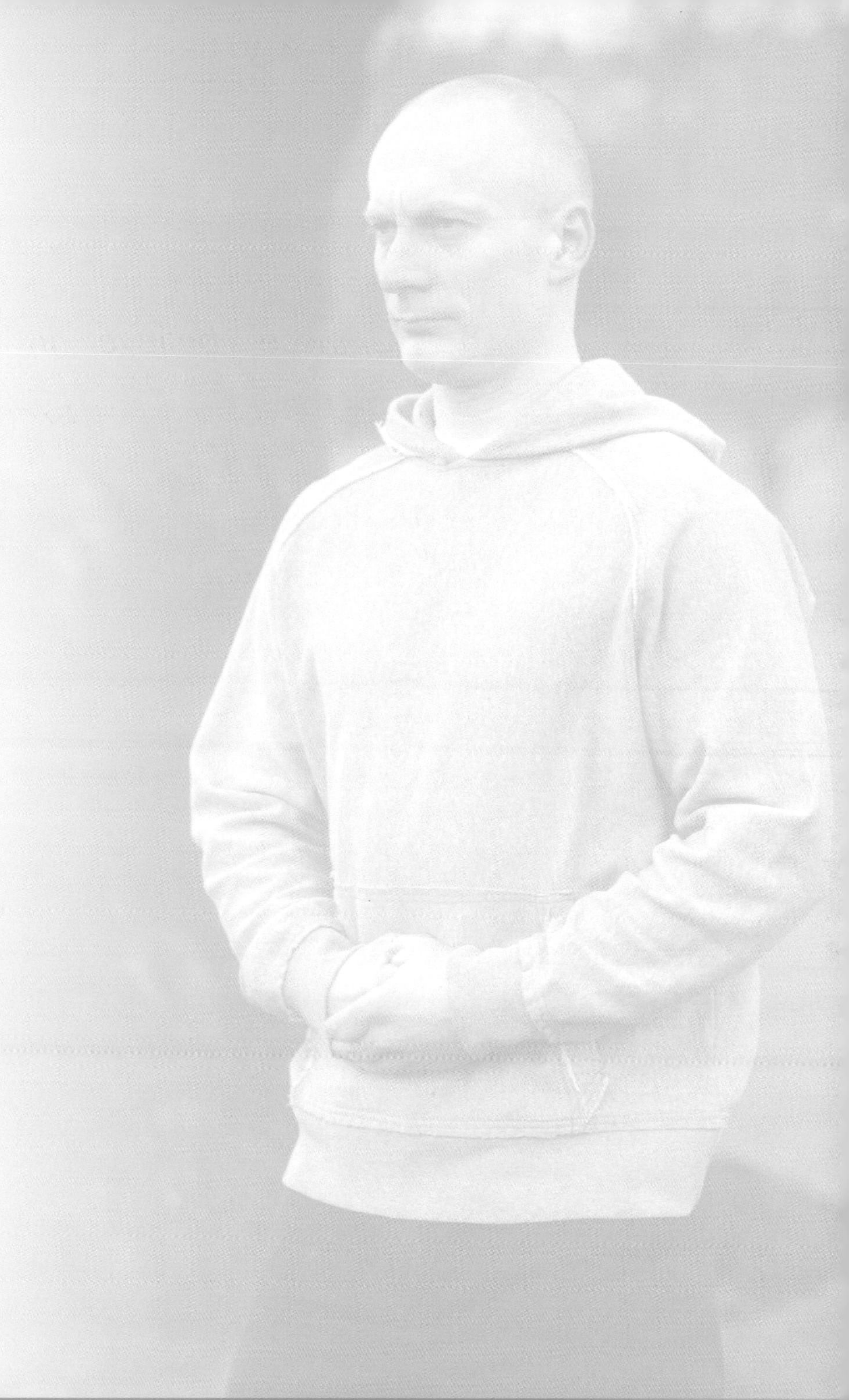

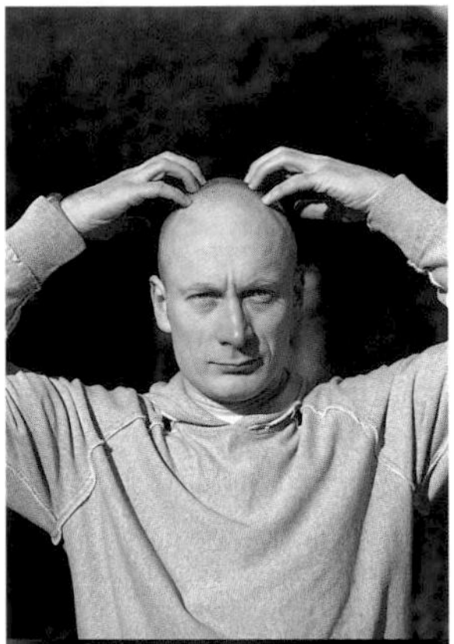

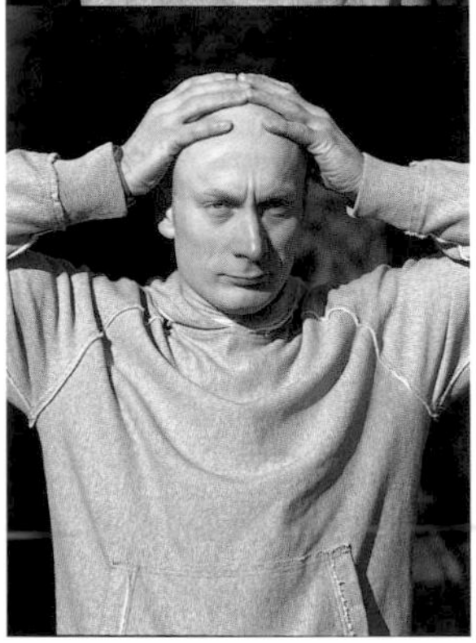

## Qi gong slap

Do this exercise every morning when you wake up to start your day with a boost of energy.

**1** Tap your head with your fingertips and gently pat your head all over with your hands. Then stroke your hair (or head), neck and shoulders.

**2** Pat your hands down the inside of each arm (one at a time) starting at the armpit and making your way down to your fingertips.

**3** Now pat up the outside of each arm (one at a time) from your fingertips up to your shoulders.

**4** Gently tap and pat your upper chest and down your breast bone and round to your hips.

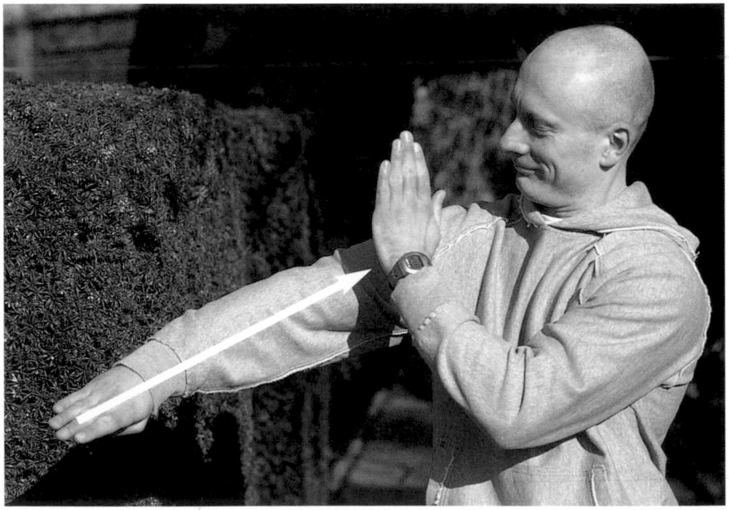

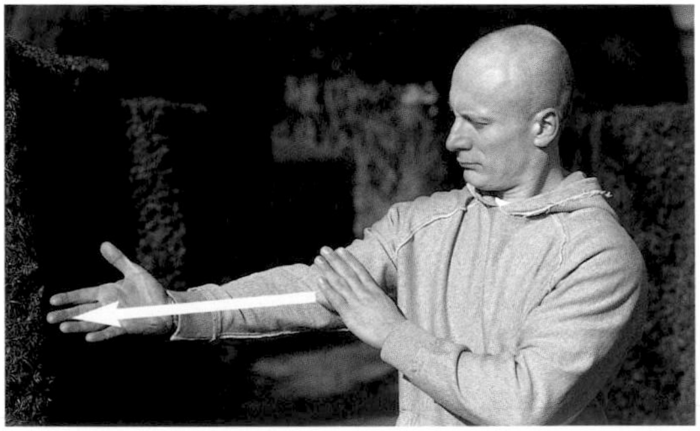

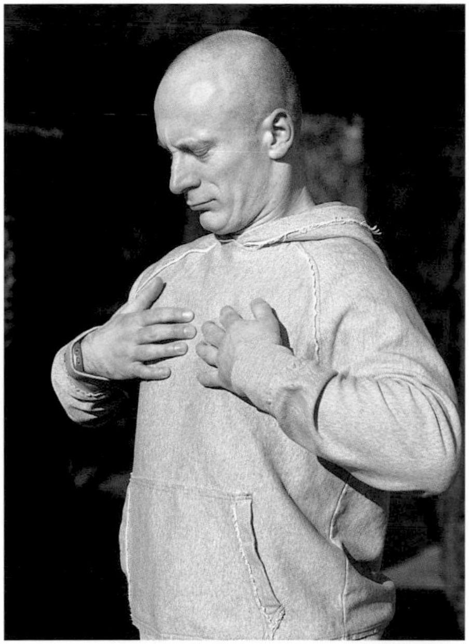

**5** Pat your hips and down the outside of both legs then brush your feet.

**6** Continue patting up the insides of both legs, round to the back.

**7** Pat the lower back (this is very good for the kidneys).

**8** Repeat the whole exercise ten times. On the tenth time let your hands rest on the kidneys for a minute, then circle your hands around to your stomach and let your hands settle (for a minute) one hand over the other just under your belly button (on your dantien).

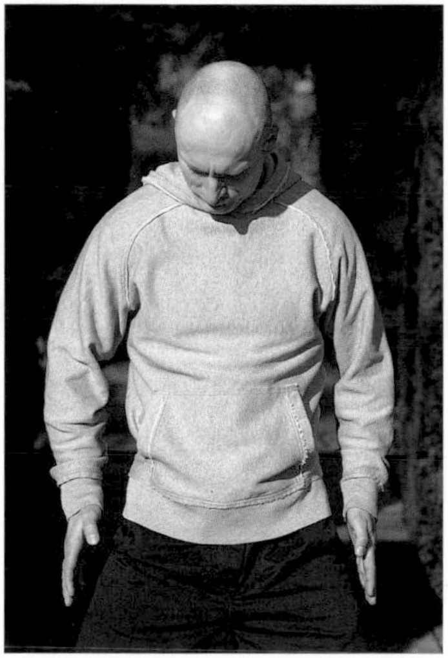

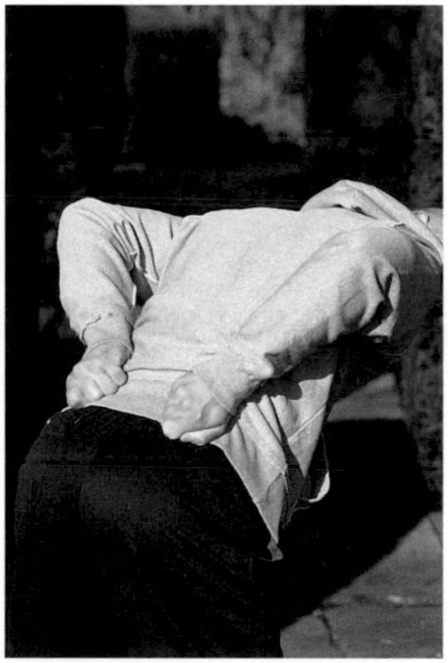

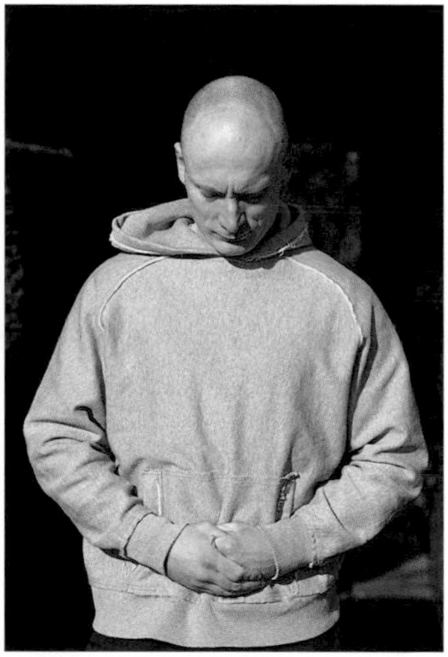

## Balancing the energy

Our bodies are often out of alignment. There are all sorts of things that can throw our bodies out such as always sleeping on one side, working at a computer at an awkward angle or without taking breaks, carrying a bag on one side, standing with more weight on one leg than the other. I remember experiencing neck and shoulder pain after having a baby, and eventually realised it stemmed from the way I was looking down at her lovingly while breastfeeding. Here is an exercise that can improve the body's symmetry, allowing the energy to flow more smoothly around it.

**1** Stand with your feet hip width apart and your knees slightly bent.

**2** Spread your arms out to the sides as if hugging a massive ball.

**3** Imagine the ball is full of energy then pull your hands into your chest bringing all the energy in.

**4** Let your chin drop to your chest.

**5** Repeat the whole exercise ten times.

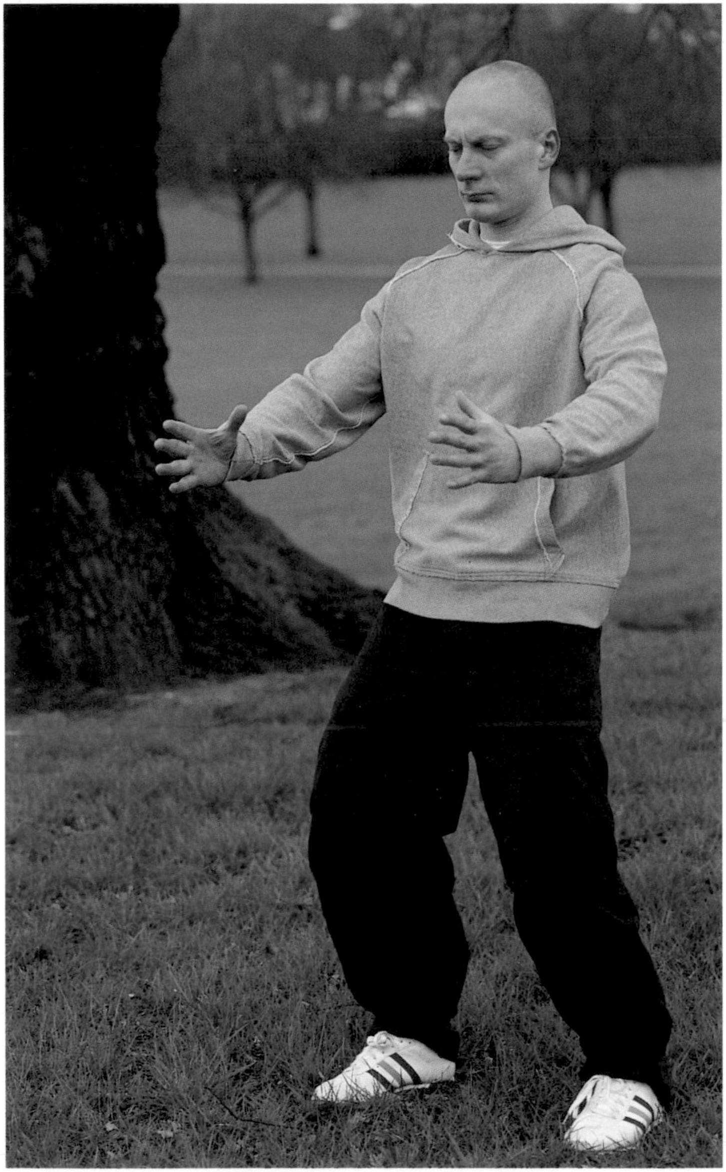

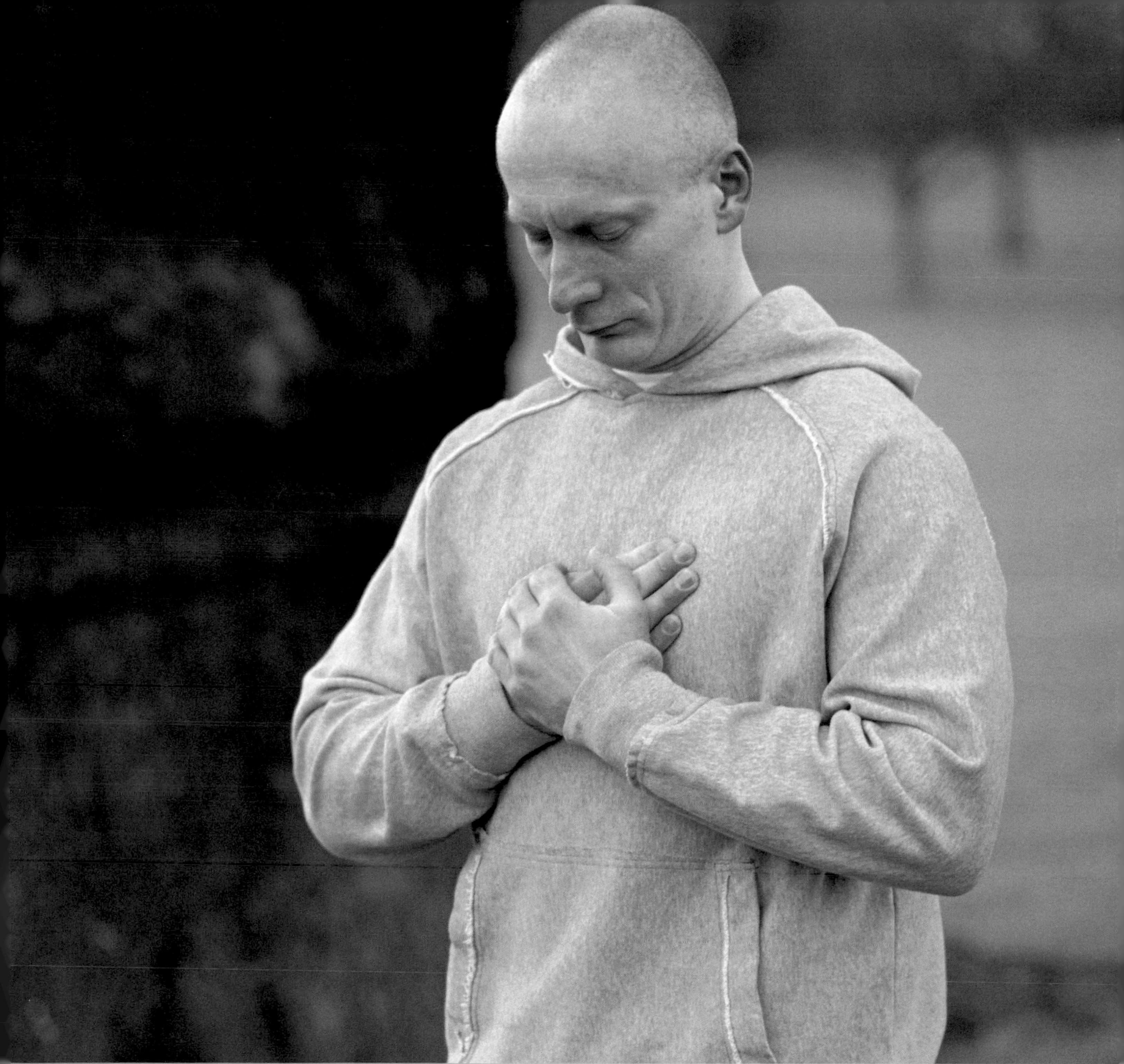

## Qi gong tree

According to the theory of qi gong, every time we place our bare feet on the ground when we walk we reconnect with the earth's vital energy.

**1** Stand with your feet hip width apart, stretch out your toes and bend your knees slightly.

**2** Gently pull up your abdominal muscles while allowing your buttocks to sink towards the floor.

**3** Drop your shoulders and allow your chin to drop slightly, relaxing your neck. You should feel your body grounded from the waist downwards.

**4** Imagine that your head is being held up by an imaginary rope.

**5** Hang your arms bent loosely by your sides as if holding on to an imaginary ball. You should feel completely relaxed; if anything hurts you should breathe it out.

**6** Imagine you are a tree and your feet grow roots deep into the ground. As you breathe in imagine that you are drawing up the earth's goodness through your roots to nourish you.

**7** With each breath in pure positive energy is taken in to stimulate the flow of qi around the body.

**8** With each breath out all negative energy, toxins and anxieties are exhaled into the earth.

**9** You should feel like all your cares have been taken away. Your mind should feel peaceful.

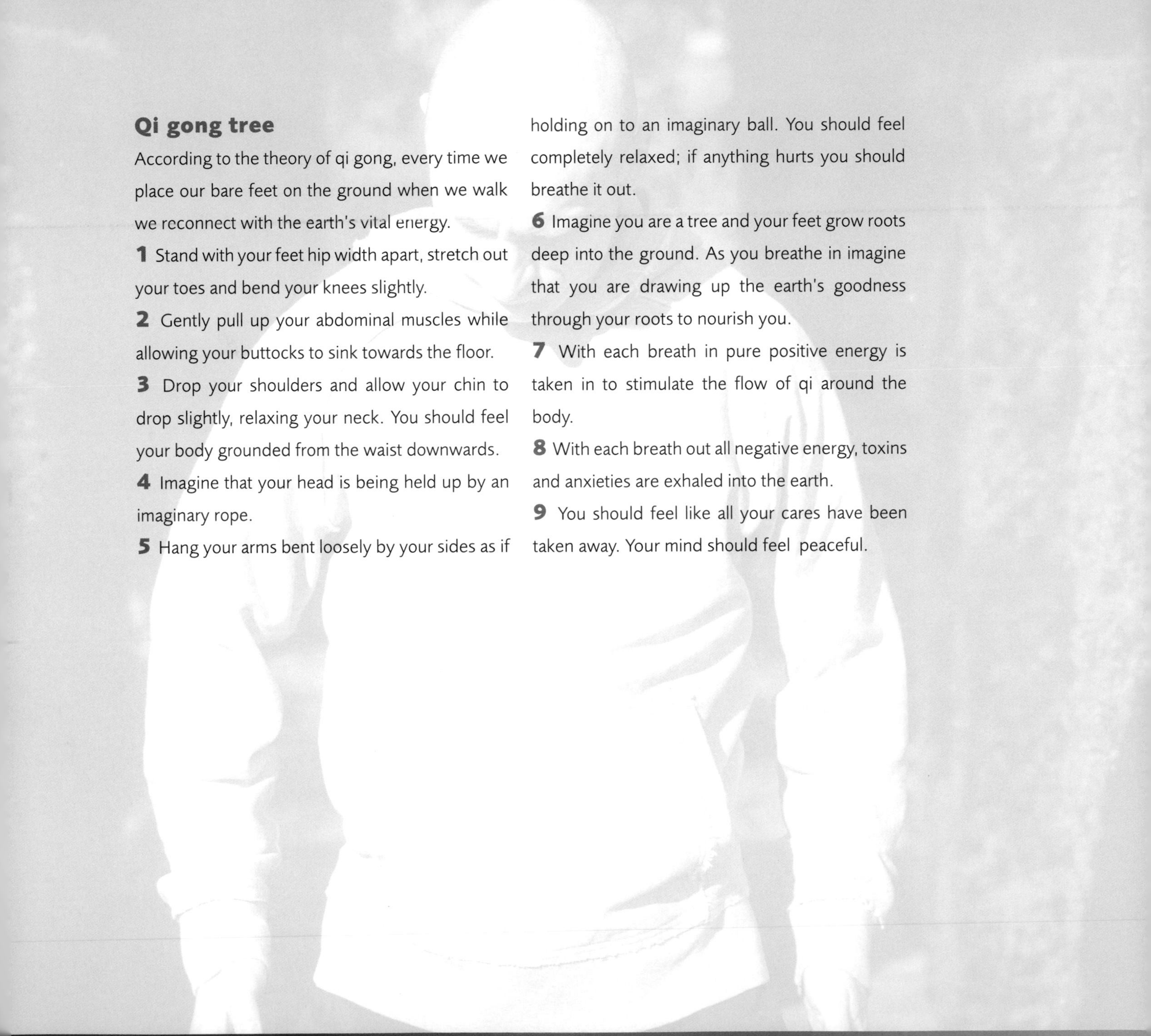

## The qi gong ball

This exercise helps to increase vitality at any time of the day. It increases the energy in the dantien where energy is stored (see page 111). After you have done this exercise you will probably feel a tingling or hot sensation in your hands.

**1** Stand with your feet hip width apart, your knees slightly bent and your hands in front of your abdomen (dantien) with your palms facing inward.

**2** Imagine that a ball of energy is coming from your abdomen (dantien) and filling your hands.

**3** Slowly, move your hands apart so that you are holding the growing ball of energy in your palms.

**4** Once the ball has grown to the size of a big beach ball hold it for a few minutes.

**5** Imagine that the ball of energy contracts when your hands move closer and expands when they are farther apart. Repeat several times contracting and expanding the energy ball.

**6** Now bring your palms back to your abdomen (dantien) letting the ball contract back into the abdomen until it just feels like a spark. Hold your hands there for a minute.

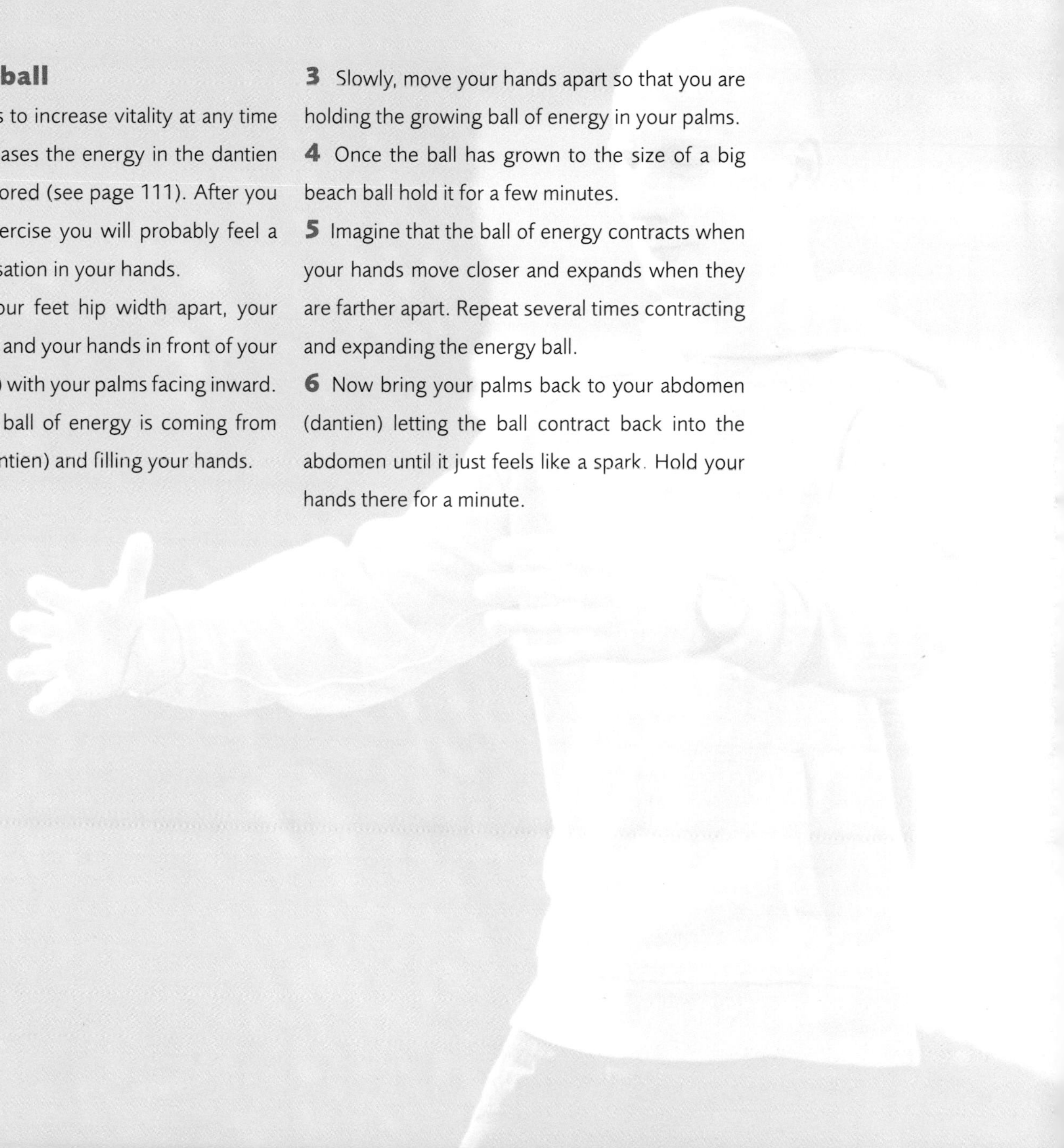

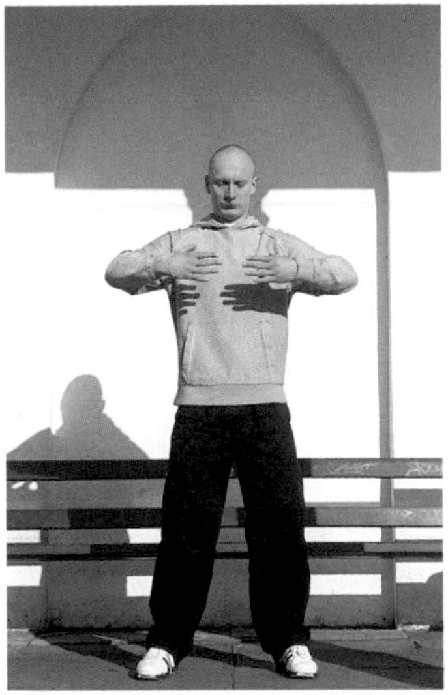

## The energy sweep

This exercise stimulates the flow of energy in all the meridians especially the gall bladder, large intestine, liver, kidneys and spleen. Sweep as fast or as slow as you like and you will feel the energy starting to flow.

**1** Stand with your feet hip width apart and your knees slightly bent.

**2** Lift your elbows up and bring your hands (palms inwards) into your chest.

**3** Stretch your arms out to the side and then up above your head.

**4** Bend your arms and cradle the back of your head with your hands.

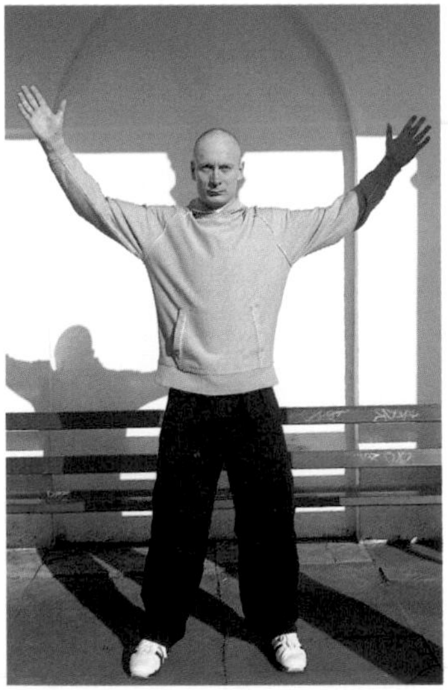

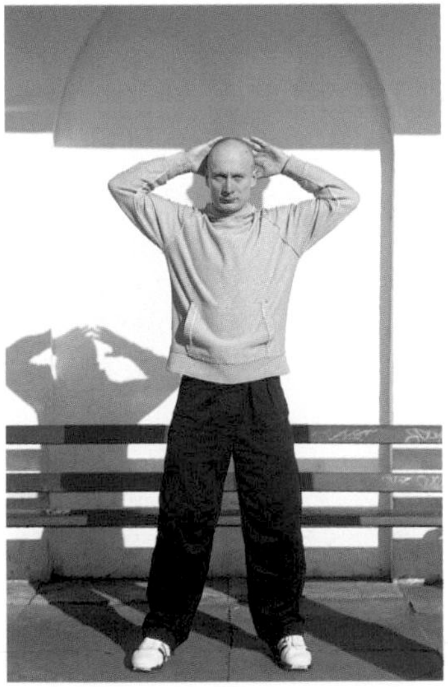

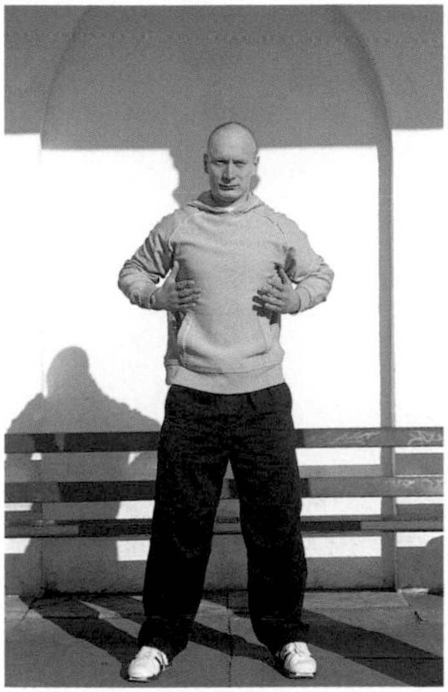

**5** Sweep your hands down your neck, over your shoulders, down your chest and rest your palms on your lower ribs.

**6** Sweep around to your back and rest one palm over each kidney.

**7** Sweep your palms over your hips and down the outside of your legs.

**8** Sweep over the feet and up the insides of your legs.

**9** Rest one hand over the other just under your belly button.

**10** Repeat ten to twenty times.

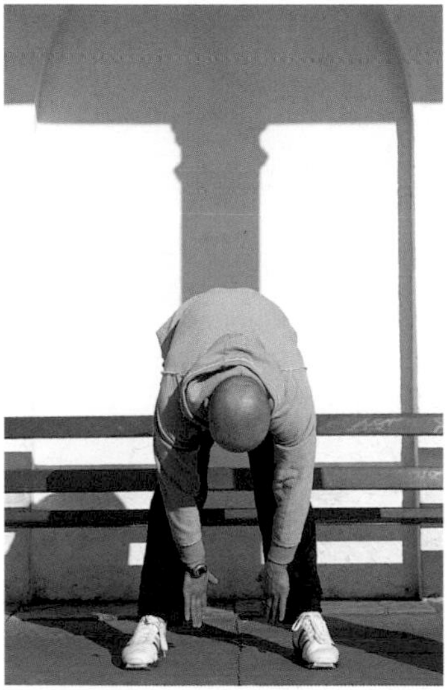

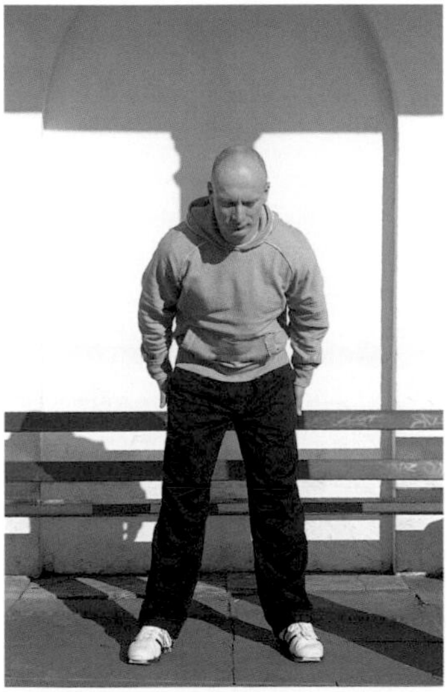

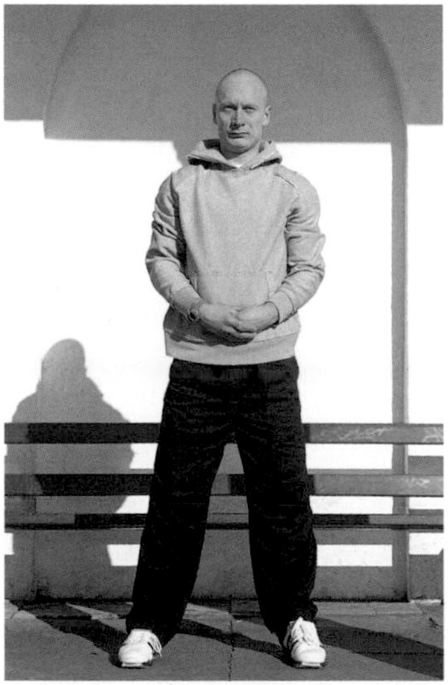

# Yoga

*Yoga originated in India about five thousand years ago and is well known for its ability to help you to relax deeply both mentally and physically.*

The yoga most often practised in the West is hatha yoga (although there are many other types) which concentrates on postures (asanas) which stretch, realign and balance the body, and breathing (pranayama) which helps you to relax and centre mind and body. It can also include meditation (dhyana) which helps to calm and focus. The result is a very relaxed, centred and well-balanced body, with a focused and refreshed mind.

Yoga helps to bring balance into your life. The word yoga means union, meaning the balance between mind, body and spirit. It is about bringing together the balance of your physical, mental and spiritual states, for example, your state of mind will affect your immune system and hormonal systems which will affect your circulation and breathing and so on. So in order to treat physical tiredness, say, you need to look at your mental, physical and spiritual needs too.

Like many of the ancient traditional medicines, yoga holds that the key to good health and happiness lies in the free flow of energy (prana) around the body. Yogis believe that if we live in harmony with nature and keep our energy balanced by learning to control our breathing and our posture we will be healthy. Yoga's precise postures work deep into the body encouraging the blood to circulate so as to give you endless energy. The blood then nourishes every organ and softens all the muscles and ligament tissue. The deep stretching of yoga brings the bones and muscles back into alignment and also lubricates the joints helping to keep you supple through to old age.

Indian medicine believes that we take in vital energy through the breath. Our breathing also helps us to get more oxygen and therefore helps with other functions such as digestion and concentration. Yoga helps you to use what you take in for energy. It will help you to store, direct and control your energy, and also to balance your chakras so that your energy can flow properly.

In yoga a restless mind is compared to a chattering monkey. If you are very stressed you will end up with your head full of racing thoughts, and can suffer from anxiety and depression, all of which will deplete your energy. Practising yoga will help to calm your mind and quieten the chattering monkey.

The benefits of yoga are numerous: it tones the body, delays ageing, helps the joints and skeleton, strengthens the circulation, heart and lungs (and therefore oxygenates the blood), and improves breathing and digestion. It not only helps posture and makes the spine more flexible, but also balances the nervous system, helping the body to relax. In addition to all that, it also balances the hormonal system, nourishes the organs and glands, balances the chakras, removes toxins and, of course, gives you energy.

## Breathing

There is a great yoga proverb that says, 'Life is in the breath; he who only half breathes half lives.' Breathing is an important medicine without which we die. It helps to feed the brain and calms the nervous system which has an effect on all the other physical systems of the body. Our lungs are our connection with the outside world: when we breathe in we take in new energy and life and when we exhale we breathe out the old, the waste and the expired. Buddhists believe that every breath in is a new life and every breath out a little death, so taking in deep joyful breaths is a way of getting a new lease of life and vitality.

Our breath becomes constricted because of trapped memories, experiences and emotions such as fear, anger, anxiety, sadness and grief. By using our breath we can slowly release these constrictions. Breathing techniques are some of the oldest, most effective and easiest ways of stimulating and balancing energy within the body.

Yoga teaches breathing techniques to improve your energy, mind, mood, physical conditions, immune system and even help slow down the ageing process.

Try not to be competitive when doing yoga. Go at your own pace and always come out of a posture very carefully. It's best to wear loose clothes and you should not eat for two hours beforehand as the digestive process uses up energy. Before doing any yoga you need to learn the breathing techniques over the page.

## Breathing the yoga way (pranayama)

Pranayama is the yogic science of breathing. It is an excellent tool as it encourages you to breathe deeply and fully, bringing oxygen deep into the cells and pulling out toxins. It also sends a surge of energy through every cell of your body.

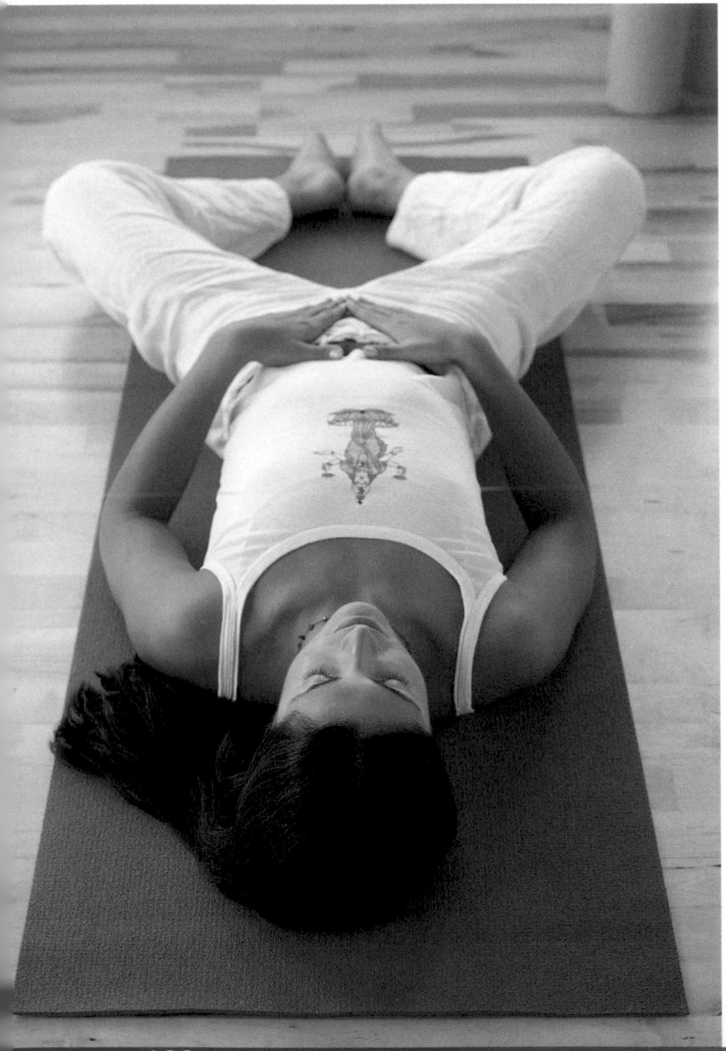

**1** Lie on your back and make yourself comfortable. Bring your feet close up to your buttocks with the soles of your feet together and allow the knees to fall apart with your hands gently resting on your abdomen. This posture stretches the lower abdomen which enhances the breathing practice. (If you find this position difficult, just lie on your back with your hands on your abdomen; with each inhalation lift your arms out and up above your head and with each exhalation bring your arms back to your sides.)

**2** Breathe in through your nose and feel your abdomen expand and contract.

**3** Breathe out through your nose and notice your abdomen flatten.

**4** If you feel comfortable you can extend the inhalation of the breath so it comes up from the abdomen into the chest, hence breathing in longer and deeper.

**5** Bring your knees back together and stretch out your legs.

**6** Repeat five to ten times.

## Alternate nostril breathing

Alternate nostril breathing stimulates both sides of the brain and helps them to be in balance. It harmonises and soothes the body and mind leaving you feeling calm. It's particularly good to do if you can't sleep.

**1** Sit in a chair and close your eyes.

**2** Place your hand on your nose with your thumb on one nostril and your ring finger on the other.

**3** Close off one nostril at a time without moving your hand.

**4** Starting with closing the right nostril, breathe out through your left nostril (always start with an exhale) then inhale through the left nostril.

**5** Swap nostrils by exhaling through the right nostril and inhaling through the right nostril.

Breathe normally, not too deeply. Don't worry if you need to blow your nose a lot.

Note: always consult a doctor if you suffer from any illness or are pregnant before doing any yoga.

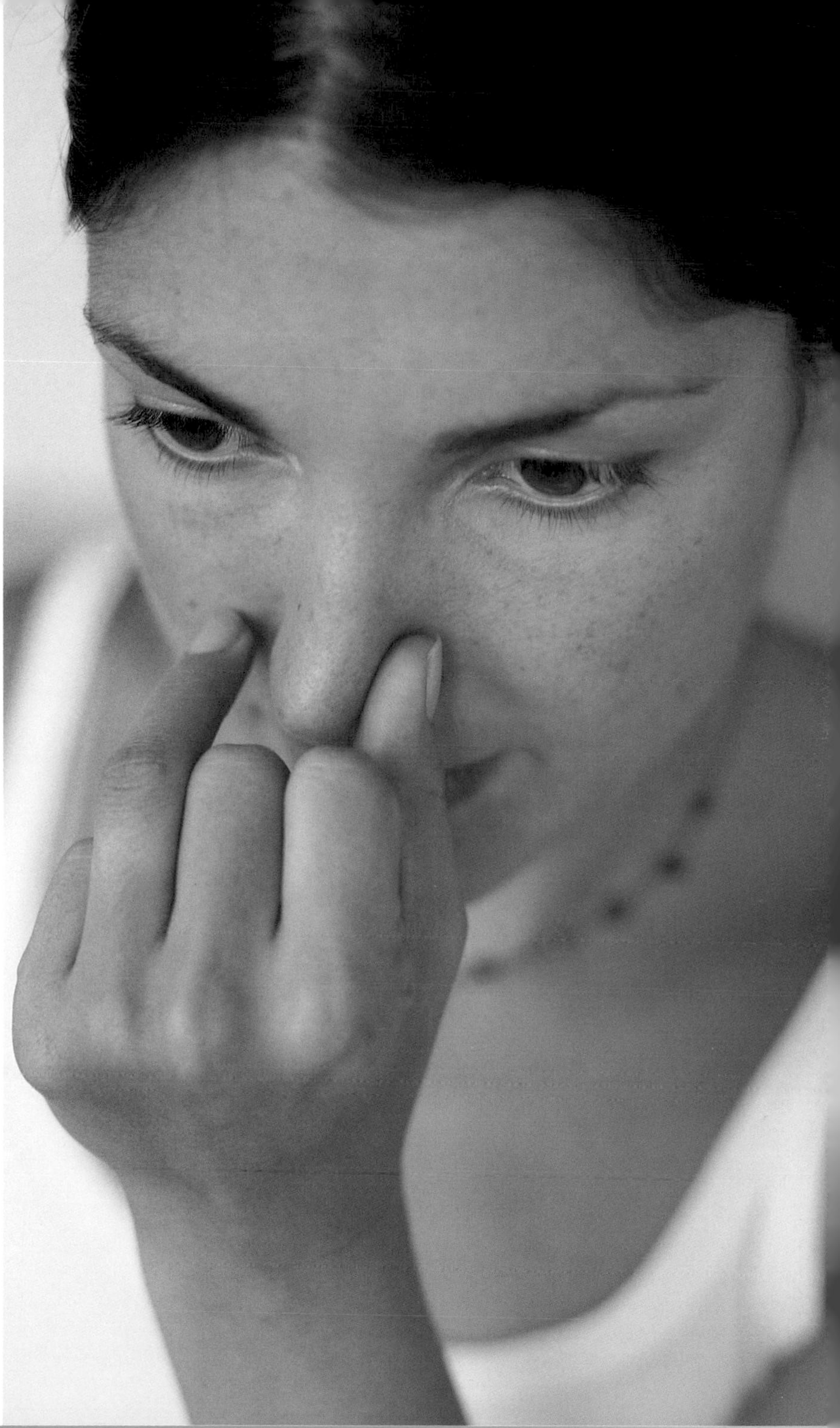

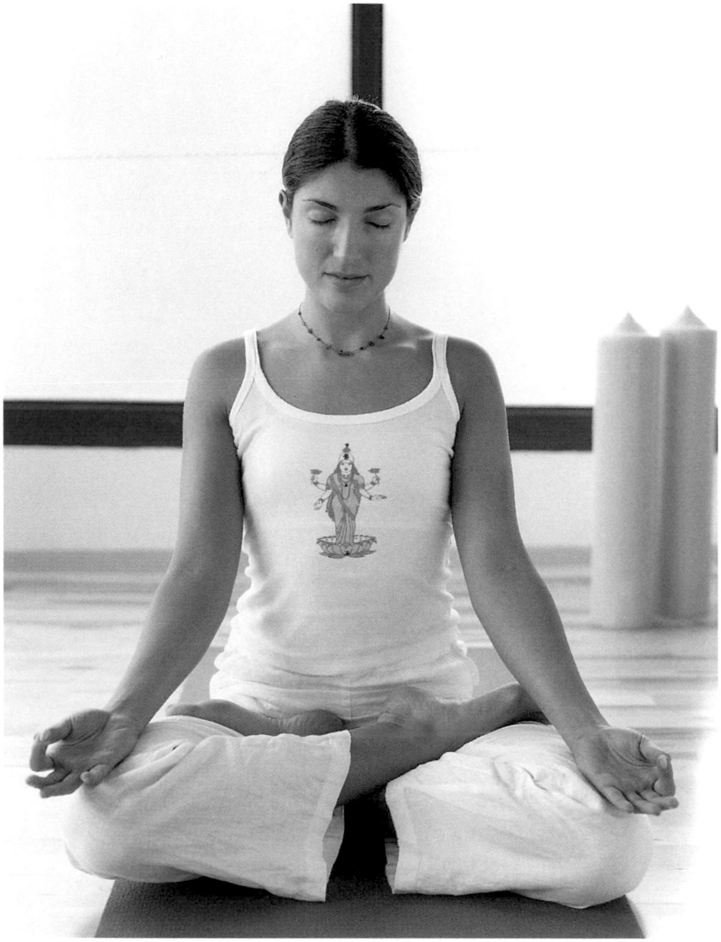

## Sitting lotus

**1** Sit with your legs crossed.

**2** Rest your feet on the opposite calves (if you find this difficult try the half lotus in which you rest just one foot on the opposite calf).

**3** Put the back of your hands on your knees with your thumb and first finger touching to make an 0.

**4** Close your eyes and concentrate on the ground beneath you.

**5** Relax your jaw and let your tongue rest on the roof of your mouth.

**6** Visualise that your spine is being stretched up to the sky.

**7** Breathe deeply and slowly through your nose whilst thinking of something positive or saying 'Om'.

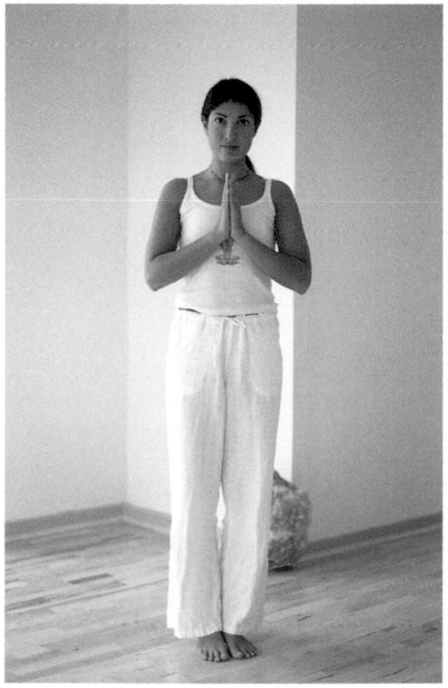

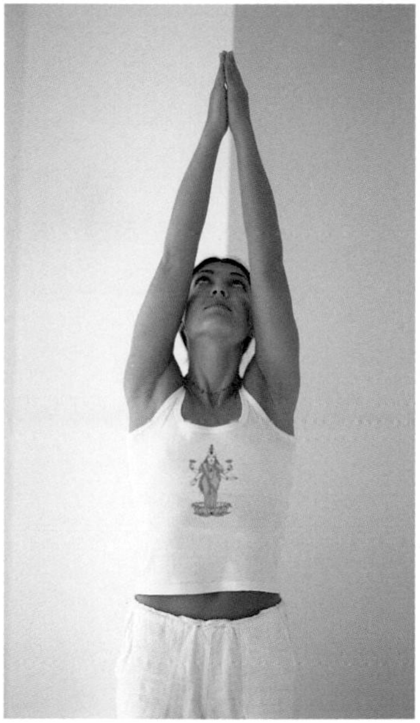

## Sun salutation

This yoga position allows energy to flow throughout the whole body. It warms and invigorates the body and increases blood flow to the head. It is also a good stretching and strengthening exercise for the arms, back, shoulders, buttocks and legs. It helps to oxygenate the body and improve circulation, relieves tension and releases energy. It also improves flexibility and body tone. Go as far as you can with each motion without strain or pain. Start by doing it once and then gradually increase to ten times.

**1** Stand with your feet together, arms by your side, looking straight ahead. Bring your hands together in a praying position at your chest and exhale.

**2** Inhale as you bring your arms straight up over your head. With your palms still together, stretch up as high as you can and look up at your thumbs.

**3** Exhale keeping your arms straight as you bend forward, allowing your hands to reach the floor either side of your feet with your head relaxed down.

**4** Inhale and step so you are in a lunge position with your left leg backwards. Keep your hands

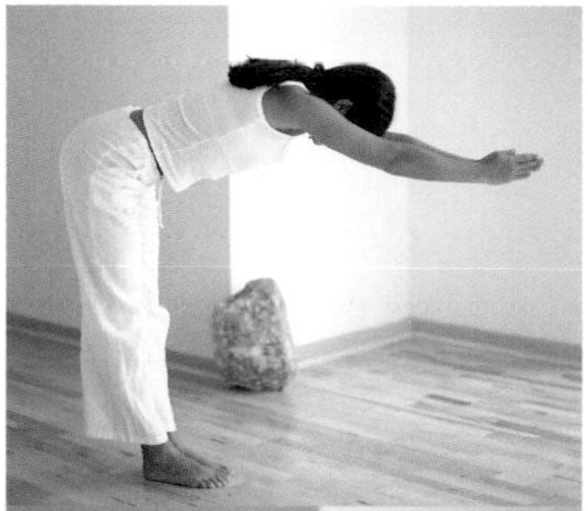

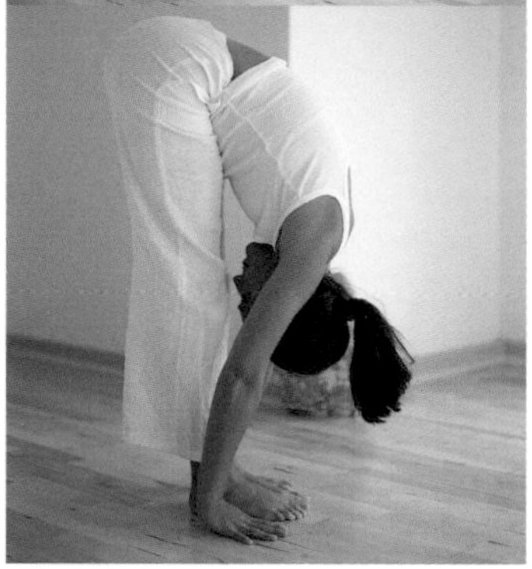

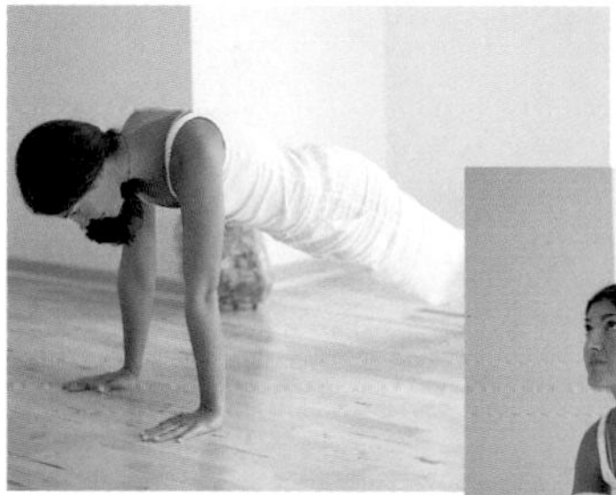

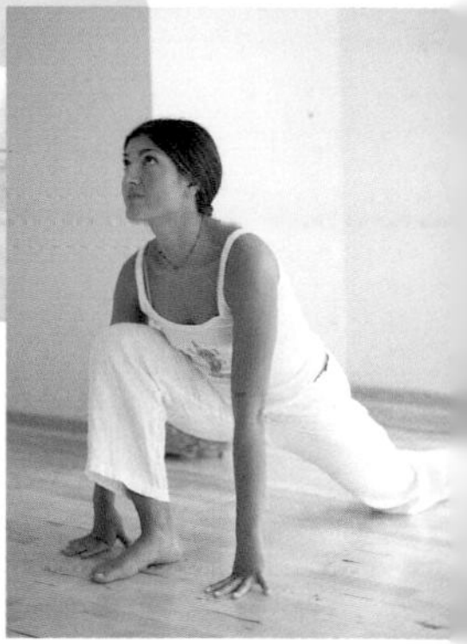

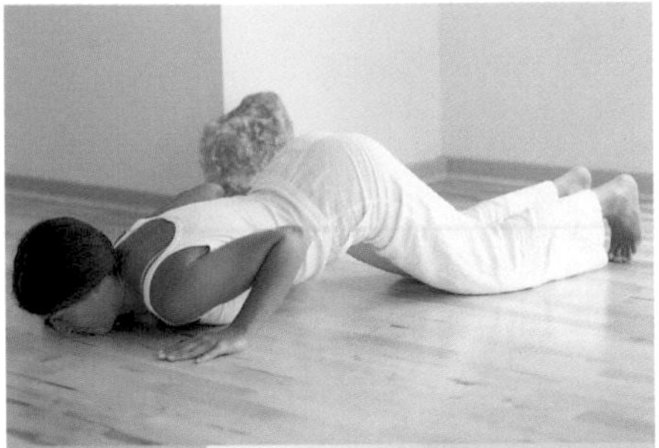

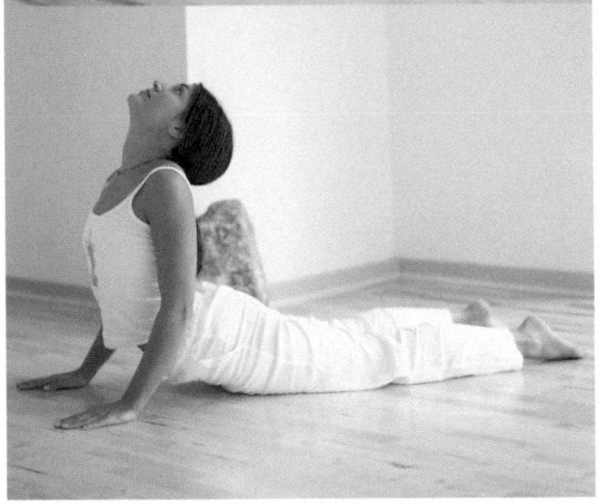

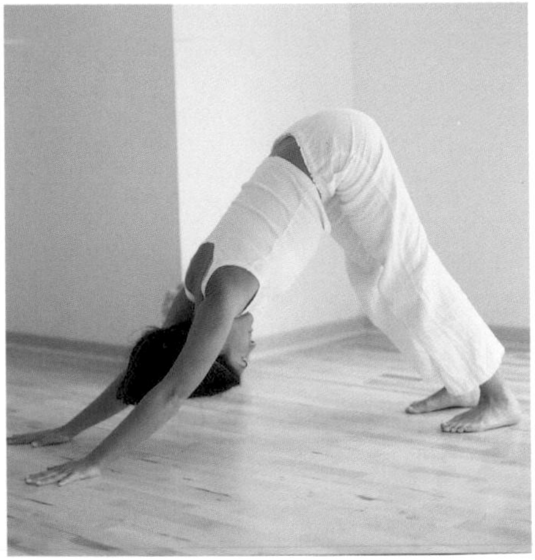

either side of your right knee and keep them firmly on the floor. Look upward stretching your back and chest. Step your right leg back.

**5** Exhale, lower your knees to the floor and then lower your chest down toward the floor with a straight back and then inhale and straighten your arms and look up while bending back as far as you can comfortably go.

**6** Exhale and push your hips up into an inverted 'v'. Your arms should be shoulder width apart and your palms facing front. Keep your feet and heels flat on the floor.

**7** Inhale and lunge forward with left leg forward between your hands and look upward stretching your back. Exhale and step your right leg forward between your hands. Keep your legs together and straighten them.

**8** Inhale. Come up vertebra by vertebra with your hands raising out to the side and then above your head meeting in a prayer position. Look up at your hands.

**9** Exhale and bring your hands in prayer position in front of chest.

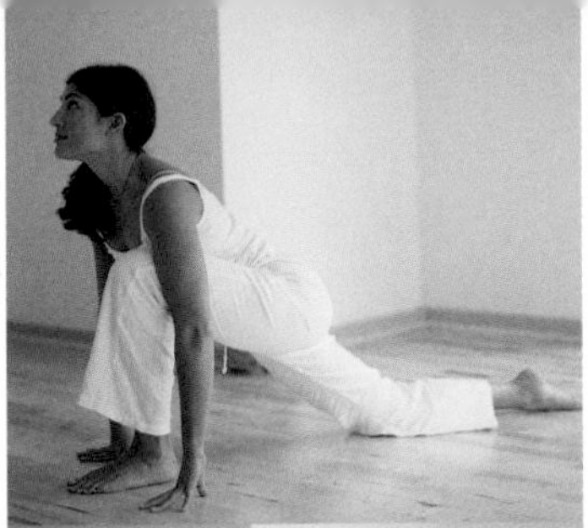

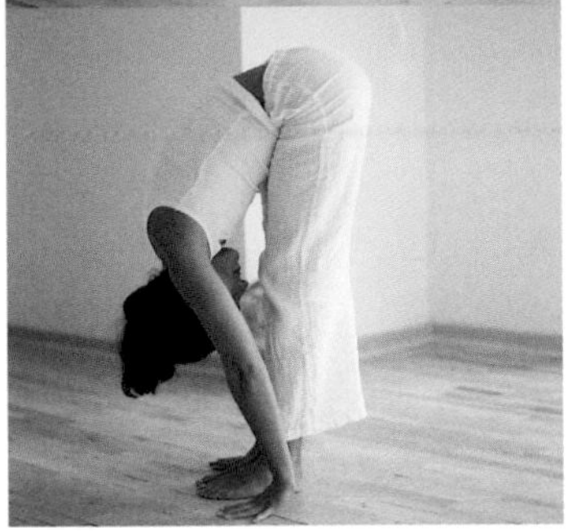

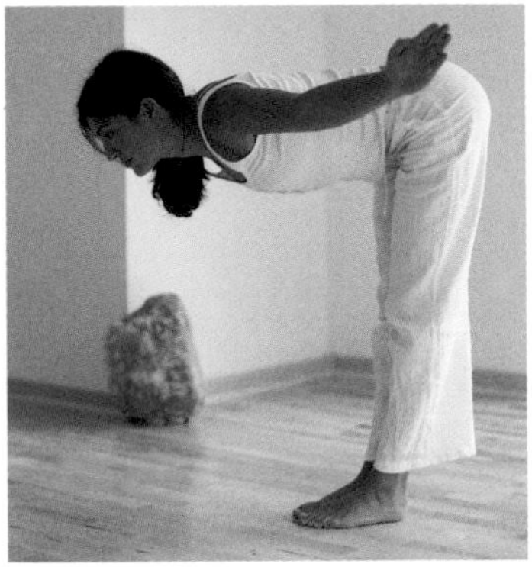

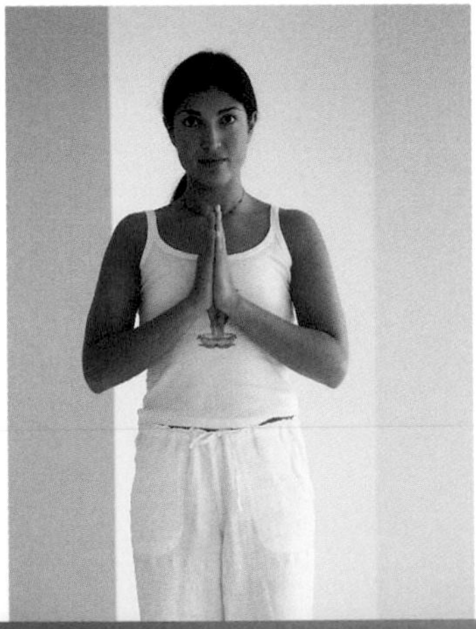

## The energy triangle

This exercise opens up the hips and shoulders and allows the energy to flow smoothly. The good news is that it also helps to shape your waist and makes you more supple.

**1** Stand with your feet apart and inhale through your nose.

**2** Stretch your arms out to the side like a star.

**3** Turn your left foot ninety degrees to the side and breathe out through your nose.

**4** Breathe in through your nose and bend down sideways until your left hand reaches to your ankle. Stretch your right hand up to the sky look up at your hand.

**5** Breathe out through your nose. Come back to standing position, turn your foot back to the front and repeat on the other side.

**6** Repeat five times.

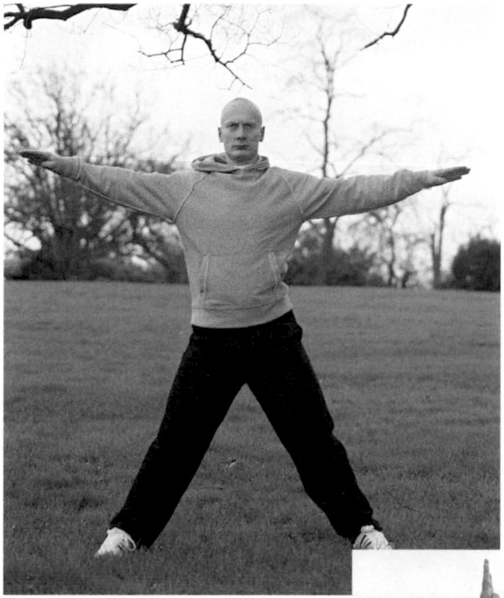

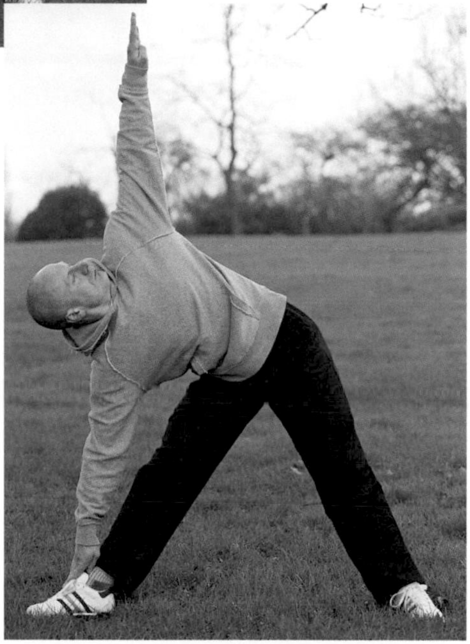

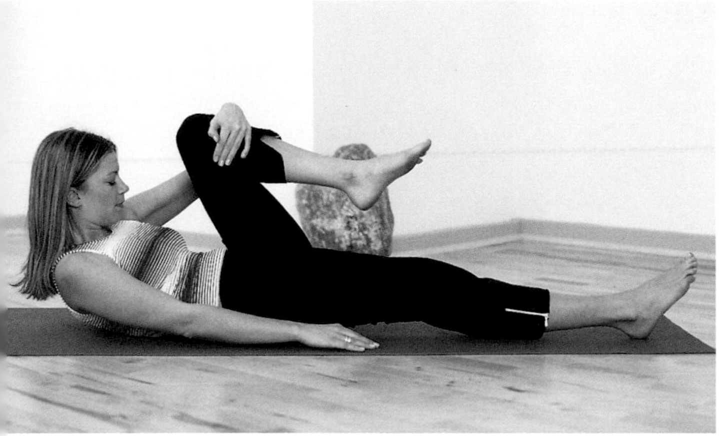

## Head to knee pose (above)

Helps with constipation and irritable bowel.

**1** Lie on your back with your legs straight.

**2** Bring your right leg bent into your chest and hug it with your right arm.

**3** Breathe in and lift your head in toward your knee. Hold and breathe.

**4** Exhale and lower your head. Inhale. Exhale and lower your leg.

**5** Repeat three times on both legs.

## Leg raises (above right)

**1** Lie on the floor with your legs straight.

**2** Inhale and lift your right leg with your foot flexed so that it is at right angles with your body but do not strain. You can bend your other leg if you find this too difficult. Exhale.

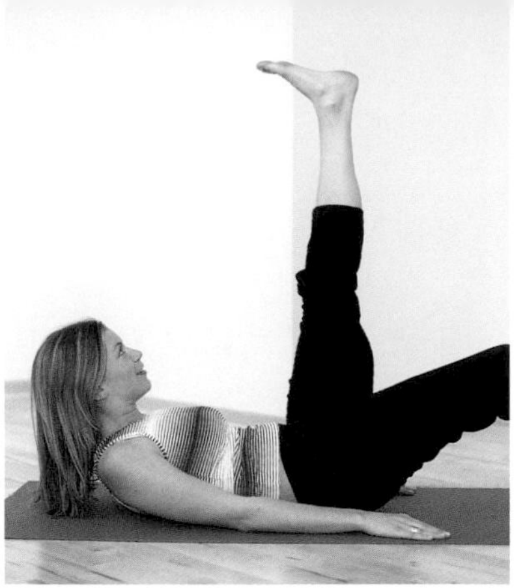

**3** Inhale and gently lift your head toward your leg.

**4** Exhale and lower your head. Inhale.

**5** Exhale and lower your leg.

**6** Repeat three times on both legs.

## The half-shoulder stand (right)

This posture is very good for increasing energy as it helps blood circulation. It also helps aching legs and low blood pressure, and elimination of waste in the bowel. The thyroid gland is also stimulated helping to produce hormones from the endocrine system (if thyroxine is low it can often cause low energy). Because it is an inverted position it gives the organs a rest. Women should **not** do this exercise during a period.

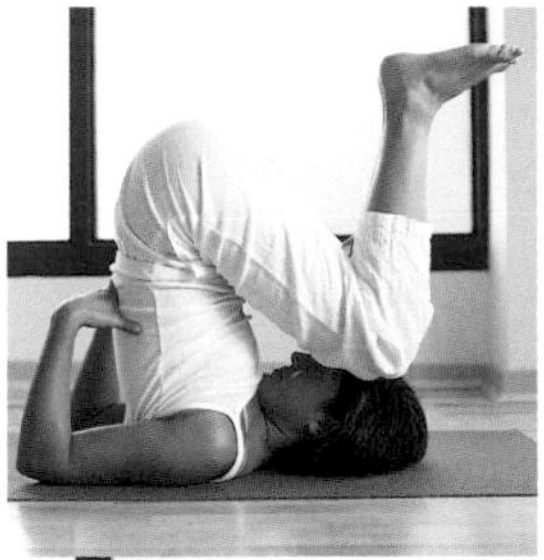

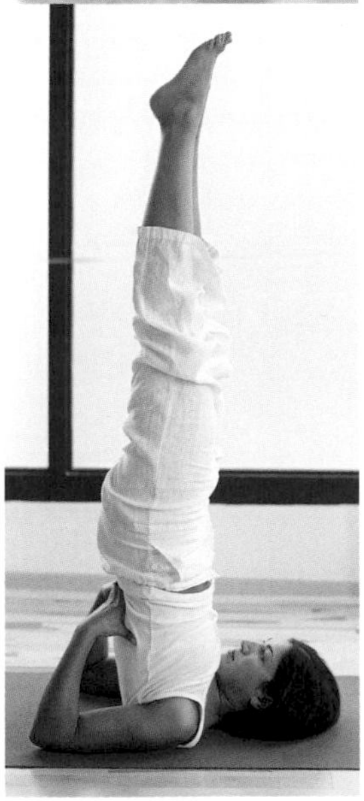

**1** Lie on your back with your arms by your side, palms down.

**2** Inhale, bringing your hips and legs off the ground supported by your hands.

**3** Bring your knees to your forehead; if you are comfortable you can extend your legs first to the ceiling and then, so that your legs are at forty-five degrees to your body. Hold the position and breathe normally. Keep your neck straight. Do not strain. Inhale.

**4** Exhale and slowly roll back on to the floor.

## The fish (below)

**1** Lie on your back with your arms by your side.

**2** Place your palms facing down under your bottom, squeeze elbows in toward each other and keep your legs straight.

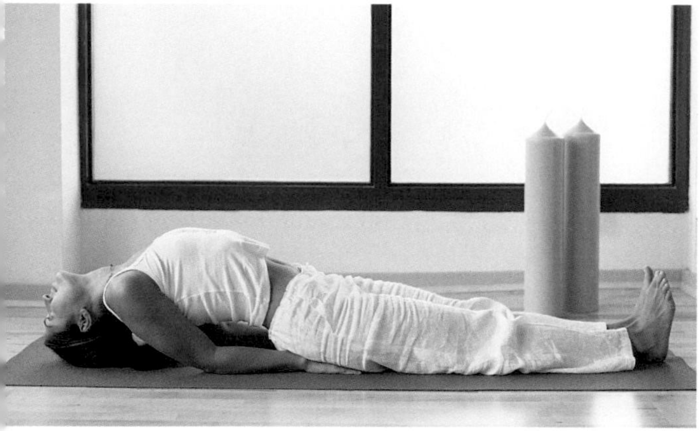

**3** Inhale and put the weight of your body on to your forearms and elbows. Keep your feet flexed.

**4** Lift your chest (arch your back) and lower your head slowly and then rest the crown of your head on the floor so that you are looking behind you. The pressure on your head should be light and the majority of the weight held by your arms.

**5** Hold for five to ten breaths, or as long as you can while breathing deeply and then exhale to come out of the posture.

## The bridge (below)

Helps to strengthen and make the spine more flexible.

**1** Lie on the floor with your knees bent, your ankles under your knees, your feet hip width apart and your arms beside you.

**2** Place your palms on the floor clasping your hands under your back and pulling your shoulders downwards.

**3** Inhale and lift your hips as high as you can so that you are resting on your shoulders making a bridge. You can put your hands under your waist to help lift you higher on to your shoulders if you like. Make sure your head, neck and feet are still flat on the floor. Use your arms and feet to support you by pushing them down into the floor. Breathe normally and hold the posture for a few seconds.

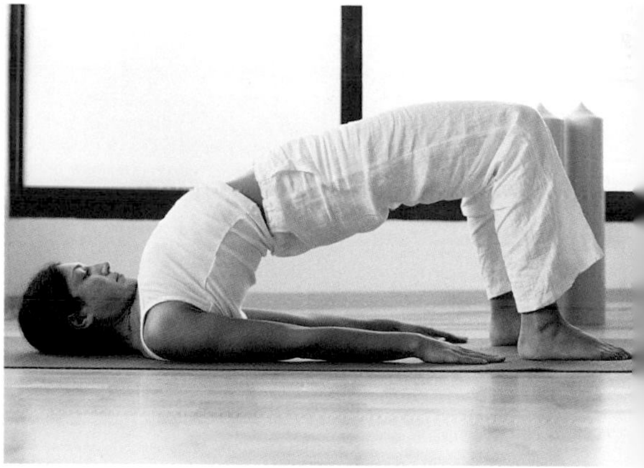

**4** Exhale and slowly lower your back vertebra by vertebra bringing your hips down last, until you are flat on the floor.

**5** Relax for a few deep breaths and then repeat twice.

## Hand clasp (below)

This posture also opens the chest, stretches the back and helps the shoulders.

**1** Kneel on the floor, sitting on your heels.

**2** Put one arm behind your back and reach up as

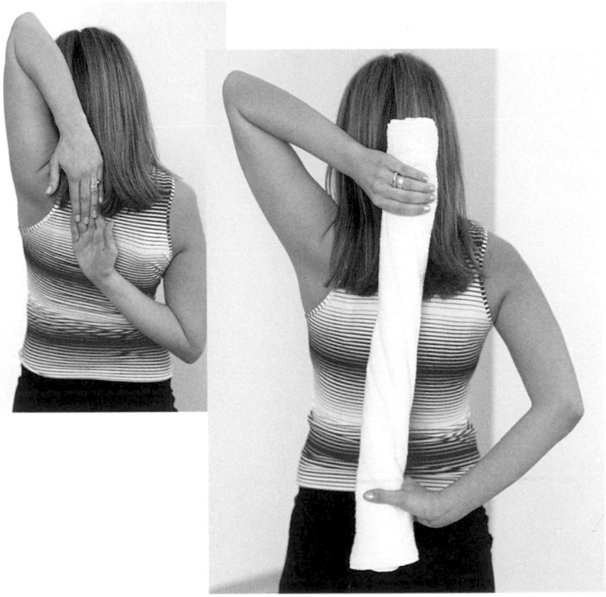

far as you can toward your shoulders with your arm bent and your palm facing outward. Bring your other arm over its shoulder so that the hands meet. Try and hold hands, but if you can't reach use a towel and hold it between your hands.

**3** Pull up and down and hold for a few seconds.

**4** Repeat with the other side.

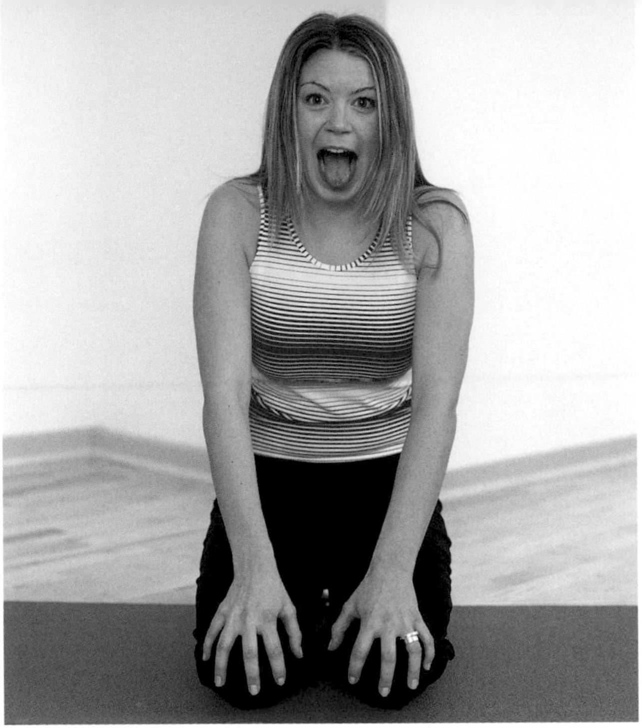

## The Lion (above)

This pose stimulates the blood and energy to the face helping you not only to feel more energised but to look it too. It's also good if you are coming down with a cold.

**1** Kneel on the floor, sitting on your heels.

**2** Put your hands on your knees, with your fingers spread. Inhale through your nose.

**3** Leaning slightly forward, exhale through your mouth and make a 'Haa' sound, while sticking your tongue out as far as it will go.

**4** Stretch out your fingers and look up at the space between your eyes. Hold for a few seconds and then close your mouth

(Don't worry if you feel a bit silly doing this pose!)

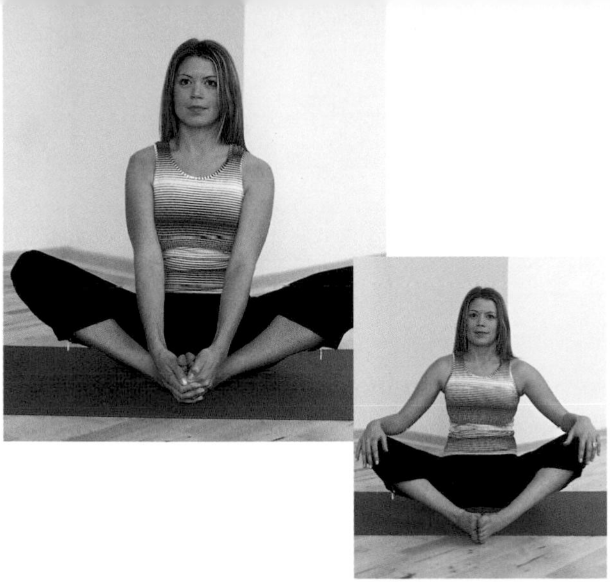

## The Butterfly (above)

**1** Sit upright with the soles of your feet together.

**2** Hold on to your feet/toes with your hands. Slowly and gently bounce your knees up and down going as close to the floor as possible.

**3** After a few minutes put your hands on your knees and gently push them down toward the floor.

## Forward stretch (below)

This helps your nervous system and solar plexus.

**1** Sit on the floor with your legs together and stretched out in front of you.

**2** Sit upright with your feet flexed.

**3** Inhale and lift your arms up over your head and look up at your hands.

**4** Exhale, lengthen the spine and bend forwards (from the hips), moving your chest toward your legs. Only go as far as you can. Try to keep your back straight and lengthened. Hold for a few seconds.

**5** Inhale and slowly come back up.

## Backward stretch (right)

This is great for increasing your energy and good to do after the forward stretch.

**1** Lie on your front.

**2** Lift your weight up on to your forearms with your elbows under your shoulders.

**3** Pull your shoulders back.

**4** Look straight ahead and hold for a few seconds. Don't forget to breathe.

**5** Exhaling, lower yourself down and rest.

**6** Repeat twice more.

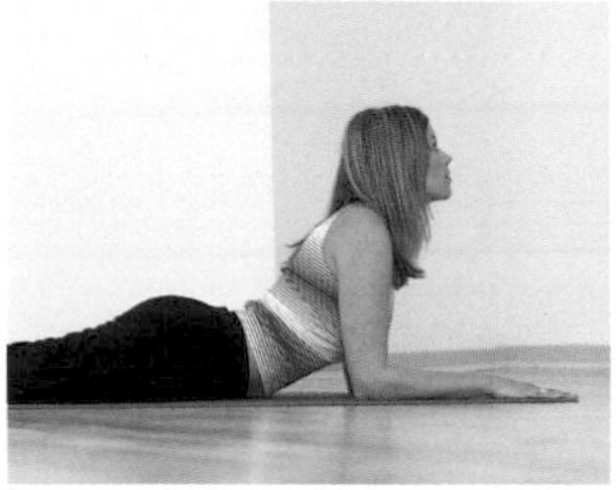

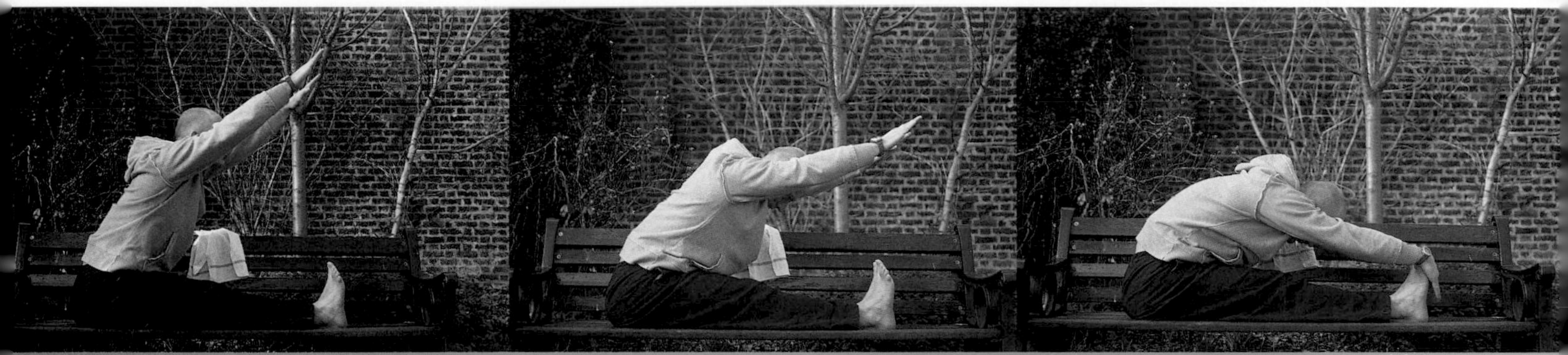

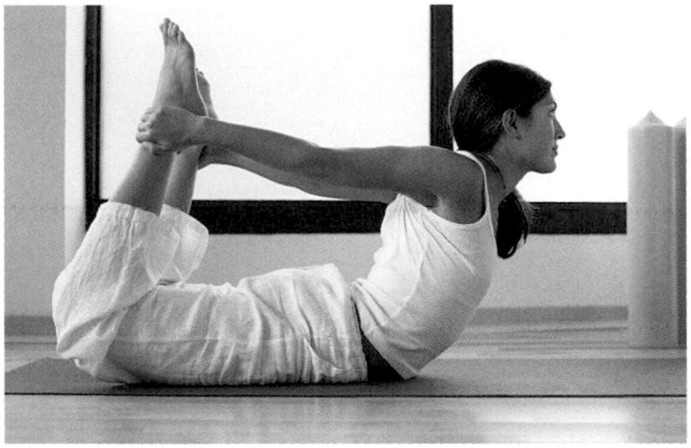

## The bow (above)

This is great for increasing energy and gives the internal organs a massage.

**1** Lie on your front and bring your feet bent back toward your bottom, knees hip width apart.

**2** Reach back with your hands to hold your ankles. Exhale.

**3** Inhale and lift your chest and head and pull your shoulders back while still holding your ankles. Also lift your knees, thighs and hips so that you are resting on your abdomen. Use your legs to pull yourself up.

**4** Arch your back and look upwards, or straight ahead if it hurts your neck.

**5** Take three deep breaths (you might rock slightly as you do so).

**6** Exhale and come slowly down and relax into the pose of a child (see right).

## The pose of a child (below)

As your head is below your heart in this pose it circulates blood to the brain and gives you energy.

**1** Kneel down with your bottom resting on your heels.

**2** Bend forward and rest your forehead on to the floor.

**3** Put your arms at your sides with your palms by your feet facing upwards.

**4** Breathe deeply and relax.

Note: sufferers from high blood pressure should not do this exercise without seeking medical advice.

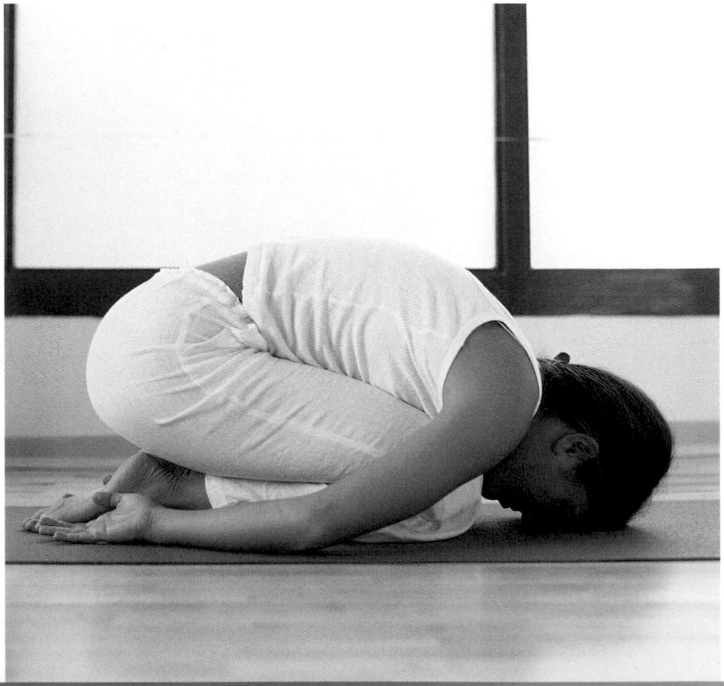

## Energy boosts during the day and at work

Sitting at a desk all day, particularly at a computer, will make your shoulders, neck and spine tense and as a result you will feel aching and tired. The lack of movement in a stuffy office also slows down the flow of blood and qi around your body. This is when most people reach for a caffeine pick-me-up or sweets.

It is all too easy to get sucked into your work, to almost become your work and forget about taking care of your body. Most of us live in our heads rather than our bodies and have no idea even how our bodies are feeling until maybe at the end of the day when we finally stop and realise how hungry, thirsty, tired, stiff and achy we feel.

Try and stop just for a minute every hour to touch base with your body. How are you feeling? Is your neck tense? Are you clenching your jaw? Are you hungry or thirsty? Do you need water or a good, nourishing meal instead of a quick, limp sandwich? Does your back or bottom ache from sitting too long? Do you need a stretch, are you tired? Do your eyes need a rest?

It's not always possible to give in to every need of the body but try to give yourself some of the quick fixes that are good for you like a glass of water, some fruit, stretching, rolling your neck, taking a break for a few minutes. You will find that it is easier to work and concentrate if you are relaxed and happy.

- Try taking regular breaks just walking around the office to get a glass of water or go to the toilet. Try walking just out to the front door (or at least to a window), take some deep breaths and then walk back in back to your desk.
- Try and get a twenty-minute walk or cycle every day by walking to work or getting off the train/bus early or parking your car farther away and walking the rest of the way.
- When you go to the toilet (or in the office if you can), do the standing yoga stretch (see overleaf). It can also be done outside if you have some outside space. It helps to relax the shoulders neck and spine and it allows the vertebrae to stretch instead of being pushed on top of each other. This, in turn, allows the spinal fluid to flow smoothly and nourishes the spinal cord and brain thus helping also with concentration and lifting your spirits.

The exercise opposite is good if you sit at a desk all day. You can do it at intervals during the day and again at the end of the day. It will relax your shoulders which are often tense from stress and from poor posture. It also strengthens the muscles either side of the spine and spreads the vertebrae apart. (Sitting at a desk pushes the vertebrae on top of each other stopping the spinal fluid from flowing properly and therefore preventing it from nourishing the brain and spinal cord.) This exercise will help to lift your spirits as well.

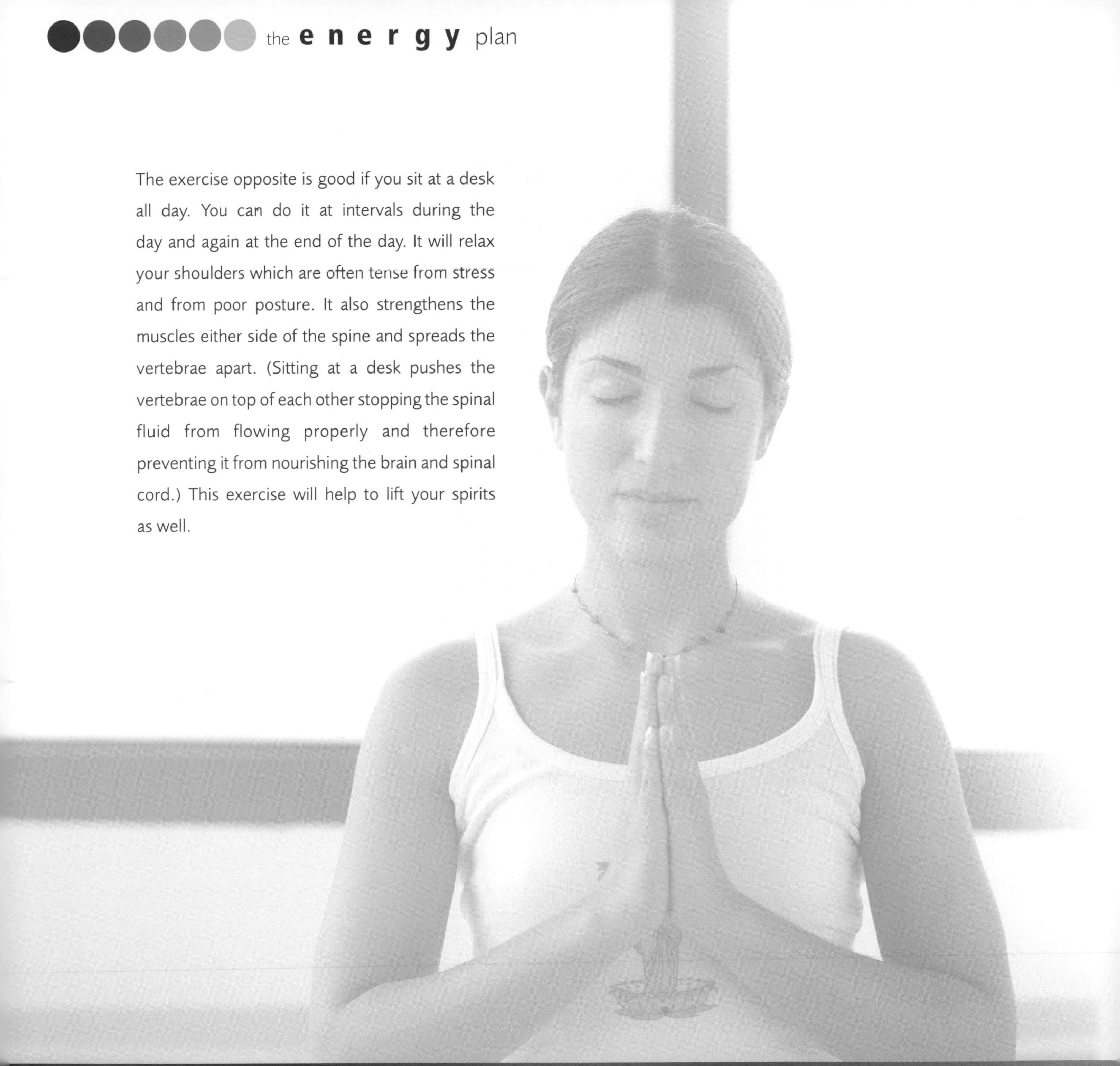

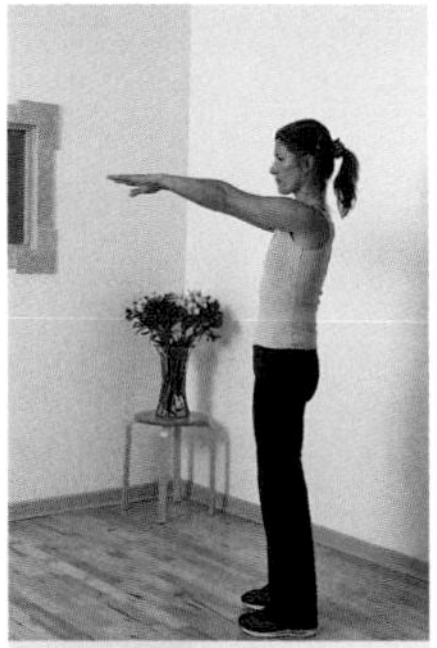

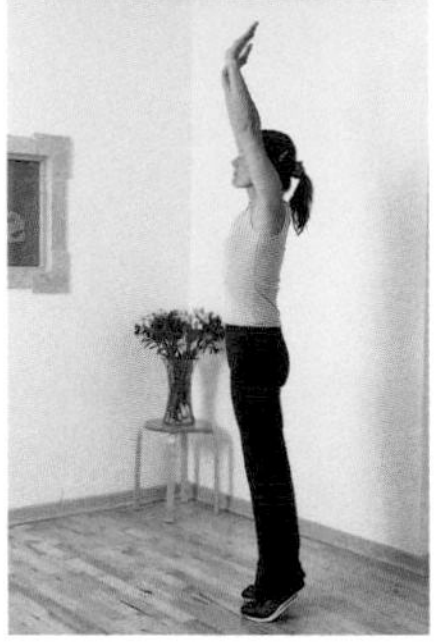

## STANDING YOGA STRETCH AT YOUR DESK

**1** Stand with your feet hip width apart and your knees slightly bent and shoulders relaxed.

**2** Inhale through your nose and lift your arms up straight in front of your body to shoulder height.

**3** Stretch your arms up to above your head with your palms facing the sky; imagine that you are pushing the sky away. Go up on to your toes.

**4** Slowly lower yourself down off your toes and firmly ground your feet.

**5** Breathe out through your nose and bend down and touch the floor/your toes. Let your body be as loose as possible.

**6** Breathe in through your nose and straighten up one vertebra at a time until you are back at the starting position.

**7** Repeat five to ten times.

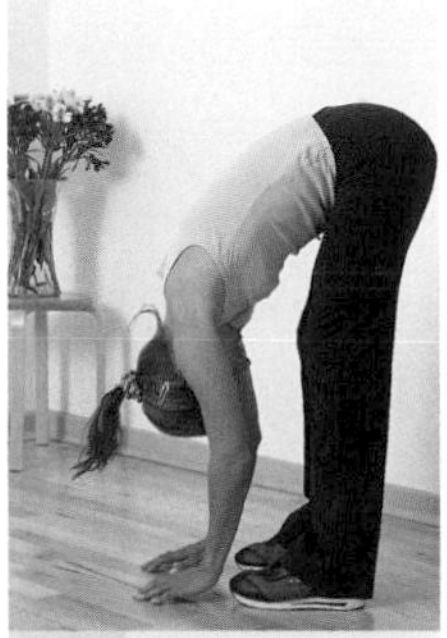

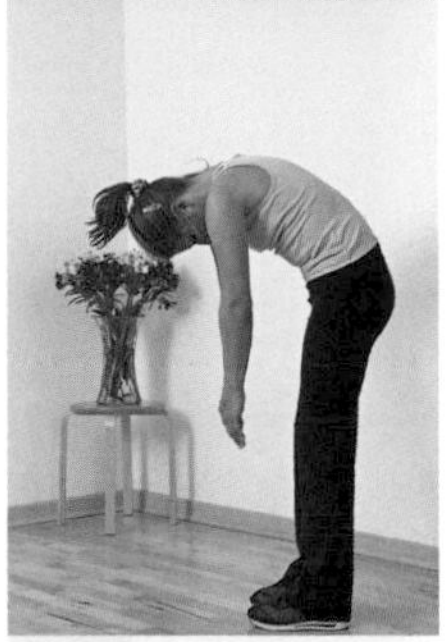

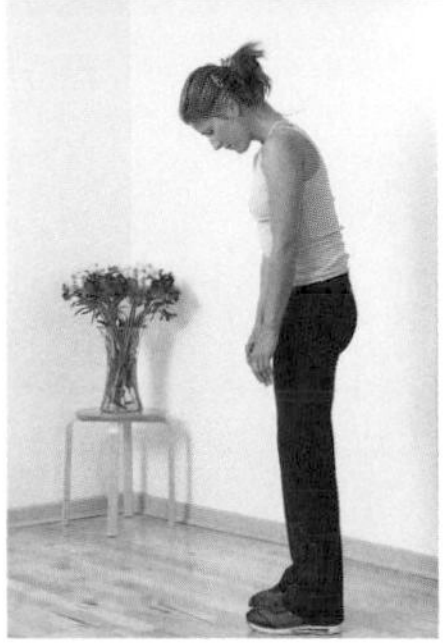

# Posture

*Our posture can affect how we feel both emotionally and physically and therefore has ramifications on our energy too.*

Posture is a very powerful thing: if you change your posture you can change your mood, and you can tell a lot about a person and how they are feeling by the way they hold themselves. The more strained or nervous you feel the more you tend to close up your body, for example by folding your arms or crossing your legs. This cuts the energy flow and the longer you stay locked in that position the more nervous you will feel. Conversely, by opening up your posture you restore energy flow and subsequently feel more relaxed.

Alexander technique is based on the close connection between posture and mood and between your posture and your physical health. When you are tired you are more likely to slump in a chair and this will make you feel more tired as you restrict many organs in the body. Your heart has to work harder and it will become harder to breathe due to the tension around your ribs.

When we are stressed we often have hunched shoulders and this hampers our breathing, creating muscle tension. In the long term, this can make the diaphragm too stiff and tense and hard to expand and stretch when you do try to relax and breathe properly.

If you sit in a slouched position your spine is sloped backward and your shoulders and the top of your back are under stress to try and keep your head up. The tension and lactic acid build-up causes sore neck and shoulders. If you sat correctly your head would balance naturally on your shoulders resulting in no tension and would allow your rib cage to expand easily when you breathe.

Similarly, if you slump at your desk at work all day with rounded shoulders you will have neck pain as again you are overworking to keep the head erect. You are also shortening and tightening the muscles across the chest preventing proper breathing. However, if you sit with a strong back and stomach and relaxed shoulders your body will be able to cope better and you will feel less tense and tired at the end of the day.

If you have had a poor posture for many years then the correct postures will feel very strange at first. Try to think about your posture throughout the day and correct it whenever you remember until it becomes second nature.

## Standing

- Stand with pelvis centred correctly.
- Use your stomach muscles to keep equilibrium.
- Keep your knees relaxed, not locked.
- Straighten your shoulders; they should be held down and relaxed (shrug them a few times to loosen them).
- Neck and head should sit comfortably on your spine; don't lean your head forwards or down.

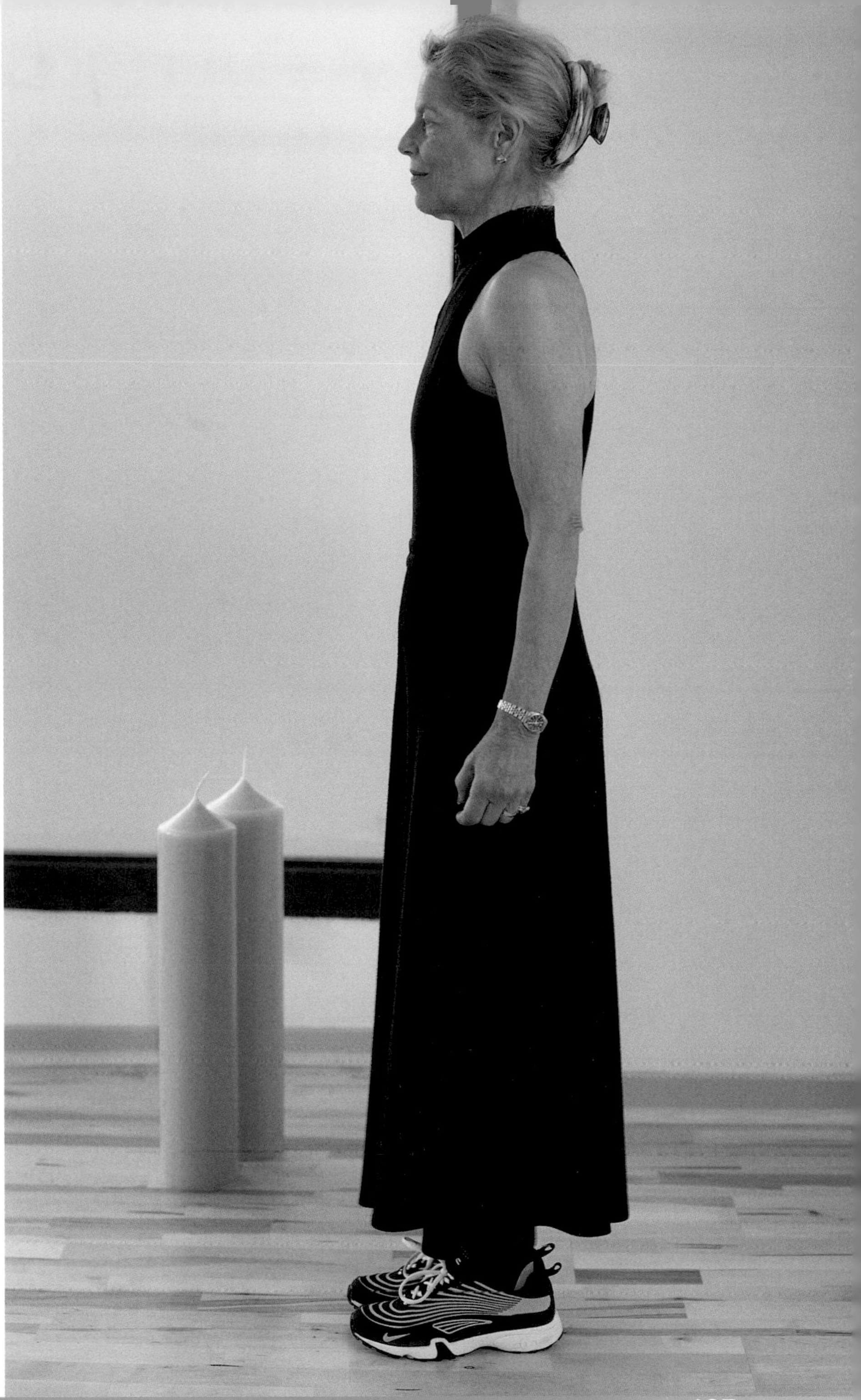

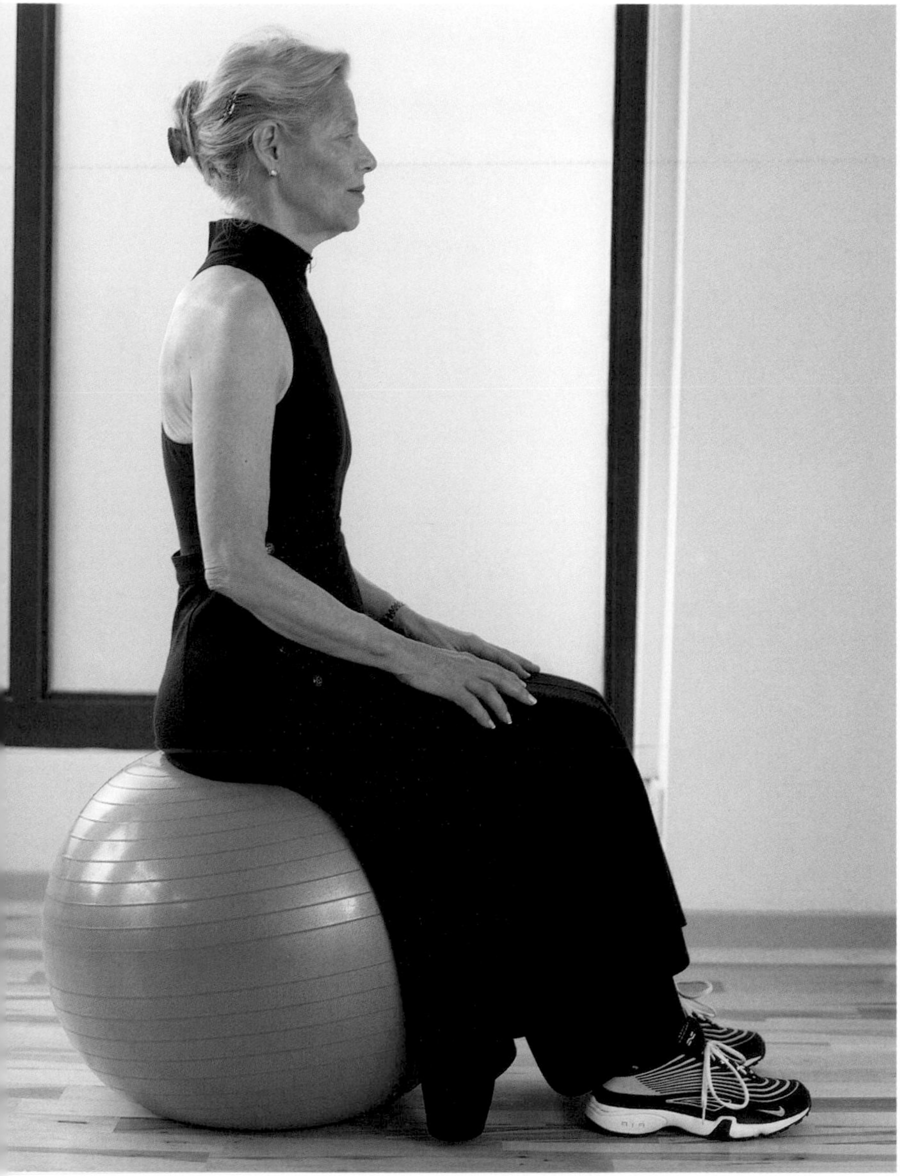

## Sitting

- Try to get a chair with good support to lower back.
- Sit with your tailbone at the back of the chair.
- Your feet should be flat on the floor; mid- and lower back need to be kept strong to avoid slumping.
- Shoulders should be relaxed and down.
- Head and neck should sit loosely (i.e. not rigid).
- Work should be at a correct height and distance away so you can keep this position.
- Take short rests every hour, walk around the room, get some fresh air or at least do some sitting stretching exercises.

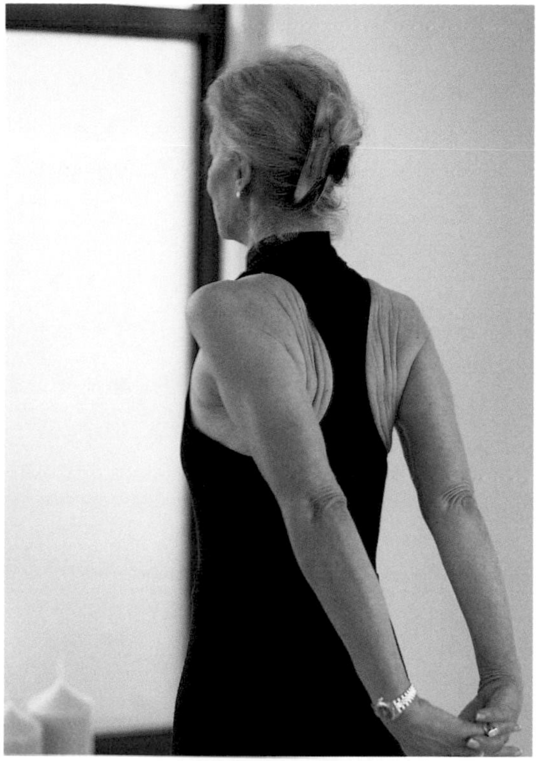

## Chest stretch (above)

This is good if your breathing is tight or if your shoulders are hunched or rounded.

**1** Stand with your hands clasped behind your back (palms facing upwards).

**2** Shoulders should be down and relaxed.

**3** Bring your hands out away from your back so you feel the stretch across your chest and shoulders.

## Spinal stretch (below)

This is very good if you are feeling stiff.

**1** Sit on a chair.

**2** Breathe out and drop your head and neck down toward your chest until you feel a stretch along your spine.

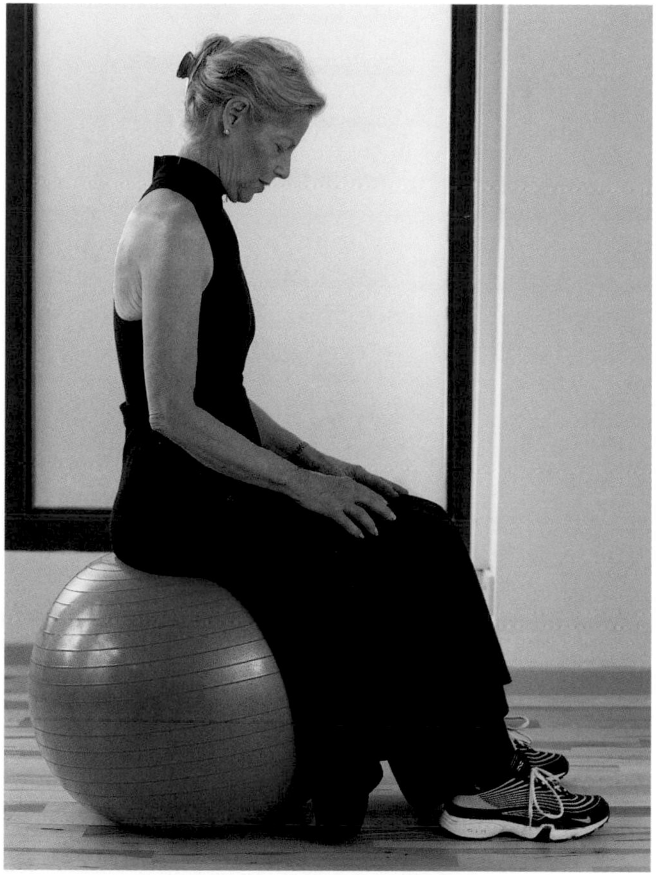

# Exercise According to Ayurveda

*Some traditions, like Ayurveda, believe that different types of people should exercise in different ways.*

## Vata

Vata people tend to be slim with an active mind. They are often restless and talk a lot. Everything they do they do quickly – walking, eating, talking etc. They find it difficult to sit still and they sleep very lightly. They learn quickly but forget quickly too and have a vivid imagination. They are very creative and sensitive.

## Exercise for vata people

Sprinters, runners and gymnasts tend to be vata people, but all sports suit vata types, especially ones that require speed and agility.

## Pitta

Pitta people usually have an average appetite and build and they walk and talk at average speed. They are natural leaders, strong-minded, fiery and quick-tempered. They have good co-ordination and are very competitive.

## Exercise for pitta people

Competitive sports suit pitta people best, so choose team or league sports, or exercise with someone else.

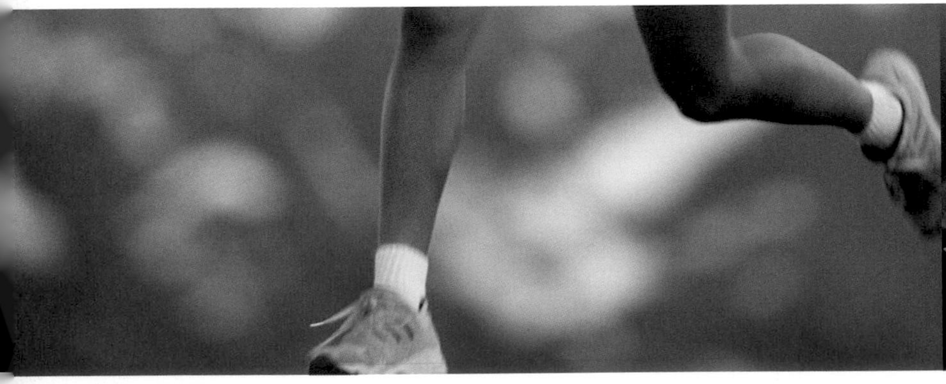

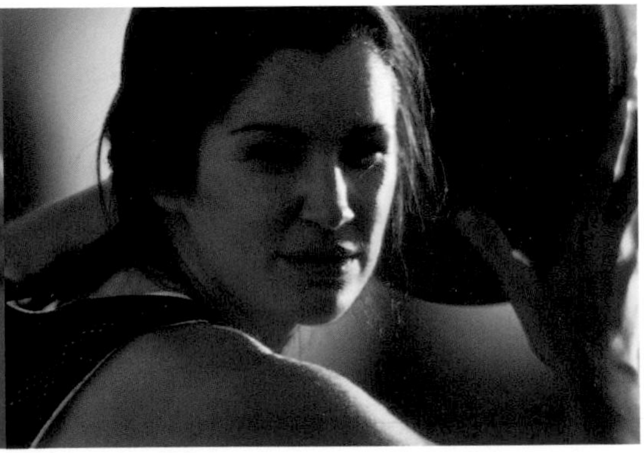

## Kapha

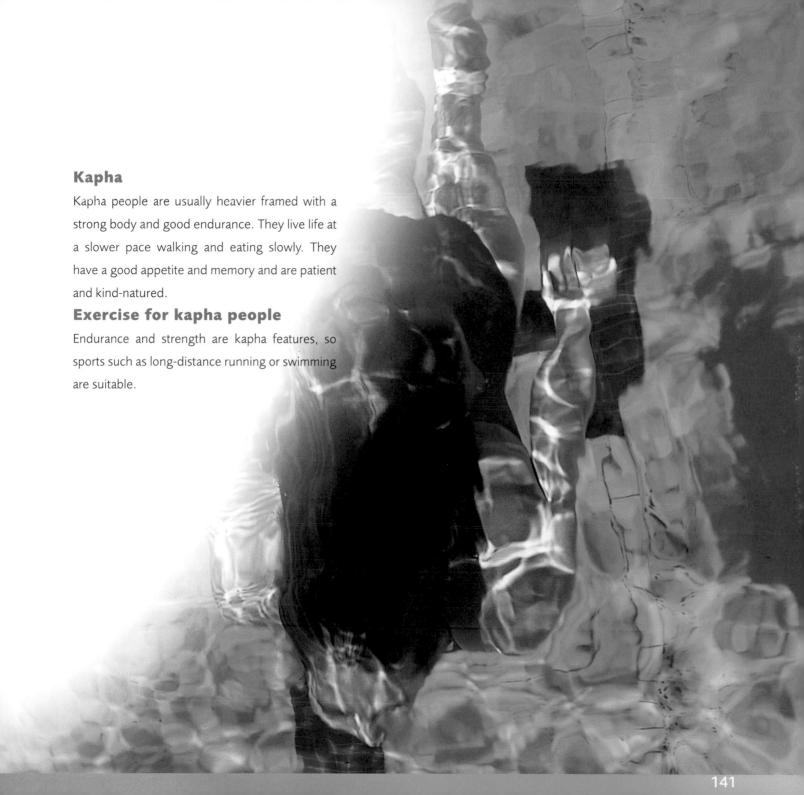

Kapha people are usually heavier framed with a strong body and good endurance. They live life at a slower pace walking and eating slowly. They have a good appetite and memory and are patient and kind-natured.

## Exercise for kapha people

Endurance and strength are kapha features, so sports such as long-distance running or swimming are suitable.

# Vibrational Energy

Many New Age philosophies believe that even if your diet is good, and you exercise regularly, you may still have no energy if the energy either around you or in your home or workplace is not right. They seek to address the non-physical, or spiritual dimension of energy, and I have included some of them in this book in order to provide the most rounded and holistic approach possible to improving your energy levels.

**Crystals** For thousands of years crystals have been used for their powers. Buddhist monks carved crystal balls out of quartz and claimed they were the gem of enlightenment. These days people use crystals for their healing qualities. They may be held, worn and placed strategically around the home or office.

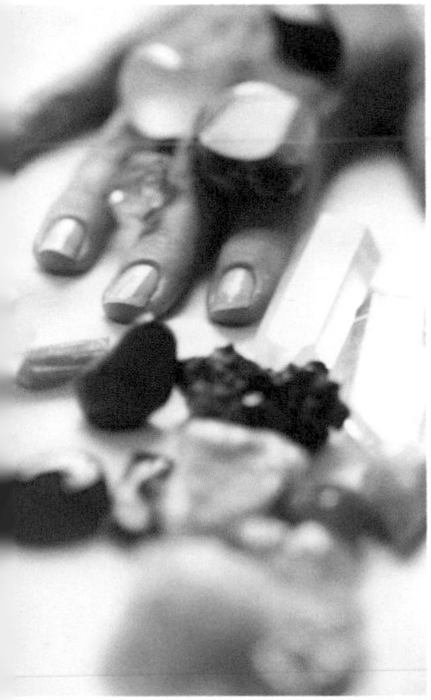

People who work with crystals say that if you work or live around a lot of electrical equipment you will start to feel irritable, low and fatigued and will possibly suffer from increasing health complaints. They say that placing quartz crystals around and on items such as computers or televisions helps to absorb some of the negative energy that they emit.

Crystals store energy from their places of origin and many have been known to have properties to help alleviate ailments such as fatigue, depression and stress. If they are kept clean and programmed they can be very invigorating whether they are used in the home or during a treatment from an experienced healer. Crystals are believed to give off positive healing energies to rebalance our bodies as they match the energy of the human aura.

Crystals generate, store and give off electromagnetic energy. Each one has its own particular energy that has a specific healing effect on mind, body and spirit. Quartz, for example, is known to generate small amounts of piezoelectricity which is used to power computers, and in healing terms it is used help you to think more clearly and speed up healing. Amber is more calming and helps with depression, while moonstone helps balance hormones and emotions, ruby helps build the blood and tiger's eye is good for beating tiredness.

If you think that you might like to wear a crystal, quartz is a good choice as it will help to keep your mind clear. However, if you find that you are particularly drawn to another type of crystal you will probably find that it is an important and relevant one to you.

## THE COLOURS OF AN AURA

**These are basic guidelines:**

| | |
|---|---|
| **Purple/violet:** | spiritual, religious, idealistic |
| **Indigo:** | inspiration, wisdom, sensitive, spiritual |
| **Blue:** | intellectual, intelligent, rational and logical thinker, intuitive |
| **Turquoise:** | dynamic, energetic, good organiser, communicator, likes to influence others |
| **Green:** | calm, balanced, kind, caring, gentle (dark green = deceit or jealousy) |
| **Yellow:** | happy, loving, full of vitality, compassionate, optimistic (dull yellow = suspicion) |
| **Orange:** | full of vitality, warm, generous, powerful, inspirational (too much orange = pride) |
| **Gold:** | well balanced, kind, generous, great spiritual leader |
| **Red:** | physical, ambitious, sensual, high sex drive (cloudy red = violent tendencies) |
| **Pink:** | true romantic, modest, shy, gentle |
| **Brown:** | unsettled, materialistic, negative or just in a bad mood |
| **Grey:** | depressed, afraid, full of morbid thoughts, low energy |
| **Black:** | deep-rooted problems (murky black = depression, anxiety, fear, illness or drugs) |
| **White:** | illness or drug abuse |

**The aura** The aura is a subtle energy that vibrates around everyone's body. Understanding auras is a key to understanding why, for example, just being around someone with an overpowering aura or personality can leave you lacking in energy.

Seeing and sensing auras gives you a unique insight into how people are feeling both physically and emotionally and interacting with others becomes much more productive. The aura cannot lie; if you feel uncomfortable around someone your aura will shrink away from them; if someone is aggressive or overpowering their aura can take over yours; if you are happy with someone your auras will meet or even merge into one.

**Seeing auras** Start by looking at the aura of a healthy tree. Look up at a tree, preferably on a clear day, and let your eyes drift slightly out of focus. You will begin to notice a faint shimmer around the tree. Do the same thing with plants against a white wall: first look at a healthy plant and compare it with one that is dying. Look at animals too and then start practising on friends, preferably against a white wall. You can also practise any time, anywhere, while in a queue, at work, on a train, in class. You can also assess your own aura by looking at yourself in a mirror.

Once you get used to seeing the aura you will notice different colours in it. If the colour is bright and clear then it usually means the person is healthy and happy. Dirty dark colours tend to mean physical illness, tiredness or an emotional problem. A flash of colour can indicate an emotion that is out of control.

**Chakras** Understanding your chakras will help you to understand your own energy. Chakras are monitors of our physical and mental wellbeing and each one relates to a particular area of the body. Your chakras spin at different frequencies. If each one spins at the correct frequency you will feel centred, energised and will radiate perfect health. Blocks in energy, however, will prevent a chakra from vibrating as it should and ill health and fatigue will result. These blocks can be cleared by visualisations, healing and exercises such as yoga which, in turn, will lead to you feeling more energised physically, emotionally and spiritually.

In Sanskrit chakra means wheel or vortex. It is a spinning wheel that takes in energy and feeds all the other areas of the physical and subtle body on a physical, emotional and spiritual level. There are seven major chakras, each of which has its own location and emotions, organs, colours, sound and level of consciousness associated with it. The chakras run in a line up the middle of the body and head and send energy along channels known as nadis. There are 72,000 nadis in the body.

The chakras emanate energy away from the body forming what is known as the aura (see previous page) which can be seen by some people as a coloured light that surrounds the body. Many healers work with their patients' chakras and aura and are able to see how a person is feeling both physically and emotionally from looking at the colours and vibrations of their electrical field of energy (the aura).

Your lower chakras relate to your more earthbound emotional states and the higher ones to your spiritual states. Your chakras are always either open or blocked; if they are closed you are dead! A blocked chakra takes in less prana (energy) resulting, as we know, in ill health and fatigue; if it is too open it will take in more energy than you are able to cope with making you feel overwhelmed.

### The seven chakras

**1** Muladhara: the root/base chakra

**2** Swadhishthana: the navel/sacral chakra

**3** Manipura: the solar plexus chakra

**4** Anahata: the heart chakra

**5** Vishuddha: the throat chakra

**6** Ajna: the third eye chakra

**7** Sahasrara: the crown chakra

### The chakra balance

**1** Stand with your feet hip width apart and imagine you have a rope from the centre of the top of your head up to the sky keeping you upright.

**2** Make sure your body is relaxed and close your eyes and concentrate on your breathing.

**3** Imagine that above your head there is a shimmering ball of violet energy and that you are breathing into it.

**4** Imagine that you are breathing in from the violet shimmering ball of energy and when you breathe out the energy moves through your body down to your feet where it exits into the earth.

**5** Repeat five times.

**6** Imagine another ball of dark red energy pulsating at a steady beat. Breathe into this red ball of energy and as you breathe in take the red energy up your feet and through the base of your spine, up to the top of your head.

**7** Repeat five times.

**8** Stand still for a minute and allow your breathing to come back to normal and slowly open your eyes.

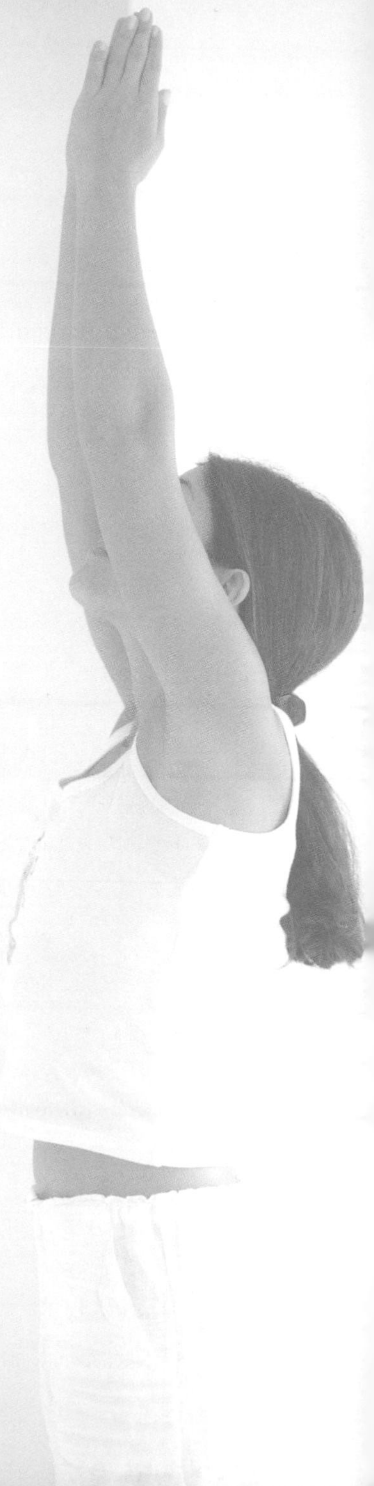

**1 The root/base chakra**

COLOUR: RED

Location: base of spine

Emotion: anchor and foundation, being in real material world, grounded in the here-and-now, will to live and wanting to be alive

Physical: adrenal system, lower bowel and system of elimination

Element : earth vibrates to a solid dense frequency

Blocked: lacking in energy, weak constitution, a feeling of being depersonalised, feel like you are not really here, live in your head, daydream, fear of letting go and opening up to your creativity

Too open: very materialistic, not spiritual

Balanced: able to accept yourself, secure, confident, lots of self-esteem, good health, lots of energy and enthusiasm for life

Healing: in order to balance this chakra it is good to do things like visualisations, for example, breathing in red light, filling your whole body with red light, imagining you are growing red roots etc. Meditation is not so good for this chakra but is better for balancing the upper chakras. It is vital to have your root chakra balanced (like the roots of a tree). Any activity that puts you in contact with the earth or helps you feel rooted in the here-and-now of the material world is good e.g. walking (especially barefoot), gardening, dancing, pottery, as is wearing red clothes below the waist (pants, trousers, skirt).

**2 The navel/sacral chakra**

COLOUR: ORANGE

Location: between the lower abdomen and navel

Emotion: creation of life, sensual energy and sexual relations

Physical: reproductive system: ovaries, uterus, testicles and prostrate, vaginal and pelvic infections, PMS, endometriosis, male infertility, fatigue

Element: water

Blocked: a disruption in your sexual relationships

Too open: envy, lust, fear, confusion, overdependence on partner

Balanced: a balance between the male and female energy (ha and tha or yin and yang), independent and whole, good sexual relationships

Healing: trust, enjoy all your senses, visualisations including all the senses, for example, smelling something nice, seeing something energising, feeling something, hearing water etc. Breathe in orange light. Pelvic tilts are good as is wearing orange from the waist downwards.

### 3 The solar plexus chakra

COLOUR: YELLOW

Location: around the solar plexus

Emotion: centre for your major emotions, wants, desires, ego and ambitions; it is where your sense of 'I am' comes from

Physical: pancreas, stomach gall bladder, spleen and small intestine, digestive disorders and eating disorders, hypoglycaemia, chronic fatigue, diabetes, pancreatic problems, indigestion, irritable bowel. Your solar plexus is your true energy centre as you get your stamina from digesting food. This is why the right food is very important for helping you to beat tiredness.

Element: fire

Blocked: selfish and unfeeling, lack of willpower and drive, depressed, exhausted and stressed

Too open: over-emotional, greedy, angry, aggressive, always looking after other peoples feelings instead of your own, over-submissive, passive, powerless which can lead to resentment and exhaustion

Balanced: feel centred, flexible not rigid, happy, warm, confident, good sense of humour, spontaneous, playful, able to express emotions

Healing: You need to learn to separate your own emotions and responsibilities from other people's. Do not block your feelings and be open to new experiences and adventures, take risks, ground yourself. Do stress management techniques such as yoga and meditation. Visualise a mirror between you and anyone who you think might drain you of energy for examplc if they are depressed and moaning to you, or very angry. Breathe gold sunlight into your solar plexus and then emanate it around the rest of your body.

### 4 The heart chakra

COLOUR: GREEN

Location: in the heart/chest

Emotion: joy and sadness, love, harmony and compassion, intimacy

Physical: blood and circulation, heart, lungs, breasts, thymus

Element: air

Blocked: difficulty in keeping up a loving relationship, detached, cold, reserved, short of breath, heart problems, immune system problems, asthma

Too open: too sensitive and worried about other people's needs till you become exhausted

Balanced: compassionate, loving, empathetic, peaceful, balanced

Healing: any exercise that helps to open the chest area. Surround yourself with nature and physical touch from loved ones. Visualise the colour green or pink pouring into the heart chakra and then emanating around the rest of your body.

### 5 The throat chakra

COLOUR: BLUE

Location: in the throat

Emotion: how you communicate and express yourself to the outside world

Physical: thyroid gland, throat and voice, ears, neck, tightness of the jaw and endocrine system

Blocked: problems with words, speak quietly, sarcastic, cynical, hostile, tiredness from not speaking your mind and trying to be someone that you are not, asthma, hyperventilation, bronchitis, hypothyroidism, throat problems, mouth ulcers and hearing problems

Too open: talkative, dominate conversations without saying anything of value

Balanced: interact with the world with

communication, talking, listening and reading, express your true feelings clearly

Healing: need to use your voice, singing, chanting, humming or shouting, sound therapy and voice work, meditation, massage

### 6 The third eye chakra

COLOUR: INDIGO BLUE

Location: in the forehead between the eyebrows

Emotion: imagination and concentration, spirituality

Physical: eyes, brain and nervous system, pineal and pituitary glands, hypothalamus

Blocked: tiredness and mental fatigue, headaches, learning difficulties, negative thinking, poor concentration, confusion, delusions, psychosis

Too open: anxiety, clairvoyant

Balanced: creative, intuitive, good at visualising

Healing: painting and drawing, write down dreams, meditation, alternate nostril breathing

### 7 The crown chakra

COLOUR: VIOLET AND WHITE

Location: in the cerebral cortex of the brain

Emotion: open-minded, thoughtful and wise, analyse and assimilate information, cynical, greedy and materialistic, intellectual, live in your head, lost touch with body

Physical: upper brain, pituitary and pineal glands

Blocked: depression, difficult to accept life, trapped in your body, no spiritual connection or direction making you feel drained and exhausted

Too open: too spiritual and unable to relate to the real world, anxiety and fear

Balanced: acceptance and peace

Healing: meditation, open to new ideas and information, look into spirituality/religion, physical exercise, massage, gardening.

The chakras in the lower half of the body create energy for the physical body and sensations to do with it whereas those located in the upper half are associated with spiritual and emotional energy.

## A Shamanic visualisation for increasing energy

**1** Close your eyes and concentrate on your breathing.

**2** Imagine that a huge and powerful eagle is in front of you looking at you with his all-seeing eye. Nod and thank him for allowing you to have his sharp far-sighted vision

**3** Now imagine a huge bear behind you. Turn and look into her eyes and notice her strength and weight and claws; she is very protective and will protect your back Thank her for her powerful presence behind you.

**4** To your right a coyote is sniffing, his tongue hanging out as if he were laughing. He is smart and quick and good at negotiating. He can help in any difficult situation but don't let him become too clever for his own good.

**5** On your left you see a buffalo, solid and dependable making you feel grounded and stable.

**6** Say thank you to your guardians (to follow tradition offer them a pinch of tobacco or cornmeal.

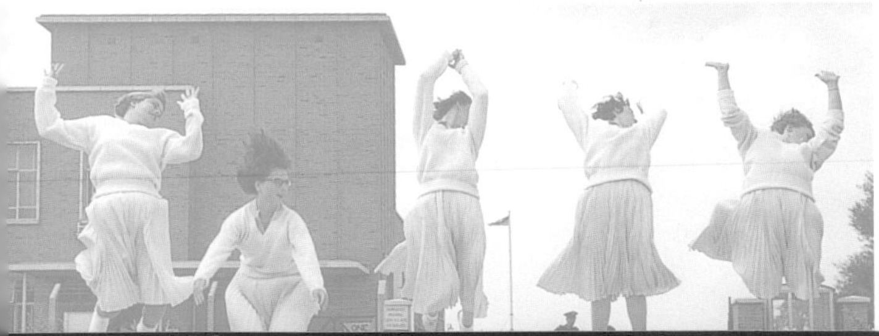

## Energy in relationships

Just as we need the energy to flow smoothly in our homes and bodies we also need it to flow smoothly in our relationships with other people. Relationships are a vital part of our lives and can be a huge source of energy or energy depletion.

Communication and interaction with people can be exhilarating, stimulating and energising. Sex is energising and it has been found that people who have a regular sex life live longer and are happier and healthier than those who don't. However, some relationships can also cause a lot of stress especially those with a partner as they can cause emotions such as jealousy, suspicion, mistrust, resentment, misunderstanding, anger, sadness, fear, depression and guilt. Small amounts of stress that can later be resolved through an argument are normal, but constant stress is draining, depressing and robs you of energy.

Most of us have noticed that different people have different effects on your energy levels: some seem to zap and drain your energy, while others seem to boost it. Obviously it is best for you to surround yourself as much as possible with people who boost your energy, encourage you and are positive toward you and your life.

Sometimes though, a relationship with a friend or family member or partner may still be very important to you and even though they drain you of all your energy, it is simply not possible to stop seeing a particular person.

In such cases it is vital at least to acknowledge that that person has this effect on you so that you can protect yourself and perhaps not see them on days when you feel particularly exhausted. When you do see them, try to imagine that you are in a protective bubble that they cannot get through, or imagine a mirror between the two of you that reflects their energy back at them.

If someone makes you very angry, instead of holding on to the anger which will later create a block in your energy try some of these techniques to let the anger out:

- go for a walk and, making sure that no one is around, shout at the top of your voice
- get a pillow and punch it with all the anger you feel instead of bottling it up
- write down what you feel either in a diary or a letter that you will never send to someone who has made you very angry
- stamp your feet while making a loud noise repeatedly until you feel better.

## Express yourself

Body workers have found that repressed emotions are stored in different parts of the body. For example, problems with your throat, jaw and mouth are due to not being able to say what you feel or not being heard. If we try to hold on to all the emotions, whether good or bad, from our past and present it is no wonder that it is hard for our energy to circulate and be at its optimum. Expressing your feelings is very important in terms of how much energy you have. Next time you see someone who is very angry or upset imagine how much energy it must take to hide their emotions away, or to keep pushing them down pretending that everything is fine. Pretending to be something or somebody that you are not is exhausting.

## Keeping energy in a relationship

- Try to pick people who energise and encourage you.
- Keep your sense of self and self-esteem (don't let others take over, dominate and engulf you; make sure you keep your own life and make your own decisions).
- Keep communicating: if you don't keep talking things through that are bothering you in a

relationship they can feel and get bigger causing you to worry and zapping your energy.

- Don't take each other for granted; try to remember what it was that you first saw in your partner.
- If things seem to have been wrong between you for a long time and you are finding it hard to resolve them, go to a relationship counsellor together.

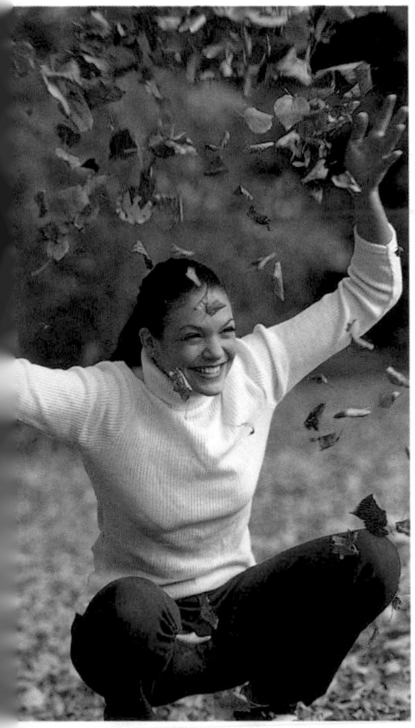

## Happiness

Happiness means different things for different people, but there is one thing that is true of everyone: when you experience what you feel is happiness, you are energised. If you are not happy with your life you will not function well. Negative emotions can reduce energy and positive emotions increase it. So by making yourself feel happy you can help to build your energy.

You can practise being happy by reacting to your day in a positive and cheerful way. Think of things that made you happy today and schedule them into your day tomorrow. Don't wait for happiness to come to you: engineer it. If you can't pinpoint what makes you happy try keeping a mood diary and write down things that made you happy, for example a chat to a stranger on the train, watching a good movie, spending time with a friend, painting, buying something for yourself.

### A few tips to keep you feeling happy:

- Remember to count your blessings regularly, and to think of the positive aspects of your life.
- Compare yourself to people who are less fortunate than you.
- Spend time with people who make you feel good and happy.
- Appreciate your surroundings.
- Watch out for moments of happiness, however brief.
- Don't indulge in self pity.
- Always try to keep a positive frame of mind.
- Try not to blame your problems on others.
- Exercise regularly (see pages 100–41) as exercise releases endorphins in your brain which make you feel happy.
- Find at least one thing a day that made you feel happy today or will make you feel happy tomorrow.

## Feng shui

Feng shui is the ancient Chinese art and science of placement and the main concept behind it is energy flow: feng shui sees your home and surroundings as acupuncture sees your body, and feng shui practitioners actually treat your home as an extension of your body. If the energy flow in your home is smooth and harmonious you will reap the benefits. If your home is very cluttered the flow of energy will be upset: where there is clutter the energy becomes stuck eventually leaving a pile of stagnant energy. Not only will it make you feel tired and possibly unwell, you will also find that things will become 'stuck' in your life and you might end up feeling very frustrated. Below right is a simple feng shui map. Place it over a map of your house, in line with the door, to work out the location of each corresponding area. You many find that a particular area is cluttered, which can cause a blockage in the corresponding energy.

So start chucking. Remove, give away, sell or throw away anything that has not been worn or used in the past year. Hoarding stops new things from coming in; you need to make space so that new energy and new things in life are able to enter. Once you have de-cluttered, have a good clean, open all the doors and windows and allow fresh air to circulate once again. Try burning some sage or other essential oils too.

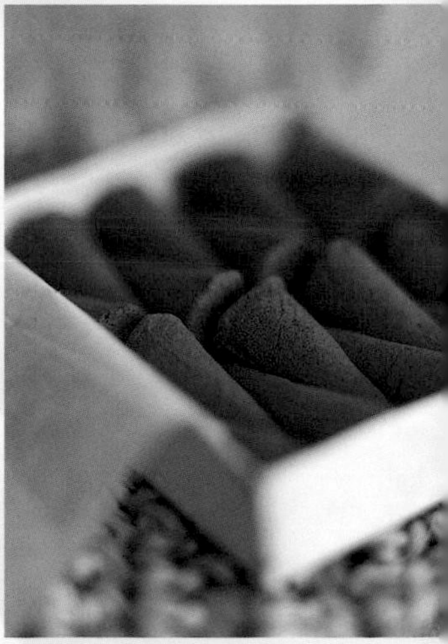

Your home should be your sanctuary giving you the strength and stability to go out and face the world. Natural light is essential for health and energy. Basement flats, homes on low ground surrounded by hills or tall trees tend to deplete energy and can make you feel depressed as there is not enough light. We need to take energy into account when decorating, choosing lighting, positioning beds and furniture. Sharp corners, for example, and angular lines can make us feel restless. Even the position of the building itself can be significant, and in China buildings are placed according to precise energetic rules.

| | | |
|---|---|---|
| **Money** | **Success** | **Relationships** |
| **Elders** | **Unity** | **Creativity** |
| **Knowledge** | **Career** | **Helpful Friends** |

← **DOOR** →

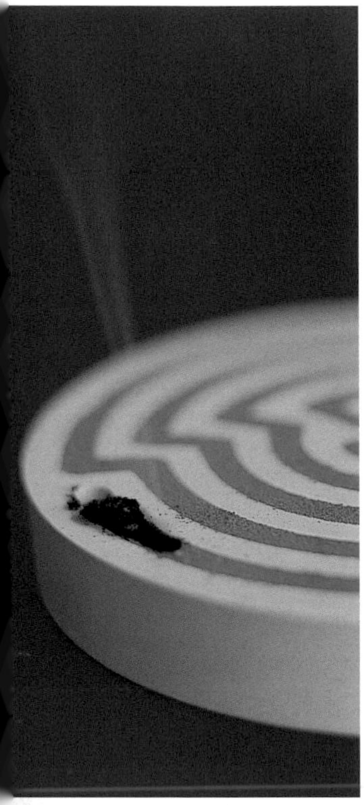

However, you don't need to be a trained feng shui practitioner to know if a house or room feels good to be in. The atmosphere in a house soaks up the energy of the people in it, so if a couple have been arguing, angry and unhappy in a house, their negative energy will be left behind like rubbish. Equally, we have all been to places where it's hard to leave as the atmosphere feels so calming and safe.

### Feng shui in the workplace

Here are a few guidelines to help you feel energised and productive at work.

- Never have your back to the door when you are sitting down – always have your desk either facing the door or preferably diagonally opposite the door. This gives you the best energy for control, authority and concentration. If for some reason you can't change the position that your desk is in and your back has to face the door then put a mirror up so that you can see people coming in to the room.
- Plants help to keep the energy clean and they can also take away the radiation effects of your computer. Make sure you look after them though.
- Always try to have fresh flowers on your desk as they stimulate mental activity as well as cleaning the atmosphere.
- Try burning a small candle or night light while you work as it helps to bring the energy of fire into the room to help enliven your own energy.

## SPACE CLEARING

Many ancient cultures have traditions of space clearing in order to move energy around houses. The Chinese have the feng shui system, the Indian culture has vastu shastra, the native American culture has smudge ceremony, the Balinese have bell ringing and flower offering ceremonies. All of these can be used to shift energy in your home. Even here in the West we have space-clearing techniques: ringing church bells on wedding days or on Sundays – clearing the air with the sound; burning incense in church or homes to cleanse the air; spring cleaning after winter (a time of hoarding).

- Try burning rosemary oil for concentration, bergamot to uplift you and citrus oil. You could use lavender if you are feeling very stressed.
- A clear quartz crystal on your desk will also help you to feel more focused and energised and can help to remove the radiation effects of your computer.
- Your attitude affects the energy of the work you do: if you are negative and bored of your work that is all it will give back to you, whereas if you are stimulated and energised by your work you will leave work at the end of each day feeling great.

### Simple remedies to help move energy

- Use an ioniser or a salt crystal to take away the positive ions which can make you feel tired and irritable. A bowl of fresh water does the same but remember to change it regularly or it will become stagnant.
- Use oils to help lift the energy of the house, for example peppermint, lemon and lemongrass or lavender for relaxing, or geranium for lifting the spirits.
- Wind chimes help to move energy.
- Pets and flowers are living energy in the house but remember to throw dead flowers away. Spider

## CLEARING RITUALS

- Clapping: clap around each corner of the room, starting at the floor and going up as high as you can. The sound might sound dull first and then should become clearer. Energy gets stuck in corners and alcoves.
- Smudging: you can buy smudge sticks (usually sage, cedar, sweetgrass) or make your own. Light the smudge stick and blow it out so that it is smoking. You can clean your aura or other people's by blowing smoke around them. Then smudge the corners of the rooms. Incense can also clean energy though smudging is more powerful.
- Bells and drums: use of sound for cleansing is very common. Go around your house using an instrument to make a noise or you can use your voice.

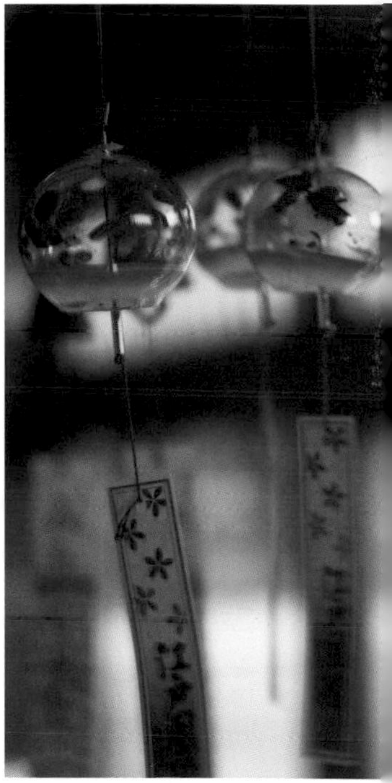

plants positioned near a computer help to soak up the radiation and ionise the air.

- A well-lit home helps to reflect the energy around the room and light up dark corners that would otherwise create a space where energy can become stuck.
- Mirrors are also good to reflect energy where it is missing in, for example, a room where a corner is cut off.

## Colours in the home

You can change the energy in your home by changing the colours of your walls – even splashes of colour help to energise areas of the house that may need it. Some people suggest that if you have two floors or more, that the downstairs should be decorated in reds, oranges and yellows. Blues are good for bedrooms and bathrooms and violets and indigos are good for bedrooms especially on the top floor.

Red is very good for increasing the energy but don't overdo it as it can be overpowering. A few red pillows and a red throw can help bring more passion into a relationship. Orange brings joy and confidence and sociability (good for entertaining rooms). Yellow lifts the spirits and helps to raise the energy which is good for many rooms in the house like the kitchen, hall living rooms and bathrooms and for rooms where you need to work as it stimulates the left side of the brain. Green helps to balance and is soothing and calming (good for troubled teenagers). Blue is relaxing and peaceful, promotes rest and helps good communication so it is a good colour to use in an office at home. In the bedroom blue can promote a good night's rest.

## Balance the elements in your home

FIRE

(= red and vibrant colours)

A real fire brings vibrant energy into the house as well as warmth, strength and peace. If you do not have a real fire you can use candles or crystals that can be hung in the windows to reflect the sunlight into your home. Mirrors serve the same purpose.

EARTH

(= browns and fawn, terracotta and brick)

Earth is grounding and strengthening. It helps us to feel stable and certain of our direction in life. Salt can be put around a room or even your bed to help earth you. Crystals can also help.

WATER

(= sea colours and river beds, very artistic with lots of paintings and clutter)

Water is purifying, cleansing and helps to rejuvenate. It is good for clearing a room of negative energies and emotions. An indoor waterfall is good to help keep the energy of the house clean, or if you can't have this a spring water mist spray is good if you want to clear the energy after an argument.

AIR

(= clean, airy, spacious, minimalist and cool)

Air transforms energy, so to enliven a room you can burn incense. Open the windows whenever you can and allow fresh air into the house even if it is only for a few minutes. Fans circulate air. And space, i.e. lack of clutter, gives a feeling of airiness; it makes you feel free with infinite possibilities.

## ENERGY CHECK LIST

In order to beat fatigue try to maintain the following:

- tune in to how you feel every day
- practise yoga postures regularly
- exercise regularly
- make sure you get some time to rest and relax as well as time for yourself
- check your posture regularly
- eat well and drink lots of water
- breathe well
- meditate for twenty minutes each day
- think positively

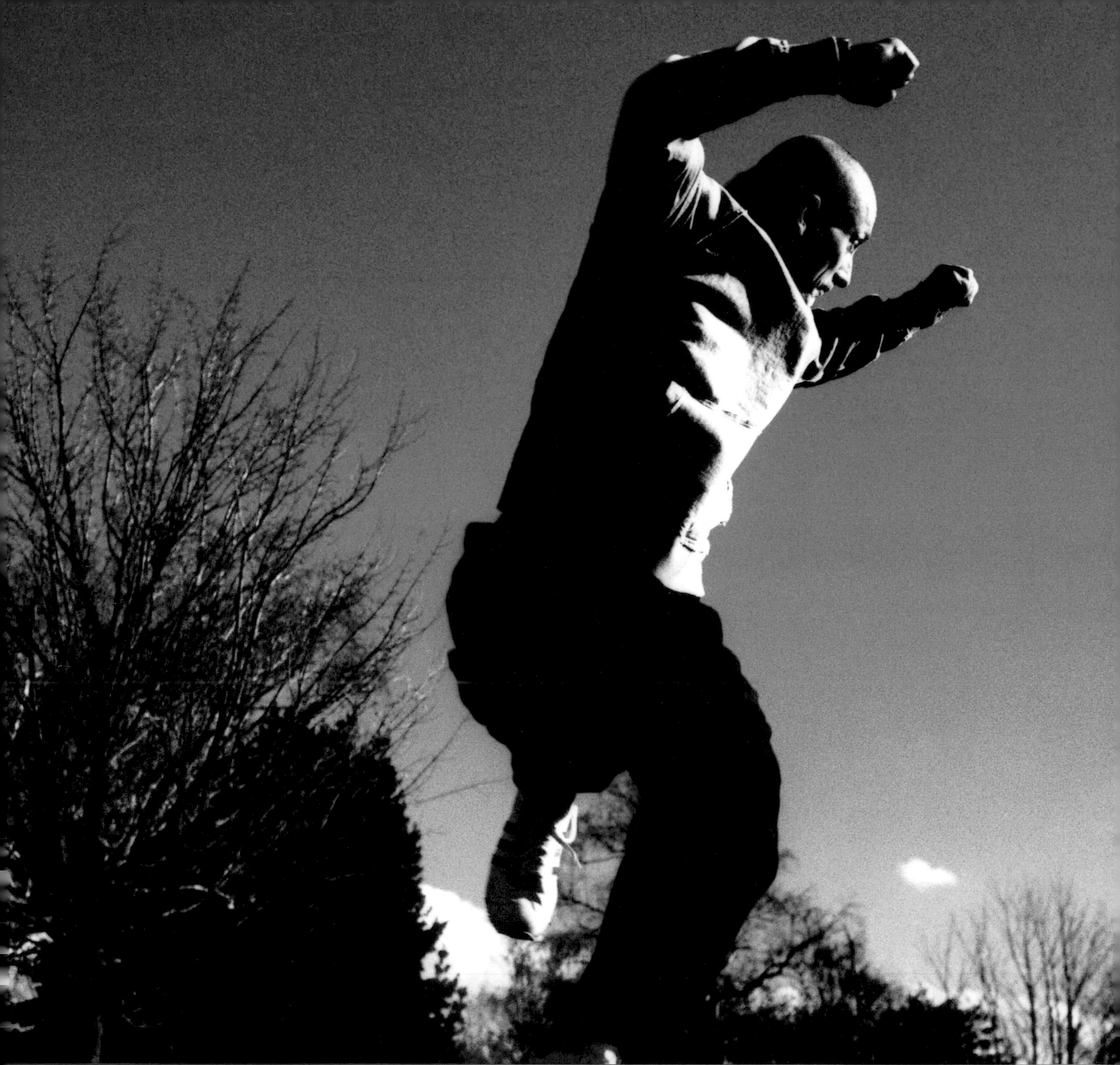

**CHAPTER 3**

# Energy Plans

*Having looked at what energy is, why we need it and how to increase it, let's now turn to some energy plans, especially designed to maximise your energy using many of the tools (therapies, diet, exercise and so on) discussed in the first two chapters. So, without further ado, let's turn the theory into practice.*

When doing any of the energy plans in this chapter it is a good idea to keep a diary of how you feel. Begin the diary a day or two before starting the plan and write down how you feel both physically and emotionally and anything else that you feel might be relevant. Keep the diary up throughout the plan and after. That way you can look back and be amazed at your progress.

## FOR BLOOD DEFICIENCY

If you are blood deficient, it is a good idea to include Floradix, iron and herbs and brewer's yeast in whichever energy plan you choose; likewise, shiitake and reishi mushrooms are particularly helpful for anyone who is run down.

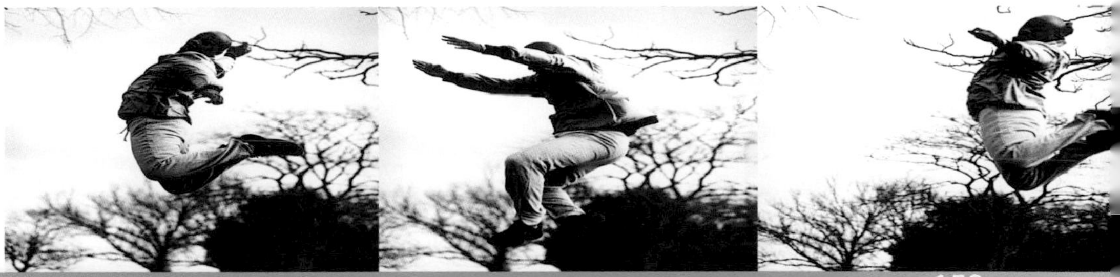

# The Seven-day Energy Plan

*This plan is specifically designed for anyone who has a heavy week ahead of them, or for people who feel that they do have energy but that they are not functioning to their optimum. If you lack energy most of the time then one of the longer plans would be more suited to you.*

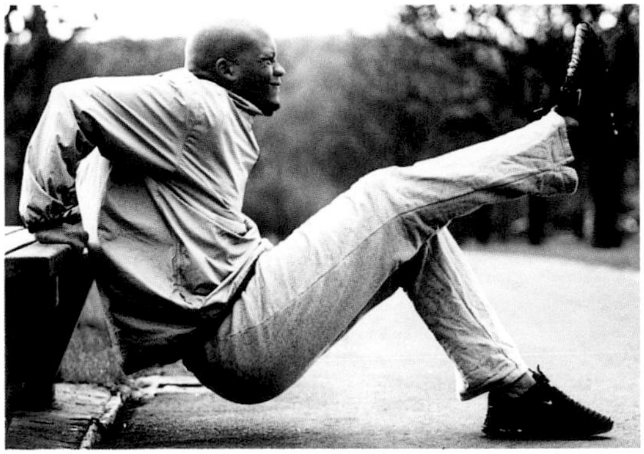

The 7-day plan is designed to provide a maximum energy boost in minimum time, so it is most effective if you can fit in all the elements every day. It consists of core features that you should do every day, with some optional extras to keep you going when you need an extra boost. You will get best results if you follow the daily routine to the letter. If, however, you miss out one or more elements on any one day, don't give up, but do as much as possible of the rest of the plan. You will still feel the difference in your energy levels.

The day before you start the plan, take the time to prepare everything. Plan your meals for the week ahead and go shopping for food, supplements and essential oils. You will find it much easier to stick to nutritious meals and snacks if you don't have to stop and plan before every mouthful. Set up the oil burner in the position you will be using it, or put the oil bottle next to the bathtub, check you have all the supplements you will be taking, and set the alarm for 15 minutes earlier than usual if you usually get up and rush out of the house in the morning without breakfast.

## The Daily Routine

- On rising, drink a glass of hot water and lemon juice to kick start your system
- Do skin-brushing (see page 168) before your shower or bath
- Burn 1–6 drops of invigorating grapefruit oil in a burner, or sprinkle into your bath
- Try to have a 30-second cold shower after your morning bath or shower. If 30 seconds is just too bracing to begin with, start with 10 seconds and build it up day by day.
- Do the Qi-gong slap (see page 112)
- For breakfast, choose one of the suggestions on page 165.
- Remember to take your supplements
- If you can, do the earth's energy visualisation (see page 78), for example on the train or bus on the way to work.
- Try to fit in a twenty-minute walk – by getting off the train or bus to work a couple of stops earlier than you normally do.
- By mid-morning, if you feel your energy flagging, do the standing yoga boost on page 135.
- Don't let yourself get too hungry – eat a snack from the list on page 170 and drink plenty of fresh water.
- At lunchtime, have one of the suggested lunches (see page 167). Most of the lunches can be quickly prepared from easily available ingredients and simply assembled at work or at home the night before.
- Go for a twenty-minute walk or cycle in your lunch hour if you haven't done so earlier in the day.
- On your way home, or when you get home, do the earth's energy visualisation if you did not do it in the morning.
- If you didn't fit twenty minutes' walk or cycle in earlier in the day, go for a walk before dinner.
- In the evening, have one of the suggested dinners (see page 171).
- Perform the foot massage on yourself, or persuade somebody else to (see page 57)
- Before going to bed, take a warm bath with a few drops of lavender oil sprinkled into it.
- In bed, or just before going to bed, do the exercise on page 80 to release the tension that has built up during the day.

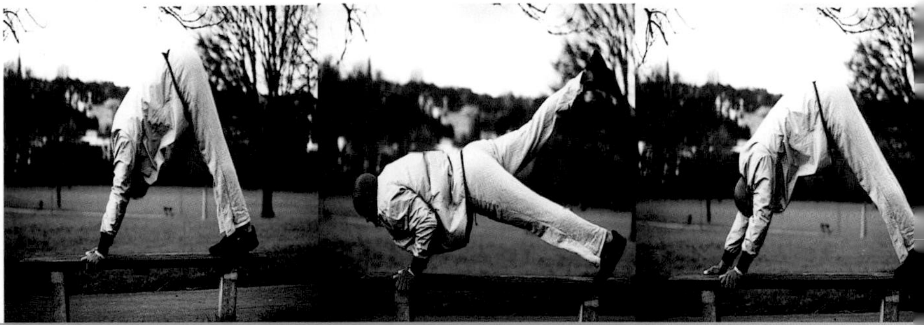

## Thirty-four-year-old female film-maker:

*'I have been tired ever since I left college about ten years ago. I guess I burned the candle at both ends: I worked very hard and went out lots; I also had a part-time job in a club which didn't close till 3 a.m. a couple of nights a week to help finance me through college. For the last six years I have been making films and still going out lots. It is a very stressful job though I do love it and wouldn't change it for the world, but the hours are hard and long and often I skip meals or eat while filming or very late.*

*I've tried to do different things to help my energy like taking ginseng, or even drinking lots of coffee; I know that isn't good for me but it gets me through the long days. When it is really busy I am sometimes so buzzing and full of energy that I can hardly sleep and I feel bad the next day. I realise that this is nervous energy and probably quite bad for me. Some people would probably describe me as always full of (nervous) energy.*

*Anyway I decided to do a seven-day plan as I had a big project ahead and had only just finished making a film a few days earlier. I was very tired and worried about being able to get through the next few weeks. I also had a week off so I thought this was going to be a good time to do it.*

# The 7-day plan

## Day 1

*Am very excited to be starting but am absolutely shattered. Miss my morning cups of coffee. Forgot to buy the stuff I needed for breakfast so cheated and had a bowl of Frosties. Will go buy food later.*

*Did the exercises and though I was dreading it, feel pretty good now. Also forgot to buy the vitamins. Ooops!*

## Day 2

*Felt tired still, have started vitamins – feels like a lot to take! Exercised and felt good afterwards again. Breakfast felt very healthy – almost forgot to take my vitamins later in the day but have found a little box to carry my daily quota in. Wanted wine but resisted.*

- If you sit down for a large part of the day, make an effort to take regular breaks – go outside for 5 minutes of fresh air, walk up and down the stairs, or even just walk round the office to fetch a glass of water.

## SUPPLEMENTS

DAY ONE and DAY TWO

- Vitamin C with bioflavonoids (1000mg, once a day)
- Multivitamin and mineral (as directed on the bottle)
- Vitamin B complex (100mg, 3 times a day with meals)
- Spirulina/blue-green algae (1 pill, 3 times a day)
- Royal jelly (2 capsules, 3 times a day)
- CoQ10 (60mg, 1 with a meal, daily)
- Bee pollen (sprinkle a few granules on your food, but stop using it if you get a rash or wheezing or any other allergic symptoms)

## EXAMPLES OF BREAKFASTS

- A bowl of fresh fruits and nuts and sunflower seeds served with natural bio yogurt
- Porridge made with hot water, chop some bananas in and sprinkle some wheatgerm on top
- Scrambled or poached eggs with smoked salmon and brown wholemeal toast
- Buckwheat pancakes with apple sauce and chopped bananas and nuts
- Muesli with lots of fruit and nuts with skimmed milk (add sunflower seeds and wheatgerm if you like)
- Boiled egg with wholemeal toasted soldiers
- Natural bio yogurt with seeds and nuts and fruit on top

## Day 3

*Still feel tired but not for so long; maybe it is just because I am sleeping more than usual. I do feel more relaxed with the relaxation exercises and I quite enjoyed the meditation. Went for a long walk today and felt great! Still find the vitamins a bit much but am doing them. Food is good. I thought I would have to eat carrot and mung beans all day!*

10 minutes' sun meditation (see page 78) will provide a quick boost whenever you need it.

## EXAMPLES OF LUNCHES

- Feta cheese, watercress, nuts, spinach and rocket salad
- Grilled chicken sandwich on mixed seed bread served with a mixed leaf salad
- Avocado and houmous and alfalfa sprout sandwich on rye bread with salad
- Butterbean and chickpea salad with couscous
- Houmous, tahini and falafel in pitta bread with a mixed leaf salad
- Grilled halloumi slices with rocket and sun-dried tomato salad sprinkled with pine nuts and sunflower seeds
- Goat's cheese salad with mixed leaves, pine nuts and sun-blushed tomatoes
- Beetroot and flageolet bean salad with barley
- Beetroot, chicory and walnut salad with couscous
- Salad of grated celeriac and carrots, with bean sprouts, sprinkled with walnuts
- Tabbouleh made with couscous or quinoa

## SUPPLEMENTS

DAY THREE and DAY FOUR

- Vitamin C with bioflavonoids (1000mg, twice a day)
- Multivitamin and mineral (as directed on the bottle)
- Vitamin B complex (100mg, 3 times a day with meals)
- Spirulina/blue-green algae (2 pills, 3 times a day)
- Royal jelly (2 capsules, 3 times a day)
- CoQ10 (60mg, 2 with a meal daily)
- Bee pollen (sprinkle a few granules on your food, but stop if you get a rash or wheezing or any other allergic symptoms)

## Day 4

*I think I am actually starting to feel pretty good. Am really enjoying the exercises and am going to try to continue when I have finished the plan to always do some exercise.*

Every morning before washing, use a pure bristle brush or loofah to dry-skin brush. Use small circular movements, and brush firmly up your arms and legs and body, always brushing in the direction of the heart.

## EVERY DAY

- Drink a glass of hot water and lemon on rising every day.
- Try to cut down on caffeine and if you do reach for it at least acknowledge that it is a time when you feel tired. If you drink a lot of caffeine I would not recommend giving it up completely for the 7-day plan as initially, when you withdraw from caffeine you feel more tired as you no longer have a stimulant pumping around your body.
- Drink lots of fresh water

## SUPPLEMENTS

- Some people say that they find it hard to remember to take supplements. If this is the case with you, try putting them by your toothbrush for the morning as you rarely forget to brush your teeth. Alternatively make it part of your meal-time routine to take out your supplements before you sit down to eat.
- Many people also feel that they don't like the idea of taking pills at all. If this is the case, you can get multivitamins and B complex in liquid form and vitamin C, blue green algae and spirulina are all available in powder form. Alternatively, some vitamins, such as C and B complex are relatively easy to find in a food source (see pages 94–5).

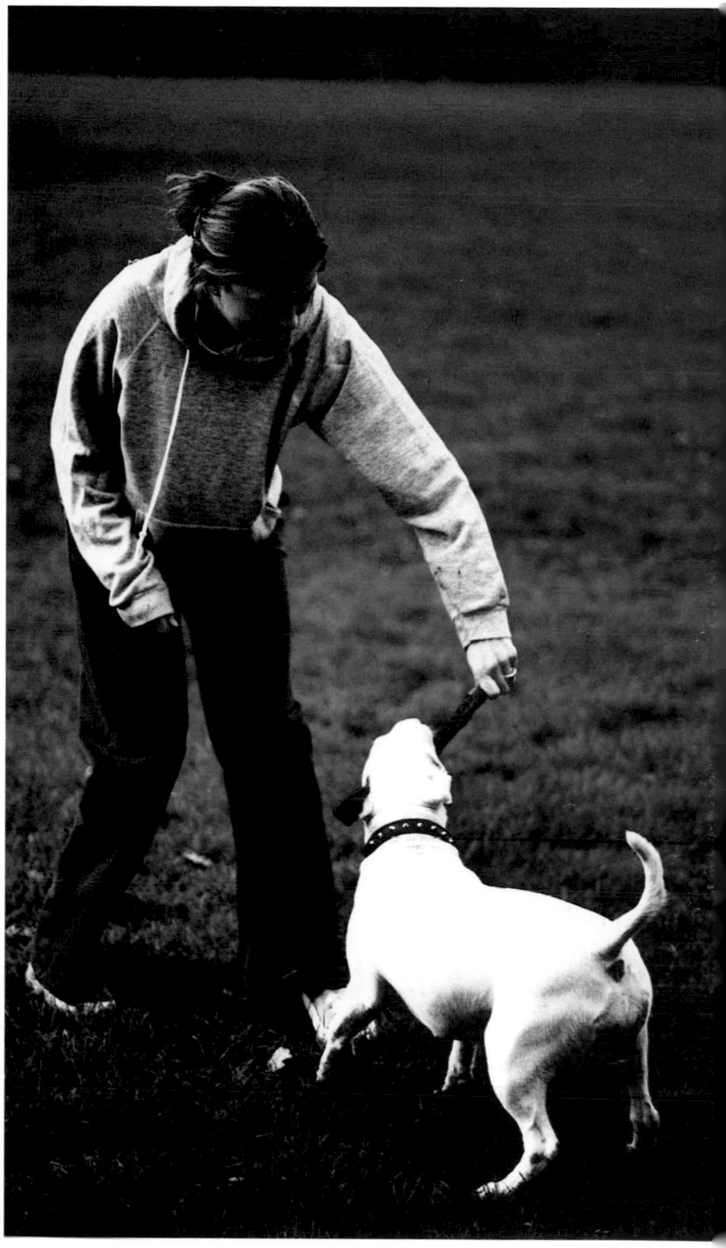

## Day 5

*Went out and drank a bit so feel a bit worse for wear but still did my exercises and felt better after it. Regret drinking; I was doing so well . . . oh well.*

### SNACKS AND DRINKS FOR EVERY DAY

- fresh fruit
- assorted bag of nuts and seeds
- bag of dried fruits, especially apricots, figs and dates
- houmous with carrot and celery sticks
- natural bio yogurt with seeds and nuts and fruit on top

## EXAMPLES OF DINNERS

- Baked potato with lentil dahl
- Stir-fried tofu and vegetables and pineapple served on a bed of brown rice
- Kebabs of marinated chicken, tofu or fish skewered with mushroom, fennel, courgette and peppers, served with rice or couscous and a green salad with avocado
- Grilled fish with steamed broccoli and spinach and baked fennel
- Warm chargrilled chicken salad with roasted parsnips and sesame seeds
- Mushroom and feta cheese omelette with Mediterranean vegetables
- Bean burger served with carrot, beetroot, buckwheat and raisin salad
- Mushroom pilaf made with brown rice sprinkled with parsley and cashew nuts
- Pumpkin pilaf made with brown rice sprinkled with parsley and pine nuts
- Barley risotto with artichoke hearts and feta cheese
- Stir fry of pak choi and shiitake mushrooms sprinkled with cashew nuts

## SUPPLEMENTS

DAY FIVE and DAY SIX

- Vitamin C with bioflavonoids (1000mg, 3 times a day)
- Multivitamin and mineral (as directed on the bottle)
- Vitamin B complex (100mg, 3 times a day with meals)
- Spirulina/blue-green algae (3 pills, 3 times a day)
- Royal jelly (2 capsules, 3 times a day)
- CoQ10 (60mg, 2 with a meal daily)
- Bee pollen (sprinkle 2 teaspoons on your food, but stop if you get a rash or wheezing or any other allergic symptoms)

## Day 6

*Back on track again. Feel good. Am in the routine of exercise, good diet, de-stressing etc. feels great and people are saying that I look a bit glowing.*

### DRINKS

- coconut, banana, pineapple and soya milk smoothie
- apricot, banana and almond milk smoothie
- freshly squeezed orange juice
- banana and date smoothie with wheatgerm sprinked on top
- apple and ginger juice
- peppermint tea
- orange, banana, pineapple and mint smoothie

## Day 7

*It wasn't so difficult. Can't believe it is seven days already. I might continue it for another seven days. I definitely feel like I have more energy and am quite relaxed too.*

**ADDITIONAL TREATMENTS**

- Work on acupressure points (see diagram on page 33), SP6, ST36, LIV3, GB34.

# The 30-day Energy Plan

*This plan is ideal for those people who have energy but would like to improve it, or people who normally feel energised but are feeling more tired than normal. It is also a good one to do if you know you have a heavy few weeks ahead of you, say before the festive season or if your workload is busier at certain times of the year than at others. If you are always tired the 60-day plan would be more appropriate for you than this one, but you can always start with this one if the longer plan seems too daunting.*

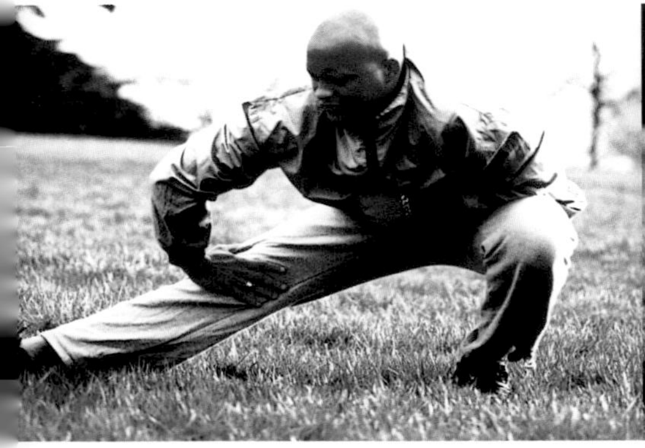

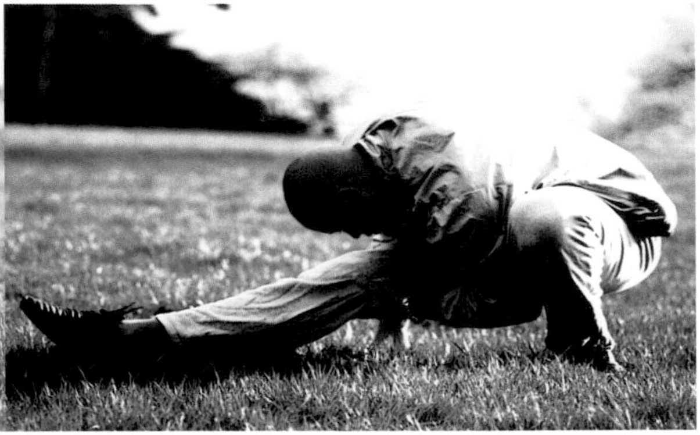

## Fifty-year-old business man

*My wife is always telling me I am an overweight couch potato – I think I'm alright although I do feel tired a lot of the time. I only agreed to do the plan because my wife and daughter bet me I'd never get through the whole month.*

*I nearly didn't make it past the first week – I had headaches and felt really tired, but I had been warned that I might feel like that due to the coffee and sugar withdrawal. So I carried on, but really only to win the bet! I did cheat a bit and didn't follow the plan 100% of the time but I did take the supplements..there's loads of them but I still take them, and I do the exercise, which I love – I'll definitely carry on with the supplements and exercise, if nothing else. I even eat better than I did before (I love cakes and biscuits and always used to have coffee and croissants for breakfast).*

*Everyone says I look great and loads of my friends have started the plan. I've lost weight and I have piles more energy, and I can't believe I don't drink coffee any more!*

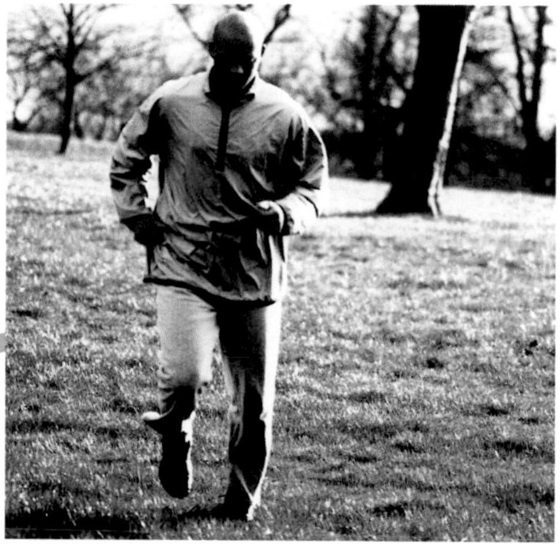

# Week 1

## Diet

If yours is a typical Western diet that is high in animal protein and fats, refined produce and additives and low in fresh natural plant foods it would be a good idea to detox (see page 179).

A week's detox programme will rid the body of all the residue from the junk food you've consumed. It will also help to reduce your sugar cravings and salt intake, and increase your intake of B vitamins (which will help you to relax) and fibre which will help the digestive process and speed up the elimination of toxins and waste matter.

You might feel slightly more tired during the first few days of detox as the toxins start to come out, but after a week you should feel calmer, brighter, more clear-headed and maybe even have a little bit more energy. (It does take at least a week as a lot of toxins lie in the fat.) With a cleaner body you will have a firmer foundation on which to build and really get to work on increasing your energy.

Eat three meals a day, as varied as possible, eating only enough to satisfy the appetite and no more. If you overeat you will not only build up toxic waste from undigested food but also become tired from the strain on the digestive system. Drink two and a half litres of water, herbal drinks or green tea, and try to be as relaxed as possible (relaxation exercises will help you to do this).

## Examples of daily menus

**1** Hot water and lemon on rising

Breakfast: fresh fruit salad with nuts and seeds and a green tea

Lunch: large salad with avocado and lots of nuts and seeds and a carrot and apple and ginger juice

Dinner: fresh salmon, poached, with broccoli, green beans, large portion of brown rice, and lots of garlic and a chamomile tea

**2** Hot water and lemon on rising

Breakfast: rye bread with mashed banana and a green tea

Lunch: lentil and carrot soup, wholemeal bread and a green leafy salad

Dinner: brown rice with roasted vegetables and pine nuts and a glass of cranberry juice

**3** Hot water and lemon on rising

Breakfast: half a melon with sunflower seeds and a banana and apple smoothie

Lunch: baby spinach, watercress, peppers, tofu and rocket salad served with rice or rye bread

Dinner: lentil shepherd's pie and green leafy salad with roasted sesame seeds and a fresh mint tea

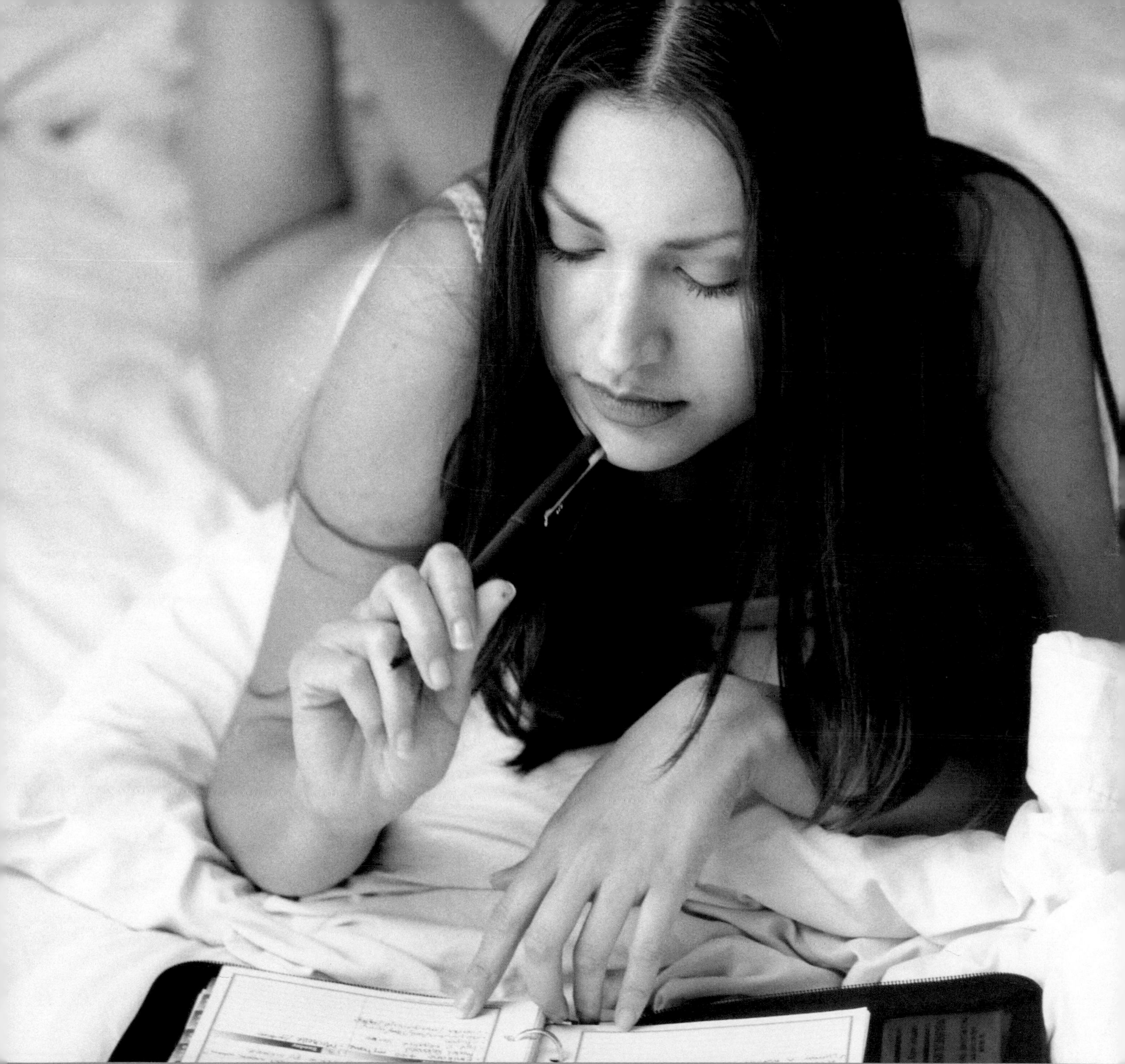

## Supplements to start you off on the energy plan

(See box opposite for detoxing supplements)

- Multivitamin and mineral (as directed on the bottle)
- Vitamin B complex (as directed on the bottle)

## Exercise

- Every morning do the windmill (page 105) and the qi gong slap (page 112) or energy sweep (see page 118)
- Three times a week do warm-up exercise, walking and cool-down exercise (see page 103), or at least one other cardio' workout from the list on page 101
- Try to do yoga postures every day or on the days that you aren't doing cardio'. (Remember to do warm up exercise before and cool down after)

## Energy boosts at work

- Do as many of these as you feel you need or can fit into your working day:
- Standing yoga stretch, and stretch at desk (see page 134)
- Relax any time, anywhere exercise and stressbuster (see page 79)
- Do ease the tension, and private release of tension (see page 80)

## Self-help and treatments

- For this week just do massage with the essential oils to help aid detoxification (see box right)
- Dry skin brushing (see page 168) followed by a cold invigorating shower for thirty seconds
- Do the posture exercises: standing, sitting, chest stretch and spinal stretch (see page 137)
- Do the breathing exercises: alternate nostril breathing and breathing the yoga way (see page 122–23)

## Relaxation and visualisations

- Every night do the Relaxing the tension exercise before bed routine (see page 73)
- Do the breath meditation once a day either in the morning, at midday or when you get back from work (see page 76)

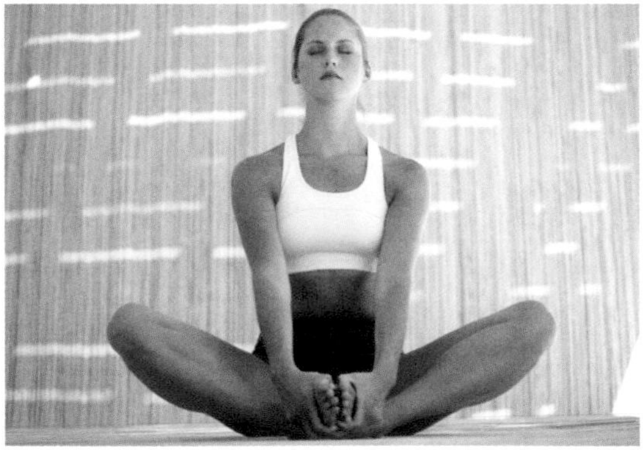

## DETOX

### Here are some of the dos and don'ts of detox:

Eat lots of: whole grains especially brown rice, leafy green vegetables, broccoli, peppers, onions, garlic, raw salads, celery, greens, cucumber, herbs, apples, pears, orange-fleshed melon, nuts and seeds (especially walnuts, brazil nuts, sunflower and pumpkin seeds), pure water, herbal drinks and green tea.

Eat some: fresh fish (not shellfish), especially mackerel, herring, trout or tuna, unsmoked organic tofu, olive oil, root vegetables, avocado, bananas, cherries, kiwi, other fruit and vegetable juices, puréed brown lentils, organic pure vinegars.

Avoid: animal foods, dairy produce, salt, sugar, refined produce, alcohol, processed foods, high salt foods, caffeine, non-organic foods and drink.

Note: all foods should be organic and as fresh as possible, eaten lightly cooked or raw.

### Supplements to speed up detox

- aloe vera (one capful a day)
- milk thistle tincture/capsules (15 drops, 3 times a day/300mg a day)
- fresh herbs: dandelion, nettle, parsley and rosemary and thyme – chop up and make an infusion to drink once or twice a day

### Treatments

- lymphatic drainage massage by a professional MLD (manual lymphatic drainage) practitioner as the lymph massage helps to get rid of toxins, and/or
- you can also self-massage essential oils into the skin after a bath to help the lymphatic system to work more efficiently (use peppermint, orange and sandalwood oils in a base oil)
- dry skin brushing (see page 168) to help keep circulation moving and to help the lymphatic system to get rid of toxins, followed by a cold invigorating shower for thirty seconds.

# Week 2

## Diet

Now that your body is cleaner your are really ready to start building your energy. The seven-day plan menus (see pages 160–73) are a template for how you should be eating to increase your energy. After trying them you can make up your own meals based on what you have learnt so far.

### Here's a brief summary:

- Unlimited fresh fruits and vegetables (not potatoes/sweet potatoes)
- Lots of water to drink (ideally around two and a half litres per day)
- Unlimited herbs, spices, garlic and vinegar
- Herbal teas, green tea
- Natural yoghurt
- Two snacks between meals of, for example, unsalted nuts (especially brazils, walnuts, almonds), seeds (sunflower or pumpkin), fresh fruit (bananas are good) and dried fruit (especially apricots, figs, dates, prunes), natural bio yoghurt with fresh fruit, oat cakes, cereals)

## Exercise

Each week try and do more and more exercise. If you that find what I suggest is too challenging start slower and build up.

- Every morning do the windmill (page 105), the qi gong slap (page 112) or energy sweep (page 118).
- Three times a week do warm-up exercise and at least a twenty-minute walk, then cool-down exercise (or at least one other cardio' workout from list on page 101).
- Do yoga postures or strengthening exercises every day, or at least on the days that you aren't doing cardio' (remember to warm up before and cool down after – page 103).

## Energy boosts at work

As for Week 1

## Self-help and treatments

- Continue to practise the posture and breathing until you feel happy that you have mastered them.
- Practise qi gong exercises: holding the dantien (page 110) or vital energy (see page 111)
- Repeat affirmations daily like: 'I can have energy, I want to have energy, I will have energy.'
- Dry skin brush every morning followed by a cold invigorating shower for thirty seconds.
- Do shiatsu pressure points: SP6, KID1, DU20, LI10, REN4,ST36 or the exercises for beating fatigue and no more blues every other day (see page 62)
- Do your to-do lists (see page 82)

## Relaxation and visualisations

- Do Relaxing the tension before bed (see page 73) every night
- Do mantra meditation (see page 76) or continue with breath meditation if you prefer
- Do earth's energy visualisation (page 78) whenever you like, especially if you are feeling very tired

## Supplements

When increasing your vitamins make sure that you go slowly and if you have any reactions (loose stools, for example) then decrease again and increase more slowly

- Vitamin C with bioflavonoids (start with 1000mg, once a day and increase to 1000mg, 3 times a day by the end of the week; continue with this dose for the rest of the plan)
- Multivitamin and mineral (as directed on the bottle)
- Vitamin B complex (100mg, 3 times a day with meals)
- Spirulina/blue-green algae (start with 1 pill, 3 times a day increasing to 3 pills, 3 times a day)
- Royal jelly (2 capsules, 3 times a day)
- CoQ10 (60mg – start with 1 with a meal daily and increase to 3)

## Extra

- Bee pollen (stop if you get a rash or wheezing or if any other allergic symptoms occur) – sprinkle a few granules on your food. If you like taking this then you can slowly increase to 2 teaspoons.
- Wheatgrass (1 teaspoon, once a day)

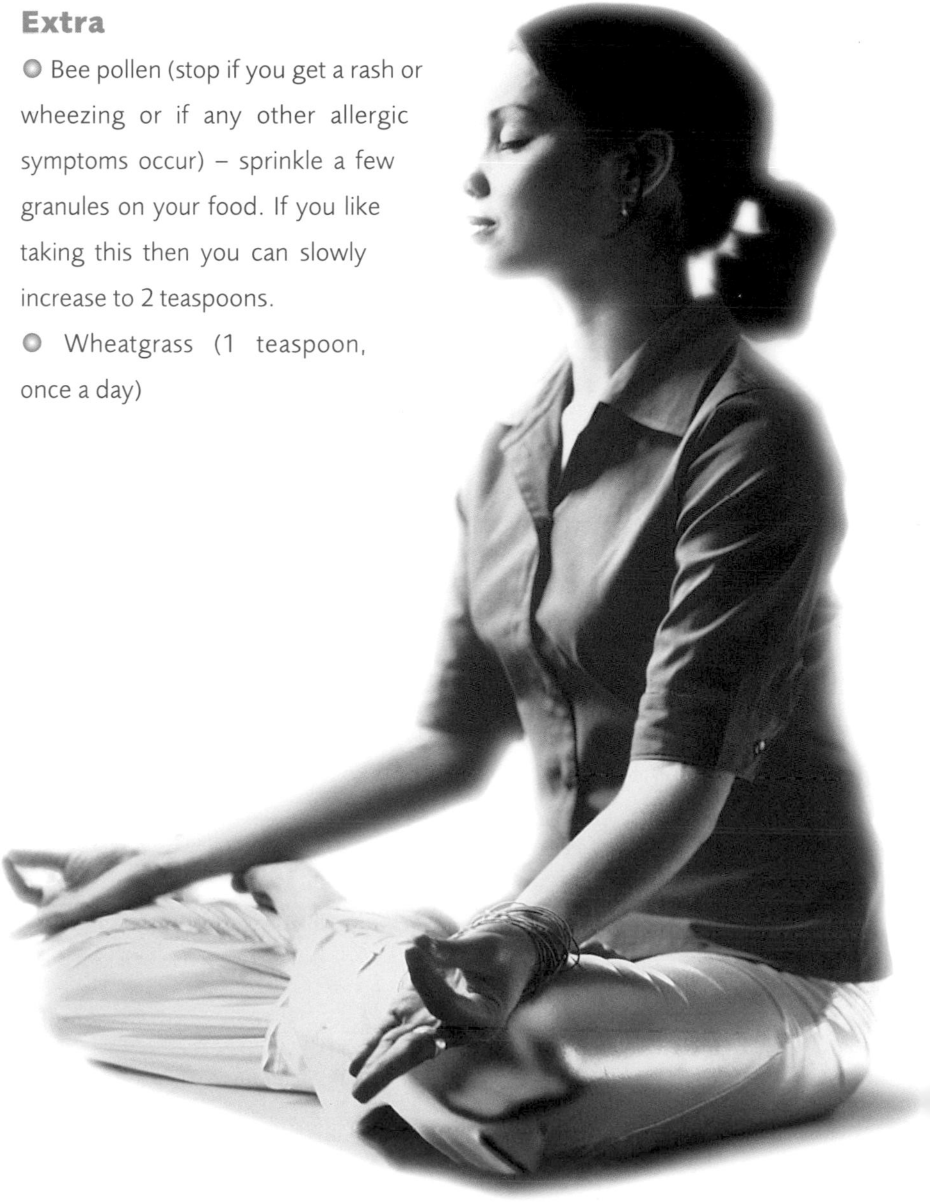

# Week 3

## Diet

As for week 2. Try to make your meals as varied and interesting as possible so that you don't get bored and stop your new way of eating.

## Exercise

As for week 2 but with more repetitions.

## Energy boosts at work

Do as many of these as you feel you need or can fit into your working day:

- Stretch at desk (see page 134)
- Relax any time, anywhere and stressbuster (see page 79)
- Ease the tension, and private release of tension (see page 80)
- Walk around the office and take regular breaks from your work or desk.
- Try to get some fresh air.

## Self-help and treatments

- Practise feeling the energy and you could also do some healing on yourself and/or on someone else (see page 47).
- Choose some oils to make a blend and either do a self-massage or find someone to give you a massage.
- Repeat affirmations daily like: 'I can have energy, I want to have energy, I will have energy.'
- Dry skin brush (page 168) every morning followed by a cold shower for thirty seconds.
- Do your to-do lists (see page 82).

## Relaxation and visualisations

- Do ten-minute sun visualisation (see page 78) whenever you can and you feel low in energy
- Do walking meditation or breath or mantra meditation every day (see age 76–7)

## Supplements

- Vitamin C with bioflavonoids (see week 2)
- Multivitamin and mineral (as directed on the bottle)
- Vitamin B complex (100mg, 3 times a day with meals)
- Spirulina/blue-green algae (start with 1 pill, 3 times a day increasing to 3 pills, 3 times a day)
- Royal jelly (2 capsules, 3 times a day)
- CoQ10 (60mg to start with, 1 with a meal daily and increase to 3 with food)

## Extra

- Bee pollen (stop if you get a rash or wheezing or if any other allergic symptoms occur) – sprinkle a few granules on your food ); if you like taking this then you can slowly increase to 2 teaspoons
- Wheat grass (1 teaspoon, once a day)

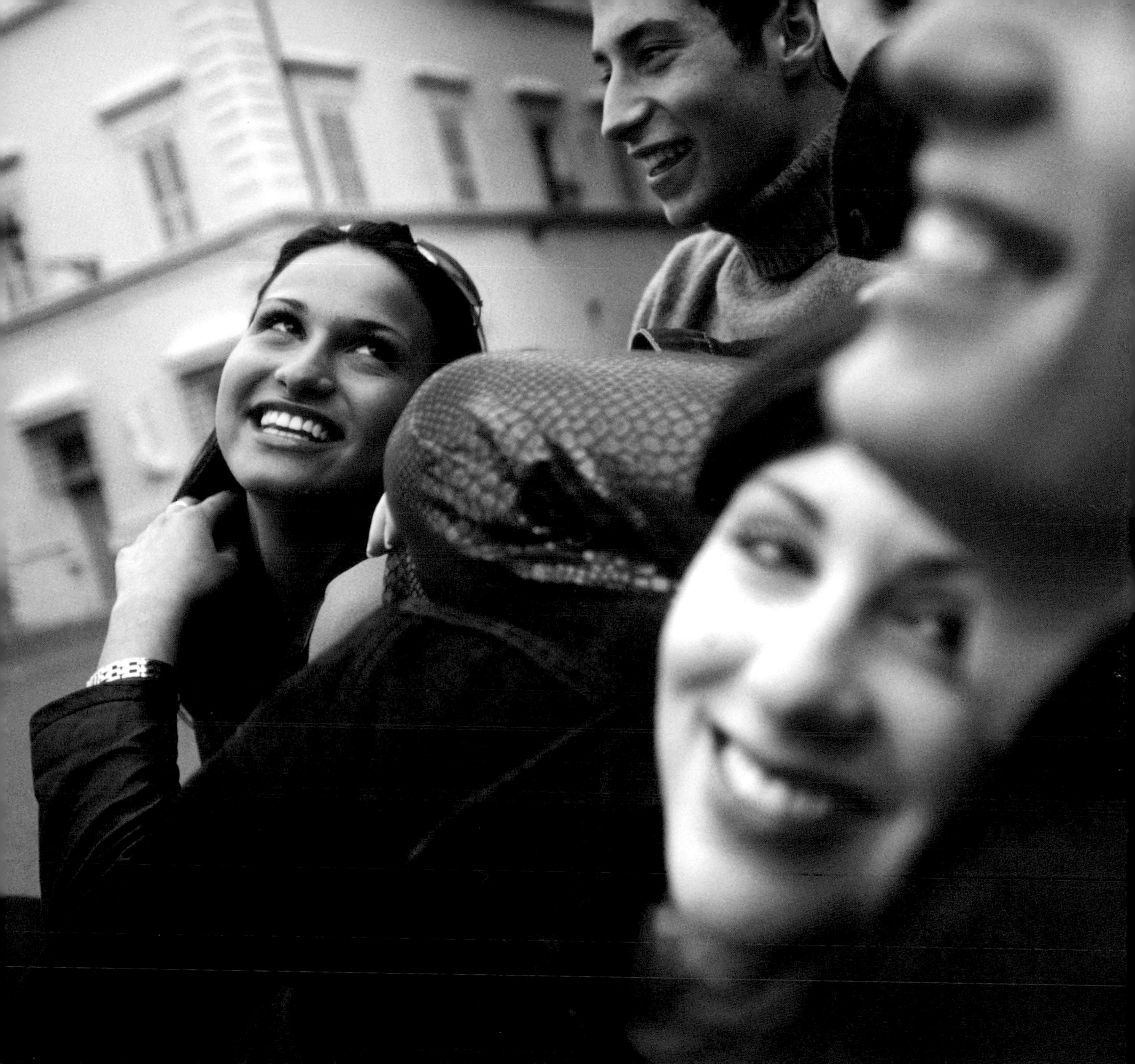

## Week 4

### Diet

As for weeks 2 and 3.

### Exercise

Note: this week do cardio' exercise with your strengthening exercises and your yoga:

- Every morning do the windmill (page 105), the qi gong slap (page 112) or the energy sweep (page 118)
- Three times a week do warm-up exercise and at least a twenty-minute walk and strengthening exercises and cool-down exercises (or at least one other cardio' workout from list on page 101).
- Do yoga postures every day or at least on the days that you aren't doing cardio' (don't forget to warm up and cool down)

### Energy boosts at work

Do as many of these as you feel you need or can fit into your working day:

- Relax any time, anywhere and stressbuster (see page 79)
- Ease the tension, and private release of tension (see page 80)

### Self-help and treatments

- Wear bright colours like red and orange to help make you feel energised
- Make yourself herbal teas (see page 65)
- Practise affirmations daily like: 'I can have energy, I want to have energy, I will have energy'
- Dry skin brush (page 168) every morning followed by a cold shower for 30 seconds
- Do your to-do lists (page 82)

### Relaxation and visualisations

- Do a meditation twice a day
- Do earth's energy or sun visualisation regularly

### Supplements

- Vitamin C with bioflavonoids (see week 2)
- Multivitamin and mineral (as directed on the bottle)
- Vitamin B complex (100mg, 3 times a day with meals)
- Spirulina/blue-green algae (start with 1 pill, 3 times a day increasing to 3 pills, 3 times a day)
- Royal jelly (2 capsules, 3 times a day)
- CoQ10 (60mg to start with, 1 with a meal daily, and increase to 3 with food)

### Extra

- Bee pollen (stop if you get a rash or wheezing or if any other allergic symptoms occur) sprinkle a few granules on your food); if you like taking this then you can slowly increase to 2 teaspoons).
- Wheat grass (1 teaspoon, once a day)

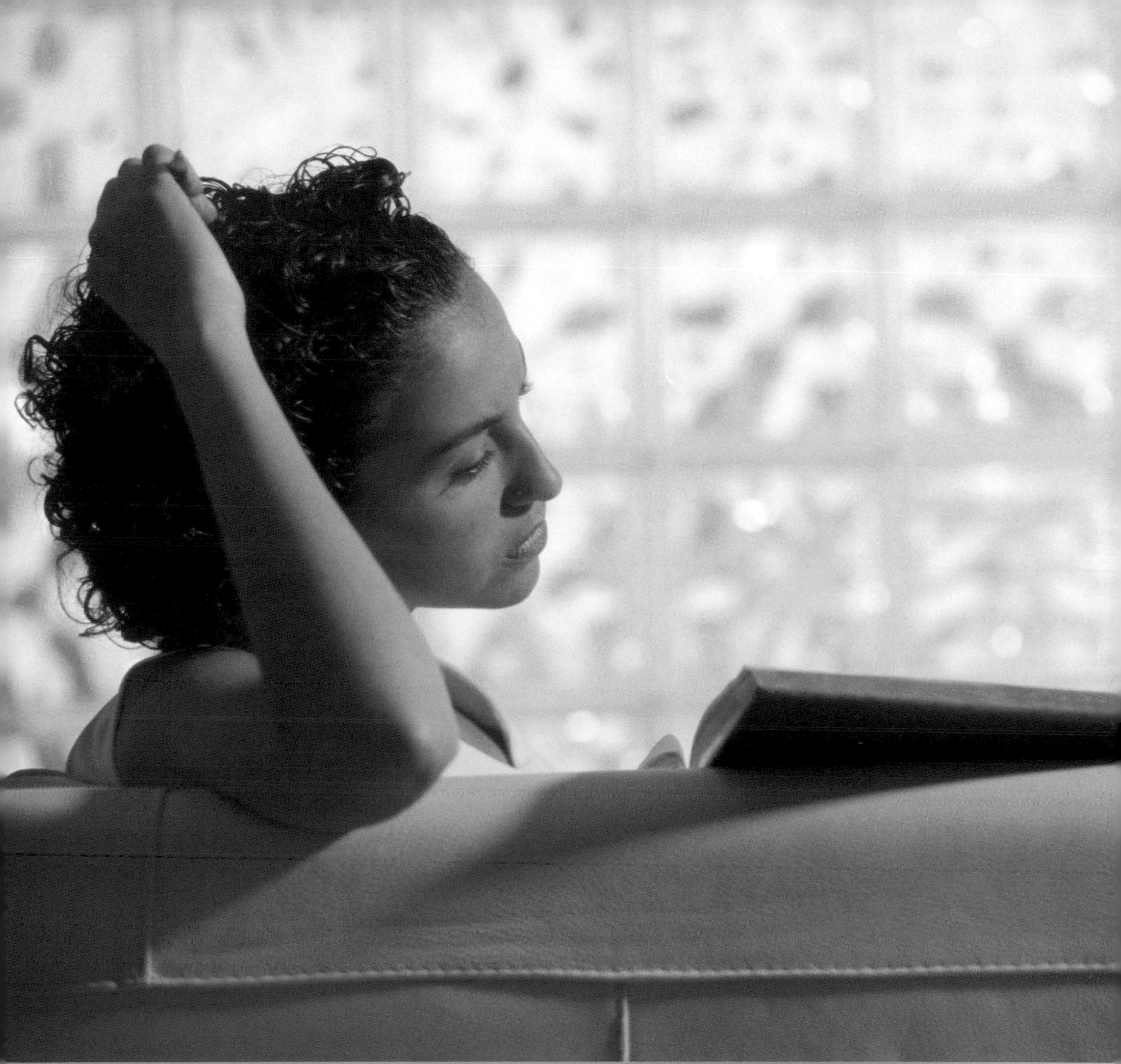

# The Six-month Energy Plan

*The six-month plan is designed for anyone who is tired all the time. It is also good as a maintenance programme for people who have enjoyed finding new energy and want to keep up their new energy levels. The idea is to build up your strength and energy and then keep them up. If you stop following the diet and exercise regimes or if you stop taking supplements or practising relaxation techniques you will slowly begin to feel sluggish and tired like you used to.*

Note: if a particular treatment, visualisation or relaxation exercise seems to suit you, don't worry about varying them as I suggest, just go with whatever is working well for you.

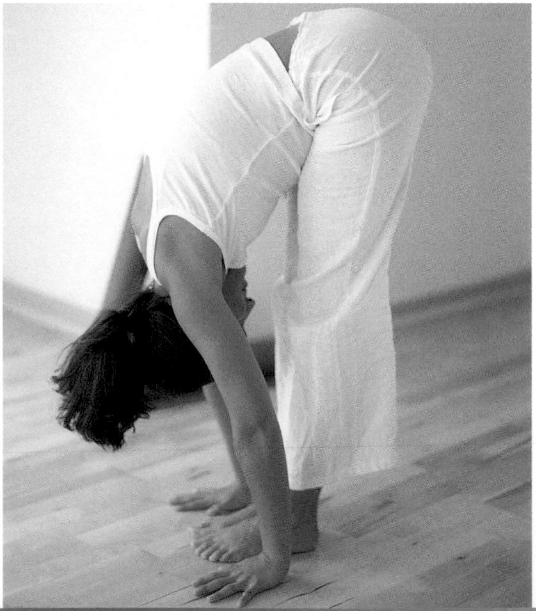

## Thirty-three-year-old business woman:

*I was always tired which I used to blame on long hours at work, but if I am honest I'd been tired ever since I can remember. I used to get especially tired after lunch and around 3pm. I always needed loads of sleep and was very lethargic which not only made me feel awful, but also ruined my social life! When Aliza asked me to do the plan I thought I'd never get through it but she told me it would be worth the effort.*

*The first few weeks were the hardest – I'm not very good at taking pills, exercising or eating properly, but Aliza told me not to worry and to carry on even if I did slip up every now and then. As for the diet I always used to be a grab-and-go type person and so I found having to plan my meals difficult. Now I can't imagine why I was worried – I just grab the right snacks instead. Once I got into the swing, it wasn't difficult to carry on for 6 months...I did think it would be harder.*

*I feel so much more energised and able to go out more – it's embarrasing to admit it, but I can't believe the difference to my social life and my libido!*

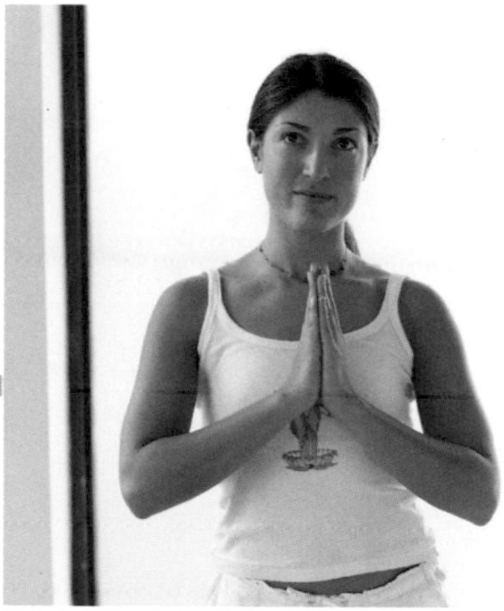

# Month 1

## Diet

As in the thirty-day plan, begin with a gentle detox for one week (see page 179) and then eat as in the seven-day plan (see page 160–173).

## Exercise

As for the thirty-day plan, starting slowly if you do not usually do much exercise, and then gradually building up to being more active.

## Energy boosts at work

Do as many of these as you feel you need or can fit into your working day:

- Standing yoga stretch, and stretch at desk (see page 134)
- Relax any time, anywhere and stressbuster (see page 79)
- Ease the tension, and private release of tension (see page 80)
- Delegate at particularly busy times; this will help to get the job get done and will also conserve your energy, ensuring that what you do yourself is also done efficiently.

## Self-help and treatments

Choose one of the following to do at least once a week:

- Diagnose yourself using acupuncture skills and then use acupressure on the appropriate points (see page 33).
- Visit an acupuncturist.
- Dry skin brush every morning (see page 168), followed by a cold invigorating shower for thirty seconds.
- Repeat affirmations daily like: 'I can have energy, I want to have energy, I will have energy.'

## Relaxation and visualisations

- Do breath meditation every day (see page 76)
- Do earth's energy visualisation (see page 78) regularly especially if you feel tired

## Supplements

- Vitamin C with bioflavonoids (start with 1000mg, once a day and increase to 1000mg, 3 times a day by the end of first week; continue with this dose for the rest of the plan)
- Multivitamin and mineral (as directed on the bottle)
- Vitamin B complex (100mg, 3 times a day with meals)
- Spirulina/blue-green algae (start with 1 pill, 3 times a day, increasing to 3 pills, 3 times a day)
- Royal jelly (2 capsules, 3 times a day)
- CoQ10 (60mg – start with 1 with a meal daily and increase to 3 with food)

## Extra

- Bee pollen (stop if you get a rash or wheezing or if any other allergic symptoms occur) – sprinkle a few granules on your food; if you like taking this then you can slowly increase to 2 teaspoons
- Wheatgrass (1 teaspoon, once a day)

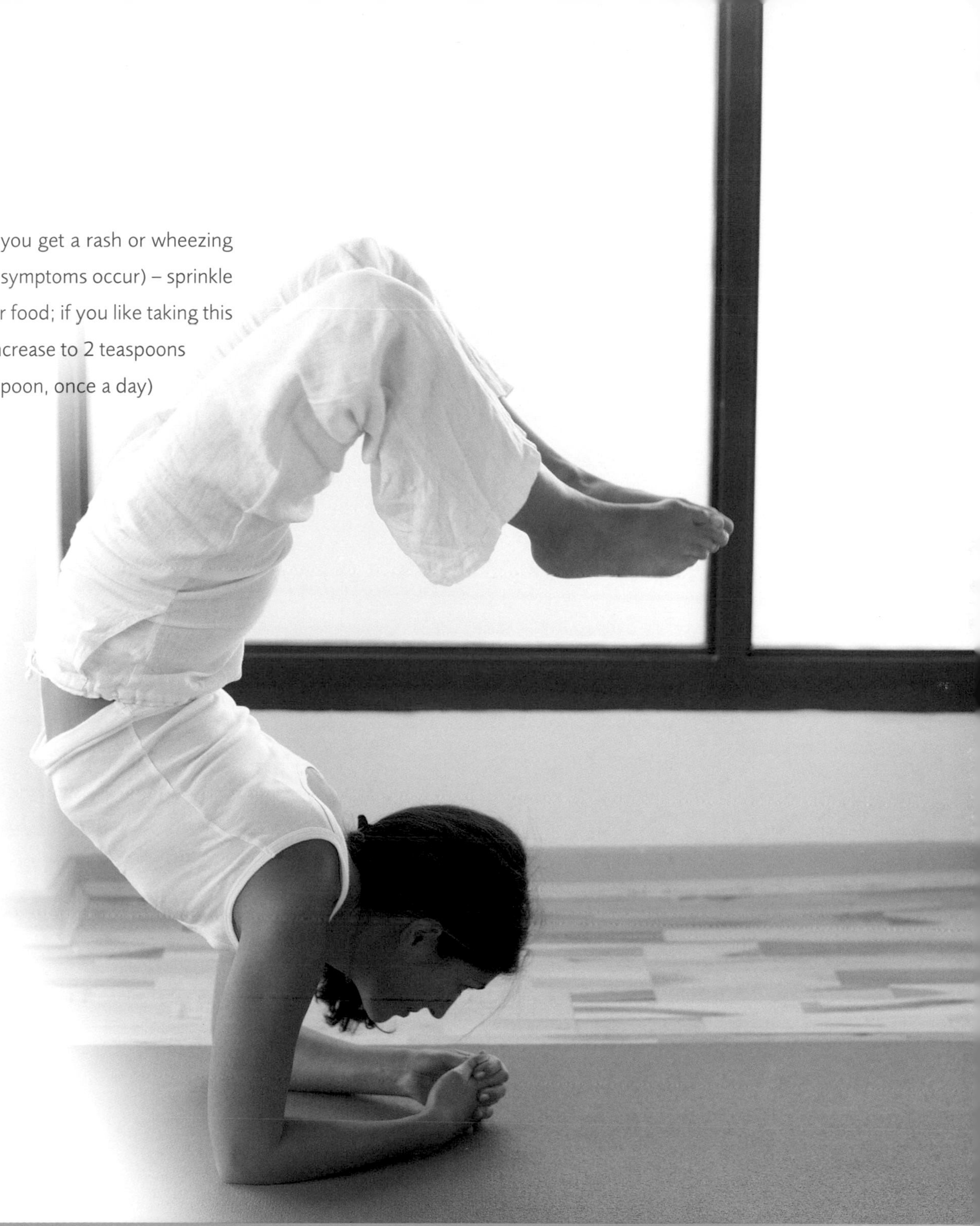

# Month 2

## Diet

As above

## Exercise

Make sure you keep challenging yourself and do more repetitions:

- Every morning do the windmill (page 105), the qi gong slap (page 112) or energy sweep (see 118)
- Three times a week do warm-up exercise and at least a 20–60-minute walk, strengthening exercises and cool-down exercises or at least one other cardio' workout from list (see page 101)
- Practise yoga postures every day or at least on the days that you aren't doing cardio' (remember to do warm-up and cool-down exercises on page 103 before and after)

## Energy boosts at work

Do as many of these as you feel you need or can fit into your working day:

- Standing yoga stretch and stretch at desk (see page 134)
- Relax any time, anywhere and stressbuster (see page 79)
- Ease the tension and private release of tension (see page 80)
- At home get your roommate or partner and kids to help with chores around the house; if you can afford it get some help around the house from a weekly cleaner

## Self-help and treatments

Choose one of the following to do at least once a week:

- Have an aromatherapy massage from a qualified aromatherapist
- Do self-massage using clary sage and lavender oils in an almond base oil (see pages 50–57)
- Repeat affirmations daily like: 'I can have energy, I want to have energy, I will have energy.'
- Write yourself to-do lists (see page 82)
- Do a dry skin brush (page 168) followed by a cold invigorating shower for thirty seconds

## Relaxation and visualisations

- Do breath meditation twice a day (see page 76)
- Do earth's energy visualisation (see page 78) regularly especially if you feel tired

## Supplements

- Vitamin C with bioflavonoids (see month 1)
- Multivitamin and mineral (as directed on the bottle)
- Vitamin B complex (100mg, 3 times a day with meals)
- Spirulina/blue-green algae (start with 1 pill, 3

times a day increasing to 3 pills, 3 times a day)

- Royal jelly (2 capsules, 3 times a day)
- CoQ10 (60mg, start with 1 with a food daily and increase to 3 with food)

## Extra

- Bee pollen (stop if you get a rash or wheezing or if any other allergic symptoms occur) – sprinkle a few granules on your food; if you like taking this then you can slowly increase to 2 teaspoons
- Wheatgrass (1 teaspoon, once a day)

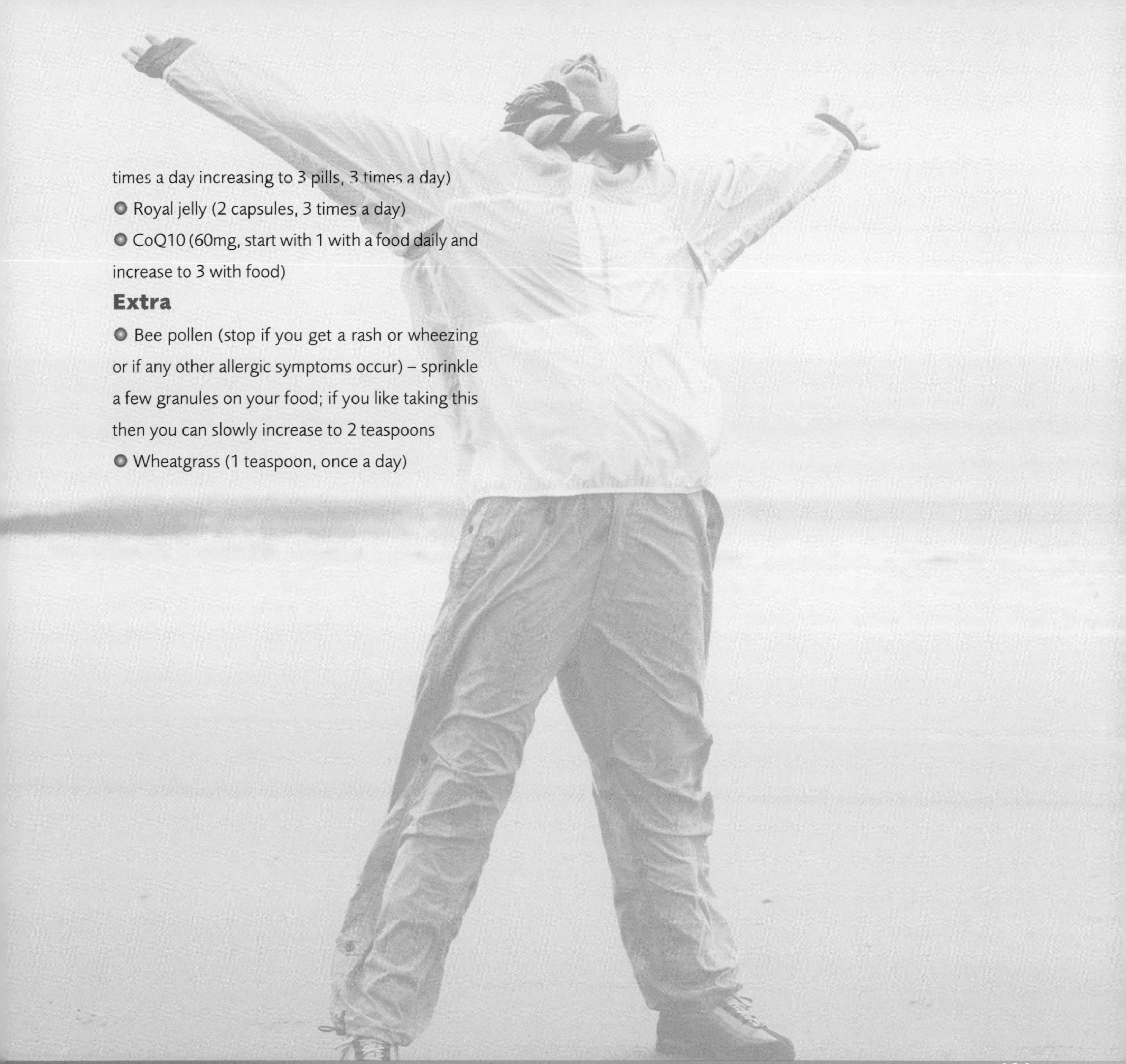

# Month 3

## Diet

As above

## Exercise

- Every morning do the windmill (page 105), the qi gong slap (page 112) or energy sweep (see page 118)
- Three times a week do warm-up exercise (page 103) and at least a twenty minutes of cardio' and strengthening exercises (see pages 101 and 100–109), followed by cool-down exercises . Do yoga postures every day or at least on the days that you aren't doing cardio' (don't forget to warm up and cool down before and after).
- Try to walk everywhere you go.

## Energy boosts at work

Do as many of these as you feel you need or can fit into your working day:

- Standing yoga stretch and stretch at desk (see page 134)
- Relax any time, anywhere and stressbuster (see page 79)
- Ease the tension and private release of tension (see page 80)
- Burn basil, peppermint and/or rosemary oil in an oil burner at work to help with mental clarity or place a few drops of one of the oils on a tissue and inhale regularly.
- Get an ioniser or a salt crystal light for work

## Self-help and treatments

Do one of the following at least once a week:

- Do feel the energy healing exercise (see page 47), then try healing yourself and other people and get them to heal you (don't try to heal anyone else if you are feeling tired; wait until you have regained all your energy)
- Go to see a healer for a treatment
- Dry skin brush every morning (see page 168) followed by a cold invigorating shower for thirty seconds
- Repeat affirmations daily like: 'I can have energy, I want to have energy, I will have energy.'
- Write out to-do lists (see page 82)

## Relaxation and visualisations

- Do breath, walking or mantra meditation twice a day (see page 76–7)
- Do shamanic visualisation for increasing energy regularly especially if you feel tired (see page 150)

## Supplements

- Vitamin C with bioflavonoids (see month 1)
- Multivitamin and mineral (as directed on the bottle)

- Vitamin B complex (100mg, 3 times a day with meals)
- Spirulina/blue green algae (start with 1 pill, 3 times a day increasing to 3 pills, 3 times a day)
- Royal jelly (2 capsules, 3 times a day)
- CoQ10 (60mg, start with 1 with a food daily and increase to 3 with food)

### Extra

- Bee pollen (stop if you get a rash or wheezing or if any other allergic symptoms occur) – sprinkle a few granules on your food); if you like taking this then you can slowly increase to 2 teaspoons
- Wheatgrass (1 teaspoon, once a day)

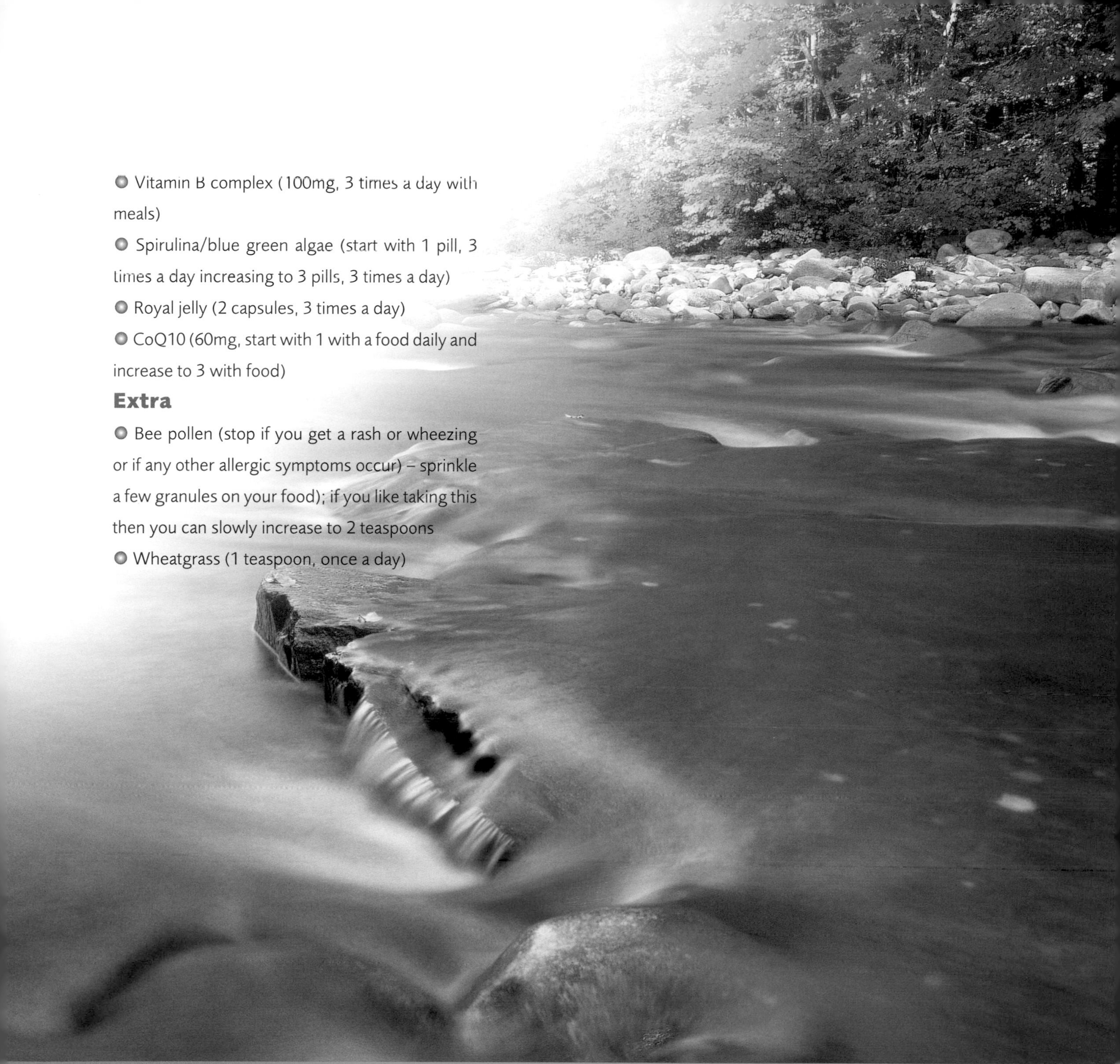

# Month 4

## Diet

As above

## Exercise

- Every morning do the windmill (page 105), the qi gong slap (page 112) or energy sweep (see page 118)
- Three times a week do warm-up exercise (page 103) and at least a 20–30 minute cardio' session and strengthening exercises (see pages 101 and 100–109), followed by cool-down exercises . Practise yoga postures every day or at least on the days that you aren't doing cardio', remembering to warm
- Try to walk everywhere you go

## Energy boosts at work

Do as many of these as you feel you need or can fit into your working day:

- Standing yoga stretch and stretch at desk (see pages 134)
- Relax any time, anywhere and stressbuster (see pages 79)
- Ease the tension and private release of tension (see page 80)
- Clean up your desk and throw clutter away. Put a plant or fresh flowers daily on it, and also hang a quartz crystal on your computer. If there is a window near your desk open it once in a while for some fresh air.

## Self-help and treatments

- Clean up the house: do one room at a time otherwise you will exhaust yourself; throw away things you don't need that are creating clutter
- Burn some incense
- Do some clapping (see page 155)
- Buy some white sage and clean the energy of your flat/house (see page 155)
- Dry skin brush every morning (see page 168) followed by a cold shower for thirty seconds
- Repeat affirmations daily like: 'I can have energy, I want to have energy, I will have energy.'
- Write out to-do lists

## Relaxation and visualisations

- Do breath, walking or mantra meditation twice a day (see pages 76–7)
- Do Shamanic visualisation (page 150) or ten-minute sun meditation (page 78) regularly, especially if you feel tired

## Supplements

- Vitamin C with bioflavonoids (see month 1)
- Multivitamin and mineral (as directed on the bottle)

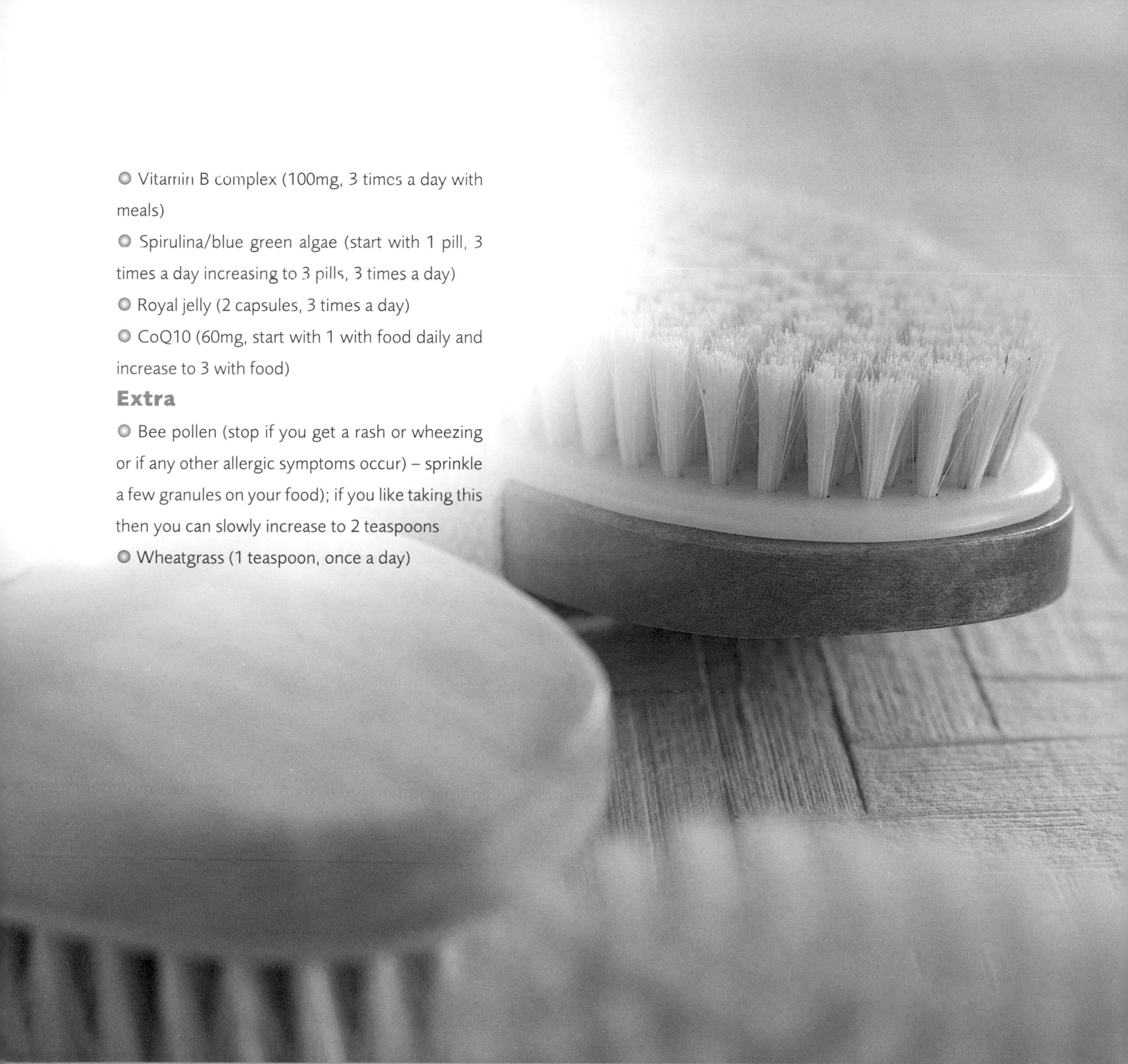

- Vitamin B complex (100mg, 3 times a day with meals)
- Spirulina/blue green algae (start with 1 pill, 3 times a day increasing to 3 pills, 3 times a day)
- Royal jelly (2 capsules, 3 times a day)
- CoQ10 (60mg, start with 1 with food daily and increase to 3 with food)

### Extra

- Bee pollen (stop if you get a rash or wheezing or if any other allergic symptoms occur) – sprinkle a few granules on your food); if you like taking this then you can slowly increase to 2 teaspoons
- Wheatgrass (1 teaspoon, once a day)

# Month 5

## Diet

As above

## Exercise

- Every morning do the windmill (page 105), the qi gong slap (page 112) or energy sweep (see page 118)
- Three times a week do warm-up exercise (page 103) followed by at least 30–40 minutes of cardio' and strengthening exercises (pages 101 and 100–109) then cool-down exercises. Do yoga postures every day or at least on the days that you aren't doing cardio'.
- Walk everywhere you go.

## Energy boosts at work

Do as many of these as you feel you need or can fit into your working day:

- Standing yoga stretch and stretch at desk (see page 134)
- Relax any time, anywhere and stressbuster (see page 79)
- Ease the tension and private release of tension exercises (see page 80)
- Buy some wind chimes and put them near a window or wherever you think the energy needs to move or is stagnant.

## Self-help and treatments

Do one of the following at least once a week:

- Try and see your aura and other people auras, and then also do the chakra balance (see page 145)
- Go and see someone who cleans auras and/or balances chakras
- Dry skin brush every morning (page 168) followed by a cold invigorating shower for thirty seconds
- Repeat affirmations daily like: 'I can have energy, I want to have energy, I will have energy.'
- Write out to-do lists (see page 82)

## Relaxation/visualisations

- Do breath, walking, mantra meditation, three times a day (see page 76–7)
- Do earth's energy visualisation (page 78), Shamanic visualisation (page 150) or ten-minute sun meditation (page 78) regularly, especially if you feel tired

## Supplements

- Vitamin C with bioflavonoids (see month 1)
- Multivitamin and mineral (as directed on the bottle)
- Vitamin B complex 100mg (3 times a day with meals)

- Spirulina/blue green algae (start with 1 pill, 3 times a day, increasing to 3 pills, 3 times a day)
- Royal jelly (2 capsules, 3 times a day)
- CoQ10 (60mg, start with 1 with a food daily and increase to 3 with food)

## Extra

- Bee pollen (stop if you get a rash or wheezing or if any other allergic symptoms occur) – sprinkle a few granules on your food) – if you like taking this then you can slowly increase to 2 teaspoons
- Wheatgrass (1 teaspoon, once a day)

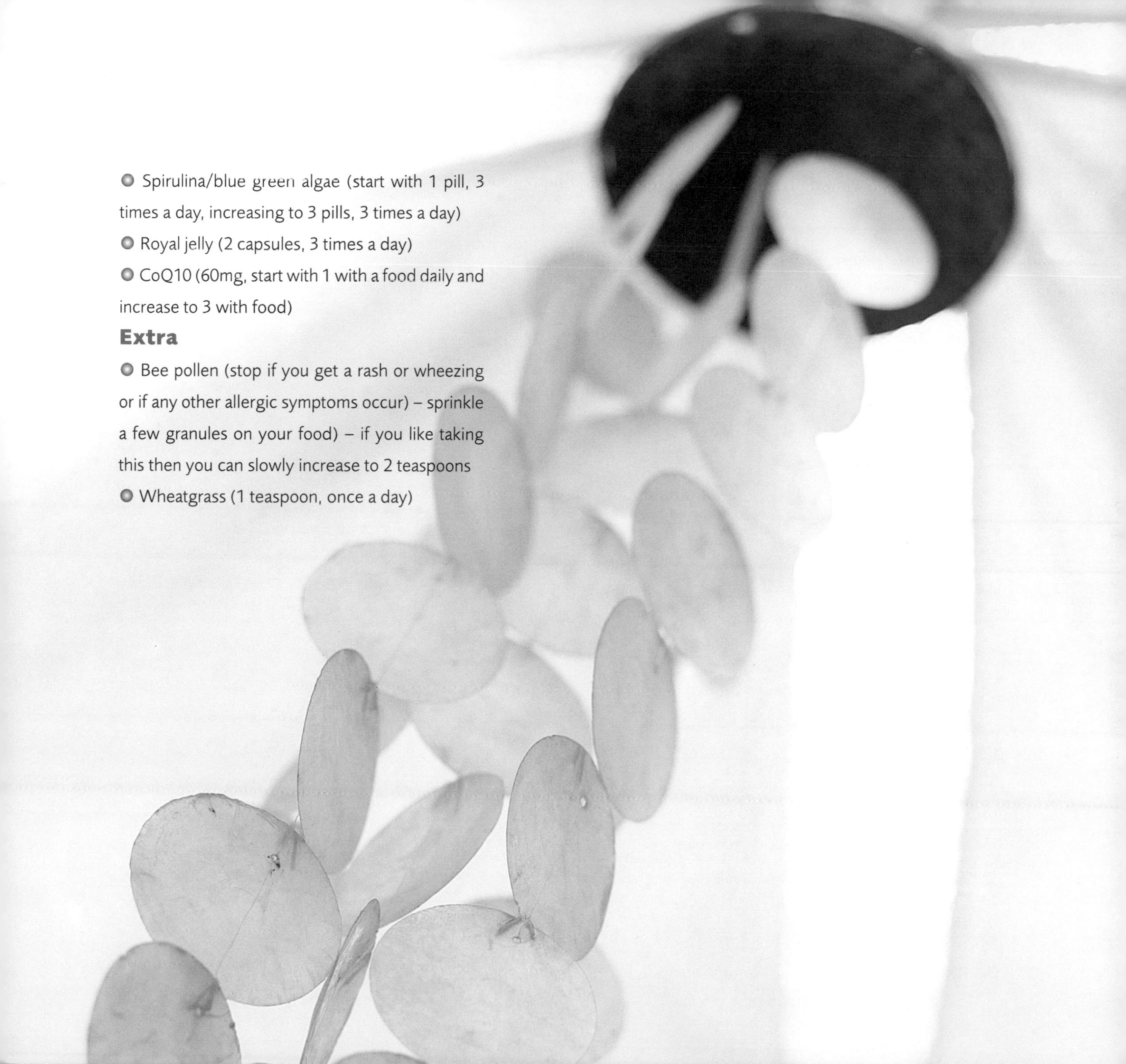

# Month 6

## Diet

As above

## Exercise

- Every morning do the windmill (page 105), the qi gong slap (page 112) or energy sweep (see page 118)
- Three times a week do warm-up exercise (page 103) followed by at least a 40–45-minute cardio' exercise and strengthening exercises (see pages 101 and 100–109) and then cool down exercises . Do yoga postures every day or at least on the days that you aren't doing cardio' (remember to warm up and cool down before and after)
- Walk everywhere you go

## Energy boosts at work

- Try and get everyone in the office laughing at least once a day; look for the funny things in life
- Do as many of these as you feel you need or can fit into your working day:
- Standing yoga stretch and stretch at desk (see page 134)
- Relax any time, anywhere and stressbuster (see page 79)
- Ease the tension and private release of tension (see page 80)

## Self-help and treatments

- Practise any of the treatments from chapter 2 that you have enjoyed or have a session with a professional. Try and do at least one a week.
- Dry skin brush every morning followed by a cold shower for thirty seconds (see page 168)
- Repeat affirmations daily like: 'I can have energy, I want to have energy, I will have energy.'
- Write out to-do lists (see page 82)

## Relaxation and visualisations

- Do breath, walking, mantra meditation, three times a day (see page 76–77)
- Do any of the visualisations that you have enjoyed, especially if you feel tired (see pages 78, 150 and 209)

## Supplements

- Vitamin C with bioflavonoids (see month 1)
- Multivitamin and mineral (as directed on the bottle)
- Vitamin B complex (100mg, 3 times a day with meals)
- Spirulina/blue-green algae (start with 1 pill 3 times a day, increasing to 3 pills, 3 times a day)
- Royal jelly (2 capsules, 3 times a day)
- CoQ10 (60mg, start with 1 with a food daily and increase to 3 with food)

## Extra

- Bee pollen (stop if you get a rash or wheezing or if any other allergic symptoms occur) – sprinkle a few granules on your food); if you like taking this then you can slowly increase to 2 teaspoons
- Wheatgrass (1 teaspoon, once a day)

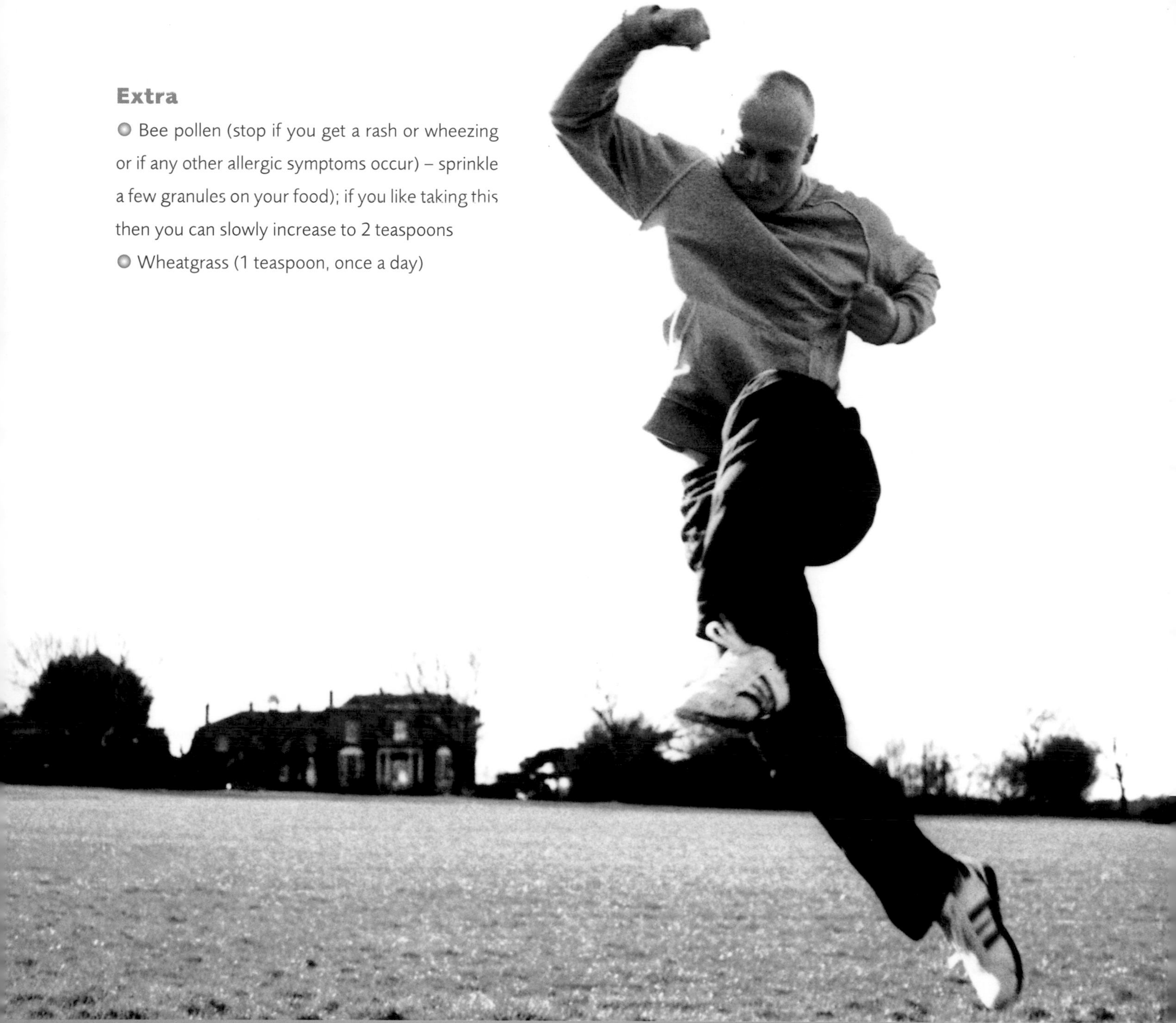

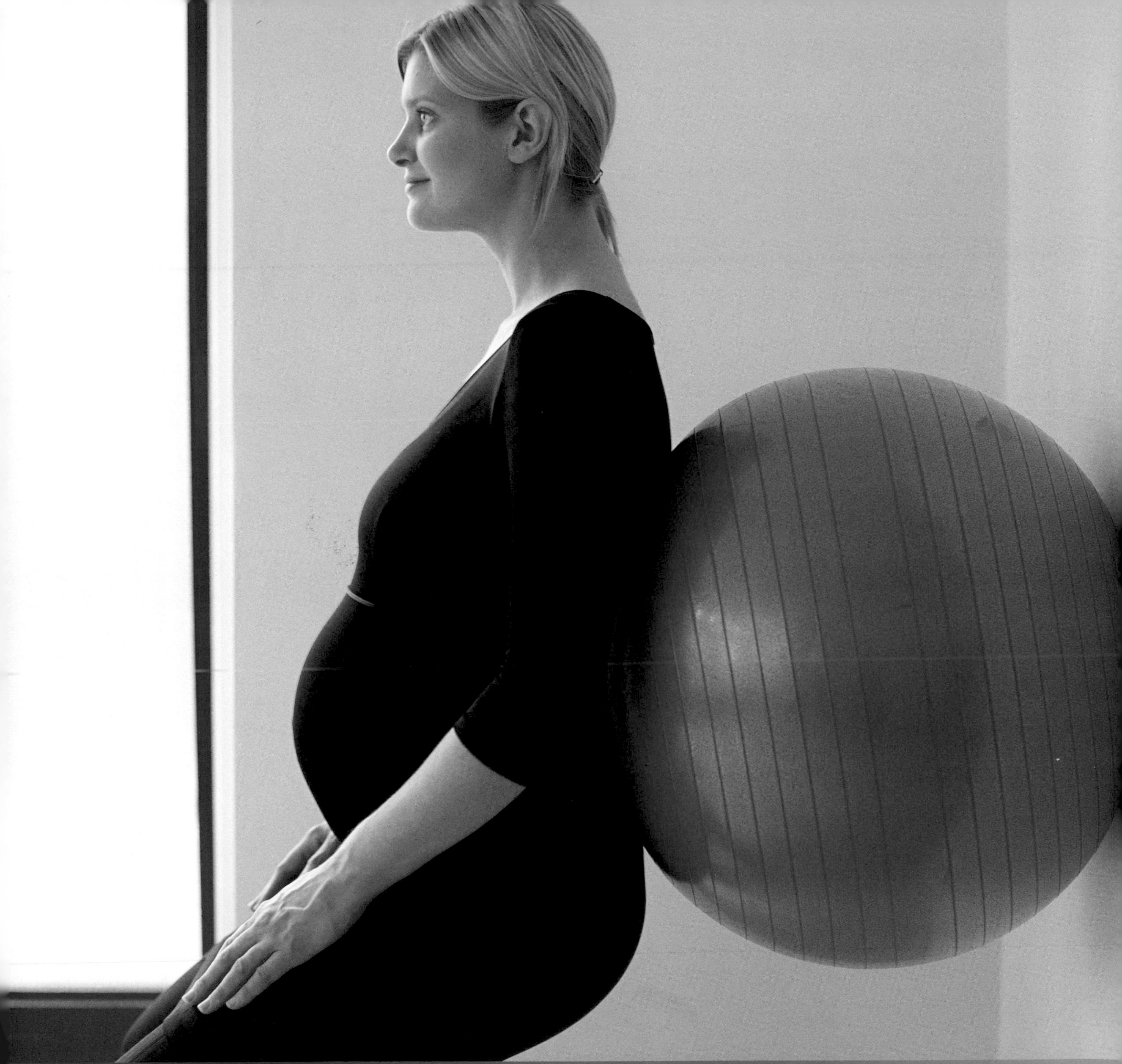

CHAPTER 4

# Energy for Life

*The first few months of pregnancy (the first trimester) are exhausting (I speak from experience, having recently had my first child). The tiredness is caused by physiological and hormonal changes – the hormone progesterone is produced by the placenta and has, among other things, a sedative effect. Hence the tiredness and the propensity to sleep, sleep and sleep some more!*

## Pregnancy

Pregnancy is not the time to start changing your exercise routine to try and increase your energy. The best thing to do is just to give in, listen to your body and get plenty of rest. As long as you eat well, rest and keep a healthy and happy positive attitude you will have as much energy as is to be expected.

After the first trimester your energy levels begin to increase and if you are eating right, exercising, getting enough sleep and feeling calm you should feel full of energy.

Don't undertake any of the energy plans in chapter three when you are pregnant. Instead, go for regular treatments from qualified practitioners to help overcome some of the tiredness and other annoying and sometimes unnecessary symptoms associated with pregnancy. Therapies should only be done after the first trimester and make sure that your practitioner knows that you are pregnant.

Homeopathy is especially good, as are reflexology and massage.

## Diet

Eating properly during pregnancy is very important. If your diet is lacking in nutrients the baby will feed off you, taking the nutrients from your hair, nails and bones, so that you feel extra exhausted and run down.

All the foods that are recommended for energy are excellent during pregnancy, although it is not recommended these days to eat anything containing nuts in case of nut allergy in the unborn foetus. Many people believe that a pregnant woman should follow her cravings as these are often the body's way of telling us what we are lacking. But don't allow yourself to use pregnancy as an excuse to binge on foods that you know are not good for you. Piling on the weight will not help you to feel energised and will make you feel even more tired when the baby arrives.

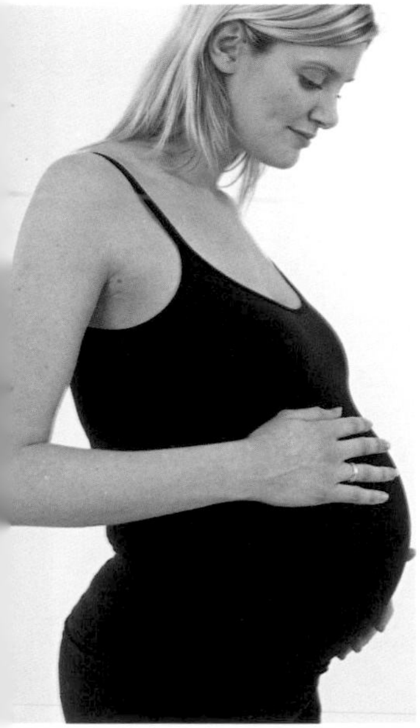

Eating regular snacks will help you to keep your energy levels up, and it is important never to miss out on a meal as this will not only make you feel tired but your baby will suffer too. Cutting out caffeine is not only good for the baby but also helps you to maintain your real energy levels.

Only take supplements or herbs during pregnancy on the advice of a fully qualified doctor, nutritionalist, naturopath or herbalist. However a good prenatal multivitamin and mineral supplement is safe, and often important, to take. (Make sure it contains folic acid.)

## Exercise in pregnancy

A pregnancy yoga class is very good as it helps the stiffness that can often make you feel tired and low. Walking is also good. I found just walking to and from work every day (a twenty-minute walk each way) was a good way to get my circulation moving and supply me with oxygen. I felt great. But always listen to your body and if you feel tired then stop and rest.

You can also do the exercises for pregnant women (opposite) every day as they are very gentle and help to keep you slightly active. If you do attempt any more vigorous exercise make sure that you do so under the guidance of an experienced trainer who knows about exercise during pregnancy. It is often advisable not to start doing exercise during pregnancy if you have never done it before, although gentle walking or swimming should be fine (but consult with your doctor first). It has been found that people who do some sort of exercise during their pregnancies tend to have a better birth than those who don't.

## Exercises

Note: exercise during pregnancy should only be done after the first three months and once your doctor has given you the all-clear. Never strain yourself when exercising and stop immediately if you feel unwell or dizzy.

- Go for a twenty-minute walk, preferably around a local park so as to get some fresh air.

**1** Kneel on the floor on your hands and knees

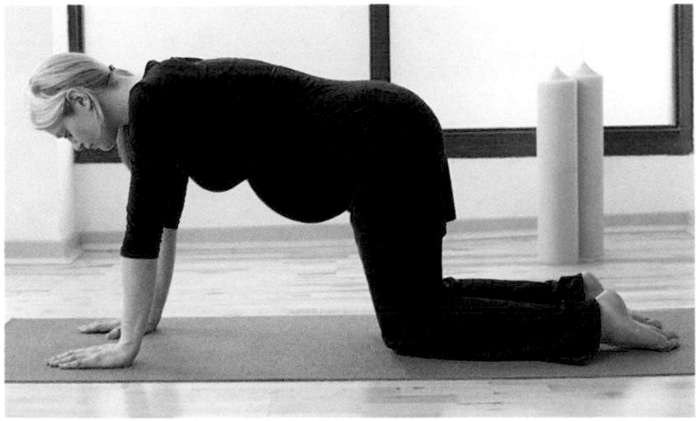

with your head in a straight line with your back.

**2** Breathe in, then exhale and suck your tummy in (the bigger you get the more this feels like an exercise!). Hold for a count of five, then breathe in and relax.

**3** Repeat ten times.

**1** Stand straight, with your right hand supported on a radiator or heavy chair/table (that won't move).

**2** Breathe in, take a step forward with your left leg. Both legs should be slightly bent.

**3** Exhale, while gently going as low as you can without straining yourself.

**4** Breathe in and return to position 1.

**5** Now, repeat with the right leg, and left hand supporting.

**6** Repeat five times for each side.

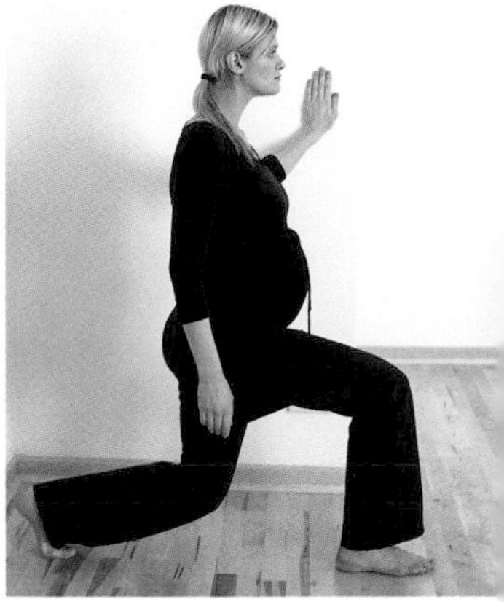

## Visualisations and relaxation

Visualisations and relaxation can help with any anxiety you may have about pregnancy and/or the birth. This is important as anxiety uses up valuable energy that you need for yourself and the baby during the pregnancy as well as during labour and once the baby has arrived.

Writing a journal can be helpful for recognising how you are feeling about the pregnancy or how your partner is behaving. It can also be a nice memento to look back on years later.

Many women get surges of energy during the day and it is important to learn to pace yourself if this is the case. It is quite common for women to overdo it during the day, returning home in the

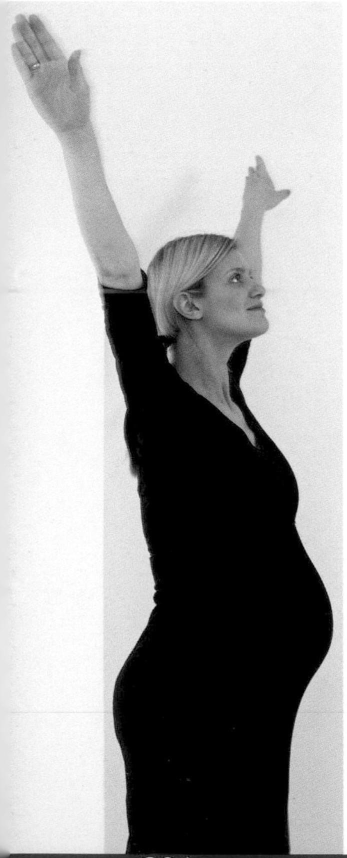

evening absolutely exhausted. Try and also find some time for yourself before the baby arrives because as soon as she/he is here your needs quickly disappear into the background.

As for the anxiety before the birth it is good to try and regularly do some visualisations:

**1** Find a time to be on your own with the lights low/off and the phone switched off, and get into a comfortable position either sitting with your feet up or lying on a bed.

**2** Try to think about what it is that is worrying you the most and think what would you like to happen. For example, if it is the birth that is worrying you because you are scared of pain then imagine your birth as you would like it to be. Make the picture as clear as possible, as bright as possible and include all the noises you would like to hear (music, for example). You should imagine that you are watching a film on a big screen in your head that you are directing it. It can only be as you want it, so if there is something that you don't like in your film rewind and rewrite it as you want it.

**3** Now you have decided what you are going to visualise, close your eyes and begin to observe your breathing.

**4** Once you are feeling relaxed, start putting your visualisation into practice. So, for the example above imagine yourself going to hospital as you want it to be and the whole birth and see the beautiful baby waiting to meet you. When you are fully satisfied with the scene you have created take a mental picture and then when you are ready open your eyes.

This is a good visualisation to do regularly, maybe twice a week or more if you like.

(See also Colour Therapy, page 42, for a useful visualisation to try during labour.)

## Energy for New Mothers

Many new mothers say that they feel totally exhausted, because of the lack of sleep, because of the birth which is tiring in itself, because their hormones are all over the place and because of the new responsibilities. And that's not even counting all the visits from well-meaning friends and relatives.

It is vital during this trying yet enjoyable time to keep up your energy:

**1** Eat healthily. It is often so overwhelming at the beginning that you can't find time to shower or go to the toilet, let alone sit down to a decent meal. However, it is vital that you eat well and drink lots of water to keep up your strength and energy especially if you are breastfeeding. (If you are breastfeeding you must always sit down with a glass of water for yourself when the baby is drinking from you.) All of the guidelines in chapter 2 for eating healthily to give you energy should be followed, but if you are breastfeeding you can eat more dairy foods and fat than would normally be recommended.

**2** Take naps wherever and whenever you can. When the baby goes to sleep try and take a nap, or at least take the time to put your feet up, close your eyes and have a rest.

**3** Accept help. If you have a friend or family member who is willing to help (and you don't have too many issues with them) try and accept their offers; at first it might be the only way you are able to get to have a shower. They might also be able to take the baby for a walk or just babysit while you have some time to yourself. It is worth it as you will feel so much more energised just for having had the break.

**4** Try to keep active: go for walks with your new baby and get some fresh air, for example.

**5** It is still important to take your prenatal vitamins (if you are breastfeeding make sure that they are suitable for lactating women).

**6** Try and set yourself realistic goals, for example, to do one thing a day like meeting a friend or going to the shops. If you try to do too much you will exhaust yourself and will probably feel quite weepy and disheartened.

**7** Talk to other people who have recently had babies. It really does help to hear that what you are feeling and thinking is normal. If you are spending the whole time worrying you won't enjoy your baby and will eventually worry yourself to exhaustion.

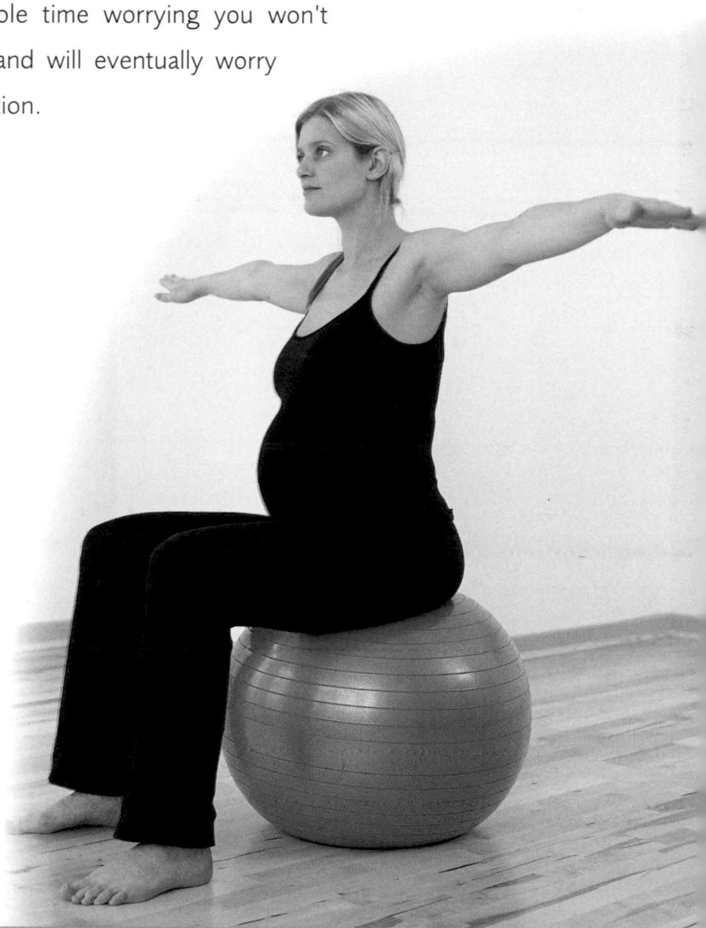

## The older person

Note: Consult your GP or therapist before following any of the advice in this section if you suffer from any medical conditions, or are in any doubt as to its suitability.

As we get older, the energy levels of our minds and bodies change dramatically. It does not mean, however, that it's time to retire from life and slump in front of the television, just because we are over fifty. Concentrate instead on what you can do to strengthen and boost your body–mind connection and your 'energy-bank', not just to keep up with life, but to be able to enjoy a good and fulfilling quality of life.

### Managing, developing and maintaining energy as you get older

In years gone by, it was commonly held that the older you get, the more muscle, strength, energy, and vitality you lose. It was said to be an inevitable part of ageing. It was also believed that once lost, these things could not be regained or restored. However, this need not be the case, and the stereotype of what it is to look, feel, and be forty, fifty, sixty, or seventy plus, has changed dramatically from what it was even twenty years ago.

The following have all been proven scientifically:

- Building strength is a great energiser.
- The stronger you are, the easier it is to move.
- Strength lifts depression, giving you the energy to tackle whatever each day throws at you – exercise releases 'feel-good' chemicals in the brain.
- As your internal muscles get stronger, your digestion improves, as does your elimination, creating a great feeling of leanness in the body, making you feel lighter.

Eating well, exercise, and a positive mental attitude are just as important in older age as they ever were before. Regular yearly checkups with your GP will enable you to deal promptly with any problem that arises before it starts to slow down your energy.

**HOURLY APPRAISALS**

So as to maintain energy levels it is especially important for the older person to do hourly appraisals/check-ins with themselves so as to become aware if they are overdoing it, while being realistic about what can be achieved.

Plenty of fresh food, fruits, and vegetables should be eaten, along with grains, nuts, seeds, pulses, fish and plant oils. Calcium, in your food or in supplements, is very important. Avoid smoking and drinking alcohol to excess, and try to maintain a reasonable body weight.

After our twenties, muscle bulk starts to decrease, so it is vital to do strengthening exercises; otherwise, muscle loss will lead to strength, stamina, and energy loss, too, and your metabolism will also slow down. Bone mass can also deteriorate after the mid-thirties, again causing the metabolism to slow down and increasing the risk of fractures, frailty and shrinkage.

## Think young

Californian health writer Deepak Chopra claims you can reverse the signs of ageing and regain the body and energy of someone fifteen years your

Controlled experiments were carried out in the 1980s and 1990s looking at factors that slowed down the ageing process and increased energy in the older person. One such experiment looked at people who exercised versus people who didn't. Half of them remained as inactive as they usually were for one year, while the others exercised with weights or did Pilates, isometric and yoga classes at least twice a week for a year. All of the volunteers were post-menopausal women and not on any hormone treatments. After a year, the inactive group had aged a great deal in terms of muscle, bone, limb stiffness and weakness. They were substantially less active and less energetic than they had been a year earlier. The women in the group that had exercised were fifteen to twenty years younger in terms of their energy, vitality, and the physical body. They also found that that their self-image changed too. They looked better, felt better and were emotionally far more self-confident. It was found that their outlook changed as their inner picture of themselves changed. They were more ready to tackle the full range of challenges that would face older people in the twenty-first century.

junior in just ten weeks. Read on to learn how to turn the emotional and physical clock back by learning new habits, activities and ways of thinking.

1 Exercise daily. Try walking a little more quickly, or park your car further from your destination than you need to. Swim once a week, walk in the park enjoying the scenery and fresh air. You can even walk briskly around your favourite shopping centre. Do floor exercises once or twice a week.

2 Practice ageless meditation three times a day.

3 Eat foods that are healthy and that you enjoy.

4 Consult a nutritionalist, health shop assistant, or your doctor for a good multivitamin and mineral supplement to protect against age-related illnesses and find out about supplements for joints and memory, such as glucosamine, chondroitin and gingko biloba.

5 Laugh as often as possible! Laughter can help to wake up your immune system.

6 Remain curious to keep your mind young, vibrant and dynamic.

7 Challenge yourself with new experiences, new places, new trends or new areas of study.

8 Make space for love (not bitterness) in your new life.

9 Stop worrying!

It is important to retrain your mind to feel younger, fitter and more energised, too. Remember, it is you who will create the new inner picture of yourself and your own idea of the energy you have. Your mind will dictate to your body, and your body will work with your mind. It only takes practice.

### Ageless meditation

1 Close your eyes, focus on your breathing, and start to relax.

2 When you are ready, pick an age from your past that you would like to be or that you really feel you are. Make sure you feel happy and comfortable to be this age and, if you don't, choose another one.

3 Repeat the age to yourself over and over again, and begin to believe it, feel it; visualise yourself and your energy at that age. Think about how your body feels, what you can do, and what your attitudes are.

4 Repeat to yourself, 'I am a healthy, active, energetic X-year old and I look and feel and act X years old'.

5 Once you feel that age and believe you can feel that age, take a mental snapshot that you can take out whenever you slip back into old patterns or someone says something that makes you feel old.

Repeat this visualisation at least three times a day.

## VISUALISATION TO INCREASE ENERGY

To help you 'see' your energy and change your inner picture of yourself as an ageless person, try meditation and deep breathing first thing in the morning and last thing at night. Don't be afraid of the word 'meditation' – it only means that you are giving your mind and body a small space of time to relax and put aside any stress of the day.

**1** Lie on your bed or sit comfortably in a quiet place (you can even do this on an aeroplane wearing headphones with the sound turned off).

**2** Take five deep breaths and, letting go of all other thoughts that enter your mind, concentrate on the noise of your breathing (in through your nose and out through your mouth). Follow in your mind or 'see' the air as you breathe it down the pathway of your spine. Start with the air going down from your neck right down to the base of your spine – that is the coccyx.

This quiet time will relieve stress, over-reactions to situations of all sorts and help you preserve and maintain the valuable energy you will need both night and day.

### Sleep and ageing

Many people complain that, as they age, they don't sleep as well as they used to. This is often due to anxiety and stress or poor physical health. Regular activity and more energy will help you be able to sleep better, as has been proven by studies at the Respiratory Sciences and Sleep Disorders Center at the University of Arizona.

### Ageing with fewer injuries

The more active and flexible you become, the less likely you will be to suffer the recurring injuries often associated with old age. You will also find that if you do suffer an injury, poor health or have to undergo an operation, you will heal more quickly than you used to if you have managed to remain physically active. Even if you have an injury in one area of your body, you can still exercise other parts to increase your circulation and therefore help promote healing to the affected area. Even gentle exercise will help you recover more quickly from any illness, injury, accident, or operation.

### Energy through the menopause

Regular exercise will minimise the effects of the menopause on your body and mind. Many women who have been exercising regularly up to menopause age do not experience hot flushes or depression.

Even a fast walk during a lunch hour or dancing to the radio or a CD in the privacy of your own home can help. Exercise can be so effective in the context of the menopause that some active women are never really certain whether they have gone through menopause at all. This is because they have no symptoms (besides the giveaway sign of losing their periods), and their energy levels remain high if not higher than they were in childbearing years.

A regular programme of exercises provides focus, has a calming effect and gives energy and a feeling of emotional wellbeing during the menopause just as at other times of your life.

### The correct time to exercise: your own biorhythms for bioenergy

Chronobiology is the study of the relationship between your internal body clock, mood and behaviour. This relationship can affect the biological rhythms that make you feel high (energetic) or low (lazy, sleepy) – the unique patterns inside you that dictate when you should sleep, wake up, do exercise, or have energy to tackle complex activities.

It has become increasingly accepted by doctors that biorhythms can have a huge influence on your actions, habits and how you look at yourself. Dr. Michael Hastings, an expert in chronobiology at Cambridge University, claims that 'everything from blood pressure, heart-rate, to strength and brain power can change according to the time of day ... and your genes determine how your body clock works'.

Listen to your body clock and how your mind works. Be aware of your energy levels at different times during the day. Maybe you are exercising or doing energetic activity in the morning, but this does not suit your mind; restructuring your exercise schedule to keep in tune with your internal clock could help you get the best results.

## BENEFITS OF EXERCISE IN OLDER AGE

Studies have shown that exercise can:

- reduce the number of free radicals in your body
- improve cardiovascular health
- stave off diabetes
- increase your energy
- help to prevent osteoporosis
- protect against cancer
- help you to think more clearly and focus better

Furthermore, according to a study from the University of Illinois, a group 60–75-year-olds who walked at a rapid pace for forty-five minutes, three times a week, increased their ability to process information and successfully complete tasks. Other research has also shown that aerobic exercise improved high-level brain function in people aged between fifty and seventy-seven. Exercise has also been shown to be as effective as some drugs in treating clinical depression, due to the endorphins (feel-good chemicals) released by the brain during physical activity.

### General timings for exercise

- 6 a.m.–noon: low-impact exercise/activity
- noon–2p.m.: low-impact activity/exercise including walking. After lunch, let food be digested, since digestion requires energy
- 3–6p.m.: energetic exercise or activities (adrenalin production is at its highest)
- 6–8p.m.: a good time to swim or do stretching exercises since the muscles are warm and flexible (adrenalin peaks)
- after 7p.m.: the body clock is winding down and you might be disturbing your body clock's natural biorhythms if you demand energetic activity of it at this time; your metabolism will also be slowing down.

Watch your mind and body reactions. Forcing your body to be active when it doesn't want to be will not give you more energy. (Don't mistake this for being out of practice with exercise though.) Just try to tune into your own body's natural

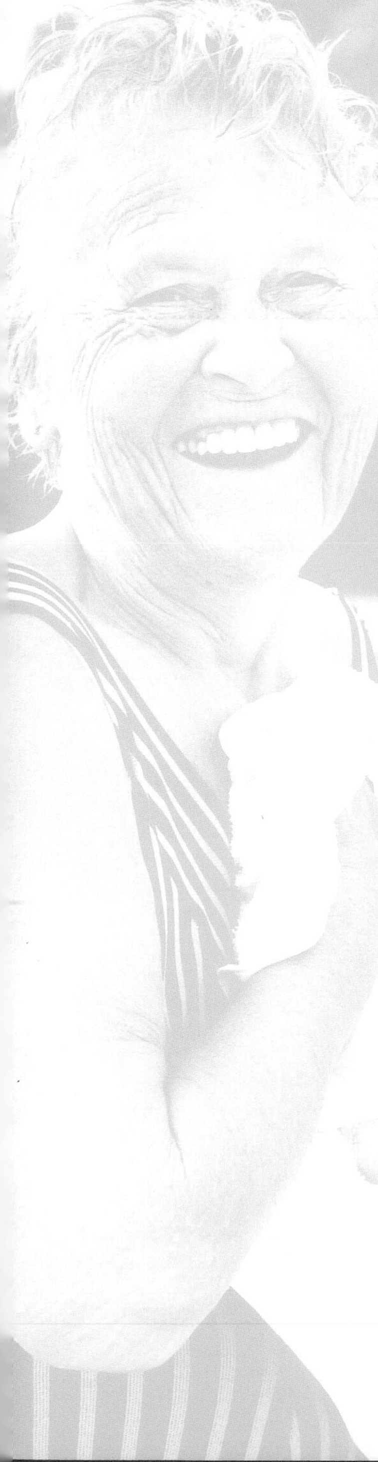

preference. Then you'll get the most out of your mind and body's natural reserve of energy. Don't be afraid to catch up on your sleep with 'catnaps' either if this is what your body clock and mind dictate; a ten-minute nap will instantly re-energise you. Learn how to make your energy work for you.

What and when you eat should also be taken into account when listening to your body clock. A qualified nutritionalist can offer advice on what you eat, when, and in what quantities to help you reach your most energetic, healthy level of fitness and to help overcome or avoid any complaint or illness. Most feel that you should eat your largest (and heaviest) meal at lunchtime, since your digestive powers are at their peak between noon and 1p.m. A light supper should then be eaten before 7p.m., after which time the body needs all its energy for repairing cells and tissues.

### Energy for life

The exercises for the older person aim to improve the circulation of oxygen around your body giving you more energy. They also help combat stress, which is a big energy robber. Even if you don't feel like doing the exercises to begin with, once you start, you will feel better immediately as you rid yourself of tension. You forget all your problems as you focus on your breathing and the exercise. Also endorphins are released when you exercise, making you feel happier and full of energy. Try to exercise once a day or once every other day.

### Brain training in the 'mind gym'

Anyone practicing meditation, visualisation, crossword puzzles, or mathematical games is already using the mind gym.

The brain can become stale if you don't challenge it, just as your muscles can become sluggish and stiff when you don't exercise. Try changing your pattern of thinking and acting to alter your mental processes and keep you alert and feeling energetic.

Society's expectations of grandparents (of either sex) and even great-grandparents have grown considerably in recent years. Scientists teach us that our brains can continue to develop throughout life and therefore more is now demanded of older people than ever before.

To help you to keep up with these increasing demands, the 'mind tricks' opposite (based on NLP, or neurolinguistic programming) can help you change not only how you think but how you communicate and act, to get what you want from life.

## MIND TRICKS FOR ENERGY

- Play memory games, bridge, chess and games that make you think ahead.
- Use the time when you are inactive (such as on a bus or train) but not necessarily relaxing. Don't just sit there.
- Change the way that you usually do a routine activity or chore.
- Practise visualisations (such as visualising a new place or activity).
- Try to make better decisions. Challenge yourself in a new way (make yourself decide things more quickly if you are usually slow, or train yourself be more careful and thorough if you are usually quick to decide things).
- Focus on detail when walking or meditating. Concentrating on things is a very good mind trick.

Just reading this book is a way of bringing your mind to the mind gym. By reprogramming your memory or altering a belief system, it is possible to change your thought process. The more difficult it is for you to alter your mind map, the more good you are probably doing as far as your brain–energy is concerned. A regular challenge should make your brain sweat like your body would if you were exercising.

Stress can cause the brain to function below par. This may be why yoga and meditation are often practiced twice a day: in the early morning and in the evening, in order to help the mind counterbalance the stresses of the day and to prepare it to cope with the stresses of the day ahead.

Eating the 'right' foods can help your brain to function. Researchers at Harvard University found that people who only (or predominantly) ate carbohydrates in the morning were less mentally alert than those who ate only protein. Protein provides the amino acids phenylalanine and tyrosine, both of which are needed to produce neurotransmitters such as noradrenalin required for concentration.

Give your mind a daily workout, and challenge yourself with new and different experiences.

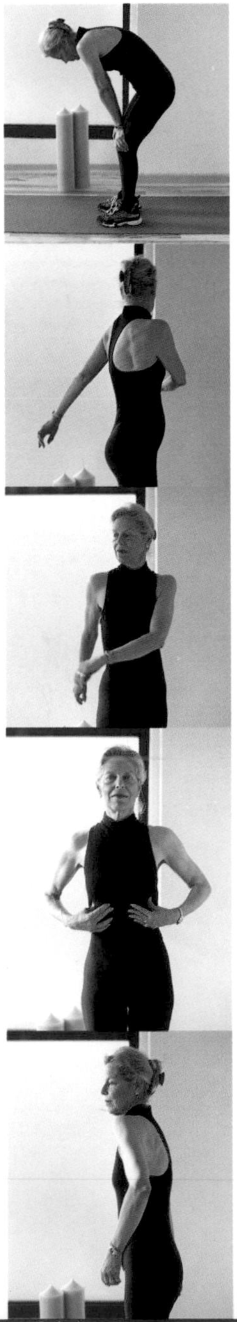

## WARM-UP/COOL-DOWN EXERCISES

Anyone of any age should always warm up and cool down before and after exercise:

- Stand with your feet slightly apart and arms straight.
- Put your hands on your knees.
- Bend your knees and push your bottom out while squeezing it tight. You should be looking down at the floor.
- Repeat ten times.
- Stand with your head up, swing your arms from side to side in front of your body and look over your right shoulder while your arms swing to the right.
- Repeat twice.
- Stand straight. Put your hands on your ribs and pull/stretch them up as you stand tall.
- Stand tall again, looking at eye level, and roll your right shoulder forward five times and back five times.
- Repeat with the left shoulder.
- Now do both shoulders together five times.
- Kneel on the floor on your hands and knees.
- Make sure that your hands are under your shoulders.
- Look at the floor and make sure that your neck is in line with your back.
- Pull your bottom inward, forming a hump back, then push your bottom back out again so that your back is straight.
- Repeat five times.

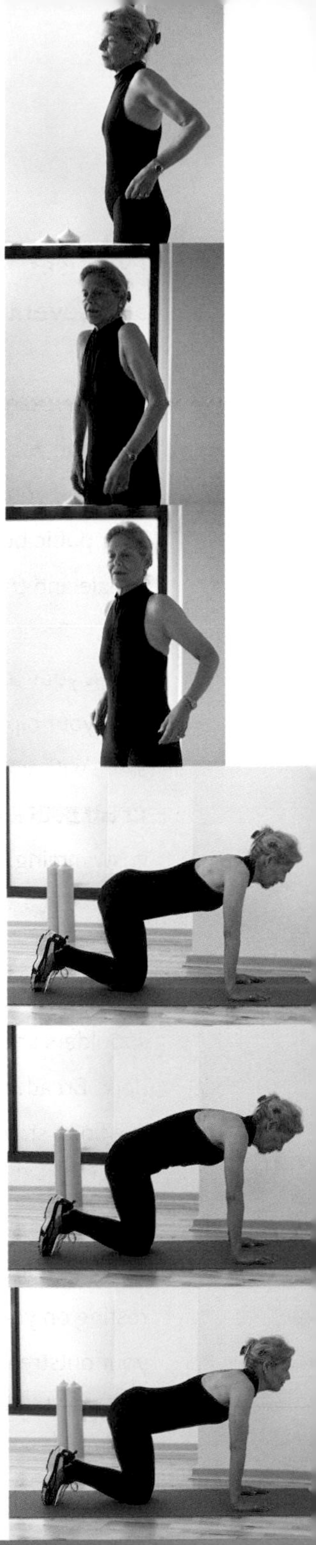

## Exercises for people aged between fifty and seventy-five

Always warm up and cool down before and after exercise. Start slowly; build up repetitions gradually.

- Lie on your stomach with your head on the floor and your hands under your stomach. Push your pubic bone to the floor, breathe in, then exhale and try and lift your stomach off your hands. Breathe in and relax. Repeat 10 times
- Lift your straight leg up and down, (no higher than your hip) keeping your bottom tight. Do the same with your other leg. Repeat up to 20 times
- Lift both legs off the floor and do little kicks as if swimming. Keep your bottom tight. Start with 20, and build up to 200 kicks
- Mini pushups: lift the top part of your body up onto your hands, keeping your hands under your shoulders and your pubic bone and legs on the floor. Breathe in and out and raise your back off the floor, straightening your arms, lower back and chin to the floor slowly. Repeat 10–20 times, building up to 50.
- Pull your body back so that your chest is resting on your knees, and your head is between your outstretched arms
- Sit-curl ups: Lie on your back with your knees up and your feet flat on the floor. Lift your bottom whilst pulling your back into the floor. With your hands behind head, lift your head to look at your breastbone, squeeze knees together tightly, and breathe in. Exhale and hold position for a count of 10. Repeat 10 times, building to 20.
- Lie on your side with your legs stretched out in line with your shoulders and hips. Rest your head on your outstretched arm. Rest your top arm straight on your hip then lift your ribs and waist off the floor. Then lift both legs off the floor and move your top leg up and down with your foot flexed. Repeat on other side. Repeat 10–20 times.
- As above but this time keep the top leg still and lift the bottom leg up and down to meet the top leg. Repeat 10–20 times.
- Roll onto your back, clasp your knees to your chest and breathe.

## Exercises for people aged over seventy

- The Windmill (see page 104)
- The Frisbee: Lift up your ribs, stretch back and stand tall. With your arms straight above your head and palms facing the sky, link your thumbs and with elbows bent a little, move hands and arms like a frisbee round and round over the top of your head. Repeat 5–10 times, changing direction.

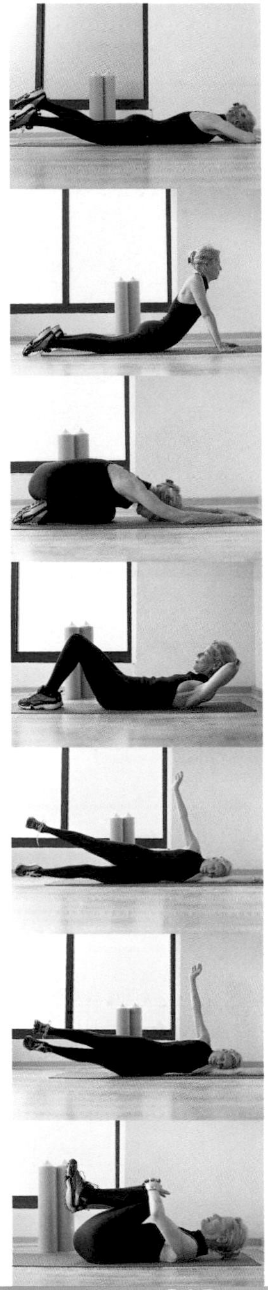

# Useful addresses

UNITED KINGDOM

Bliss
333 Portobello Road
London W10 6RE
Tel: 020 8969 3331
www.bliss.me.co.uk
*For natural products and treatments, meditation, yoga, Pilates and exercise classes.*

British Acupuncture Council
63 Jeddo Road
London W12 9HQ
020 8735 0400
www.acupuncture.org.uk

International Federation of Aromatherapy
182 Chiswick High Road
London W4 1PP
Tel: 020 8742 2605
www.int-fed-aromatherapy.co.uk

Ayurvedic Medical Association UK
9 Bilbrook Lane
Furzton
Milton Keynes MK4 1AW
Tel: 01908 524282

British Register of Complementary Practitioners
PO Box 194
London SE16 7QZ
Tel: 020 7237 5175
*Including colour therapy*

The Edward Bach Centre
Mount Vernon
Bakers Lane
Sotwell
Wallingford
Oxon OX10 OPZ
01491 834 678
*Flower remedies*

The General Council and Register of Consultant Herbalists
31 King Edwards Road
Swansea SA1 4LL
Tel: 01792 655886

The British Homeopathy Association
15 Clerkenwell Close
London EC1R OAA
Tel: 020 7566 7800
www.trusthomeopathy.org

Central Register of Advanced Hypnotherapists
28 Finsbury Park Road
London N4 2JX
Tel: 020 7359 6991

The T'ai Chi Union of Great Britain
102 Felsham Road
London SW15 1DQ
Tel: 020 7352 7716

British Federation of Massage Practitioners
78 Meadow Street
65A Adelphi Street
Preston PR1 1TS
Tel: 01772 881 063
www.bfmp.co.uk

The General Council and Register of Naturopaths
6 Netherhall Gardens
London NW3 5RR
Tel: 020 7435 8738

Dietary Therapy Society
33 Priory Gardens
London N6 5QU
Tel: 020 8341 7260

International Institute of Reflexology UK
255 Turleigh
Bradford-upon-Avon
Wiltshire BA15 2HG
Tel: 01225 865 899
www.reflexology-uk.co.uk

The Yoga for Health Foundation
Ickwell Bury
Biggleswade
Bedfordshire SG18 9EF
Tel: 01767 627 271

## AUSTRALIA & NEW ZEALAND

Australian Acupuncture Association Ltd.
PO Box 5142
West End, Brisbane 4101
Australia
073846 5866
Email: aaca@eis.net.au

International Federation of Aromatherapists
1/390 Burwood Road
Hawthorn, VIC 3122
Australia
Tel: 03 9853 1356

Maharishi Ayurveda
579 Punt Road
South Yarra, VIC 3141
Australia
Tel: 03 9866 1999

Self-Realization Healing Centre
2 Harbour View Road
PO Box 129
Leigh
New Zealand

Australian Federation of Homeopaths
21Bulah Close
Berowra Heights, NSW 2082
Australia

New Zealand Homeopathic Association
Box 2929
Auckland
New Zealand
Tel: 09 303 3124

The Australian Society of Clinical Hypnotherapists
200 Alexandra Parade
Fitzroy, VIC 3065
Australia
Tel: 03 9418 3920

Shiatsu Therapy Association of Australia
332 Carlisle Street
Balaclava, VIC 3183
Australia
Tel: 03 9530 0067

Association of Massage Therapists
18A Spit Road
Mosman, NSW 1088
Australia

Australian Naturopathic Practitioners
1st Floor, 609 Camberwell Road
Camberwell, VIC 3124
Australia
Tel: 03 9889 0488

Australian College of Nutritional and Environmental Medicine
13 Hilton Road
Beamaris, VIC 3193
Australia
Tel: 03 9589 6088
Reflexology World
PO Box 1032
Bondi Junction, NSW 1355
Australia
Tel: 02 9300 9391
www.reflexologyworld.com

## CANADA

Acupuncture Foundation of Canada Institute
2131 Lawrence Avenue East,
Suite 204,
Scarborough, Ont.
Tel: 416 752 3988
E-mail: info@afcinstitute.com

Osmosis Everyday Aromatherapy
502 Queen Street,
West Toronto, Ont. M5V 2B3
Tel: 416 504 7673 or 1 800 474 7375
Fax: 416 504 7243
*Essential oils and products by mail order*

Institute of Aromatherapy
300A Danforth Avenue,
Toronto, Ont.
Tel: 416 465 3882

Chinese Medicine and Acupuncture Association of Canada
154 Wellington Street,
London, Ont. N6B 2K8
Tel: 519 642 1970
Fax: 519 642 2932

Bach–Karooch Ltd.
PO Box 2465,
Peterborough, Ont. K9J 7Y8
Tel: 705 749 1894 or 1 800 375 6222
*Flower remedies*

Wellness Referral Network, Inc.
Information and referrals to doctors and healing arts providers in Canada:
Tel: 1 800 520 WELL

Health Action Network Society
202–5262 Rumble Street,
Burnaby, BC V5J 2B6
Tel: 604 435 0512
E-mail: hans@hans.org
Website: http://www.hans.org

Canadian Natural Health Product Association
550 Alden Road, Suite 205,
Markham, Ont. L3R 6A8
Tel: 905 479 6939
Fax: 905 479 1516

Hypnotherapy Clinic
208 Bloor Street West, Suite 701,
Toronto, Ont. M5S 3B4
Tel: 416 924 9483

Shiatsu School of Canada Inc.
547 College Street,
Toronto, Ont. M6G 1A9
Tel: 416 323 1818 or 1 800 263 1703
E-mail: shiatsu@istar.ca

Taoist T'ai Chi Society of Canada
1376 Bathurst Street,
Toronto, Ont. M5R 3J1
Tel: 416 656 2110

Ontario Massage Therapist Association
365 Bloor Street East, Suite 1807,
Toronto, Ont. M4W 3L4
Tel: 416 968 6487 or 1 800 668 2022
Fax: 416 968 6818
E-mail: omta@inforamp.net

Canadian Naturopathic Association
4174 Dundas Street West, Suite 304,
Etobicoke, Ont. M8X 1X3
Tel: 416 233 1043

Dieticians of Canada
488 University Avenue,
Toronto, Ont.
Tel: 416 596 0857

Canadian Mental Health Association
3rd Floor, 2160 Yonge Street,
Toronto, Ont. M4S 2Z3
Tel: 416 484 7750

Canadian Registry of Psychological Service Providers
Tel: 613 562 0900

Reflexology Association of Canada
541 Turnberry,
Brussels, Ont.
Tel: 1 519 887 9991 or 1 888 889 5394

Canadian Centre for Stress and Well-Being
141 Adelaide Street West, Suite 1506,
Toronto, Ont. M5H 3L5
Tel: 416 363 6204

# Further reading


**Agombar, Fiona**, *Beat Fatigue with Yoga*, 2002, Harper Collins

**Alexander, Jane**, *The Energy Secret*, 2001, Harper Collins

**Balch, Phyllis A. and James F. Balch**, *Prescriptions for Nutritional Healing: A to Z Guide to Supplements*, 1998, Avery Publishing Group

**Bradford, Nikki and Sullivan, Karen (Editors)**, *The Hamlyn Encyclopedia of Complementary Health*, 1996, Hamlyn

**Maxwell-Hudson, Clare**, *The Complete Book of Massage*, 1984, Ebury

**Mitchell, Emma**, *Energy Exercises*, 2000, Duncan Baird Publishers

**Murrey, Michael and Joseph E. Pizzorno**, *The Encyclopedia of Natural Medicine*, 1998, Little, Brown

**Peiffer, Vera**, *The Energy Technique: Simple Secrets for a Lifetime of Vitality and Energy*, 1999, Thorsons Publishers

**Pitchford, Paul**, *Healing with Whole Foods*, 1996, North Atlantic Books

**Proto, Louis**, *Increase Your Energy*, 1998, Piatkus Books

**Van Straten, Michael and Barbara Griggs**, *Super Fast Foods*,

**Westwood, Christine**, *Aromatherapy – A Guide for Home Use*, 1991, Amberwood Publishing

**White, Ian**, *Australian Bush Flower Essences*, 1993, Findhorn Press

**Wills, Judith**, *4 Weeks to Total Energy*, 1999, Quadrille Publishing

# Index

# Publisher's acknowledgements

The publisher would like to thank the following for their kind permission to reproduce the images on the following pages.

**1, 2–3** Getty Images; **6–7** Photonica/Cheryl Koralik; **8** Photonica/ Cheryl Koralik; **9** Photonica/Mia Klein; **10** Photonica/Mitsuru Yamaguchi; **12** Photonica/Nicholas Pavloff; **13** Getty Images; **15** Bubbles; **16** Getty Images; **18** Francesca York; **19** Powerstock **23** Getty Images; **24** Photonica/Niki Sianni; **25** Photonica/Jen Fong; **26** Getty Images; **27** Powerstock; **28** robertharding.com; **29** robertharding.com; **30** Ray Main/Mainstream; **31** Getty Images; **37** Getty Images; **41** Getty Images; **44** Clay Perry; **45** Clay Perry; **46** Photonica/Kerama; **49** Getty Images; **58** Photonica/Tulla Booth; **66** Getty Images; **67** Photonica/Neo Vision; **68** Getty Images; **70** Ray Main/Mainstream; **72** Bubbles; **88** Getty Images; **140** (running) robertharding.com, (basketball) Powerstock; **141** Powerstock; **142** Getty Images; **150** Getty Images; **151** Getty Images; **152** Bubbles; **155** Getty Images; **156** Photonica/Johner; **157** Photonica/Lisa Stancati; **177** Photonica/Paul Vozdic; **178** Getty Images; **181** Getty Images; **183** Getty Images; **185** Getty Images; **191** Getty Images; **193** Powerstock; **197** Ray Main/Mainstream; **208** Photonica/B. Schmid; **212** Photonica/Brigit Utech

The publisher would also like to thank Casalls (c/o Viva (UK) Limited, 2 Market Place, Somerton, Somerset, TA11 7LX; 01458 273394) for kindly loaning sports clothes for the photoshoots.

# Author's acknowledgements

I'd like to thank my husband Alexis and my daughter Shayna for being so patient with me and for putting up with my mood swings while I wrote this book. I would also like to thank my mum Judy (the woman with the most energy and someone I have always aspired to be like) and my good friend Helen, without whom I would not have found the time or space to write. Special thanks to both my friend Lee, who encouraged me to keep going and is always there for me, and to my brother Ash, whose wisdom never ceases to amaze me (although he has never even studied medicine) and who is able to love and support me even though he lives on the other side of the world!

Thanks to all the practitioners at Bliss for their advice and support, and for understanding my absence while I wrote this book. Special thanks to the following practitioners for their expert advise: Deepa (reflexology), Liza (naturopathy), Hari (acupuncture/qi gong), Tara (shiatsu/yoga), Muriel (flower remedies/homeopathy) and Asaf (hypnotherapy). Thanks to Pete Cohen for taking time out of his busy life write the foreword to this book. Thanks also to my mum, my husband, Hari, Tara, Lee, Nathalie, Dodd and Helen Jones for modelling, especially to those who stood out in the cold with me and my daughter for the sake of a good picture!

Thanks to Helen Woodhall and Kyle Cathie for their patience with my computer failings and to my Dad for sacrificing his own scriptwriting to lend me his laptop so I could reach my second deadline!

Lastly, I could not have written this book without the love and support of my husband, my rock, and the smiles and inspiration of my little ball of energy, my daughter!